W9-BYF-071

You Don't
Have To Live With
CYSTITIS

Avon Books are available at special quantity discounts for bulk purchases for sales promotions, premiums, fund raising or educational use. Special books, or book excerpts, can also be created to fit specific needs.

For details write or telephone the office of the Director of Special Markets, Avon Books, Dept. FP, 1350 Avenue of the Americas, New York, New York 10019, 1-800-238-0658.

You Don't Have To Live With
Cystitis

Revised and Updated

Larrian Gillespie, M.D.
with Sandra Blakeslee

AVON BOOKS ◆ NEW YORK

VISIT OUR WEBSITE AT
http://AvonBooks.com

AVON BOOKS
A division of
The Hearst Corporation
1350 Avenue of the Americas
New York, New York 10019

Copyright © 1986, 1996 by Larrian Gillespie, M.D., and Sandra Blakeslee
Published by arrangement with Rawson Associates
Library of Congress Catalog Card Number: 96-22962
ISBN: 0-380-78779-2

All rights reserved, which includes the right to reproduce this book or portions
thereof in any form whatsoever except as provided by the U.S. Copyright Law.
For information address Rawson Associates, an imprint of Simon and Schuster,
Inc., 1230 Avenue of the Americas, New York, New York 10020.

Library of Congress Cataloging in Publication Data:
Gillespie, Larrian.
    You don't have to live with cystitis / Larrian Gillespie.—Rev. and updated.
       p. cm.
    Includes index.
1. Cystitis—Popular works.   2. Women—Health and hygiene.
I. Title.
RG485.C9G55   1996   96-22962
616.6'23'082—dc20   CIP

First Avon Books Revised Trade Printing: December 1996
First Avon Books Trade Printing: April 1988

AVON TRADEMARK REG. U.S. PAT. OFF. AND IN OTHER COUNTRIES, MARCA
REGISTRADA, HECHO EN U.S.A.

Printed in the U.S.A.

OPM   10   9   8   7   6   5   4   3   2

If you purchased this book without a cover, you should be aware that
this book is stolen property. It was reported as ''unsold and destroyed''
to the publisher, and neither the author nor the publisher has received
any payment for this ''stripped book.''

*To all the women
who dared to seek a better way
and
to our families*

Contents

Acknowledgments

The process of revising a book requires the help and assistance of many people. I would like to thank Mr. Michael Korda for taking so much time from your complicated world to encourage me to do "only my best." Your advice was taken to heart.

To my first publisher, Eleanor Rawson, I bow on bended knee, for you have gone above and beyond the call as a publisher in helping me to accomplish this task. Your support and honesty will not be forgotten.

Editors must have the grace of a gazelle and the hide of an elephant in dealing with author's "precious babies." Lisa Considine has both in abundance, and her thoroughness and keen eye caught me talking "doctor speak" when I wanted to relay complicated medical information in a simple, straightforward manner.

Finally, I would like to express my appreciation to Commander Richard Turner-Warwick and his wife, Dame Margaret Turner-Warwick, for "adopting" me into their family.

LARRIAN GILLESPIE, M.D.

This book is not intended as a substitute for the
medical advice of physicians. The reader should
regularly consult a physician in matters relating to his
or her health and particularly in respect to
any symptoms that may require diagnosis or
medical attention.

The names and circumstances of clients in case
histories have been changed to protect their privacy,
except for Pamela Sue Martin.

INTRODUCTION

What This Book Will Reveal to You

Cystitis: Free at Last!

I F you accept the widely held attitude that women are fated to develop bladder infections, this book is not for you. If you think that cystitis, as such infections are called, is "no big deal," you should stop reading now. But if you reject this widely held idea, we can start to build a partnership in dealing with the problem of cystitis.

When I first wrote this book in 1985, I never anticipated the response it would receive not only from men and women but from their physicians. Letters have continued to pour in over the past ten years with stories of how the information you will find in this book encouraged individuals to insist on tests that uncovered the cause for their pain. Physicians wrote me, admitting they would never have read my book had their patient not persisted, but they too discovered support for the idea that the cause of the patient's pain didn't originate in his or her head! Ultimately though it was the heart-rending stories of women who couldn't get help that prompted me to revise this book with new insights I have gained about cystitis and pain.

This book emphatically challenges the belief that cystitis is as inevitable as the occasional menstrual cramp. As a surgeon specializing in disorders of the urinary tract, I have found that cystitis is preventable. It is not some kind of primeval female curse that we must all endure. Rather, it is an abnormal bladder condition that is more often than not caused by some functional (rather than anatomic) problem. Using common sense, its causes can be found and treated. *You don't have to live with cystitis!*

Your grandmother, however, was perhaps less fortunate. A hundred years ago, antibiotics (used so effectively today to kill bacteria in the bladder) were not known. Yet women developed cystitis then for many of the same reasons that they develop it today. In this book, you will learn both what is new and what is old about cystitis.

Over the centuries, numerous cures and palliatives were devised to treat the symptoms of cystitis. These remedies, many of which were excellent, have been passed down to us today. I will tell you why some work and others do not, which ones are valuable, and which ones lack merit. You will also, I hope, have your eyes opened about the many old wives' tales that purport to explain the causes of cystitis. For example, women are told they get bladder infections from sitting on the cold ground, from having too much sex, or from having too little sex. Such beliefs, which are total nonsense, have persisted because no factual information has ever been offered women to supplant those old wives' tales.

Probably no one has ever explained to you the many ways cystitis can develop, why it can recur, and how easy it is to prevent. This book will give you that information step by step. It is an attempt to bring women from the Dark Ages regarding cystitis into the Age of Enlightenment. It should help you discover why you are getting bladder infections or why the symptoms of cystitis won't go away. It lays out fundamental principles that you can use in getting to the cause of your problem. It tells you how to maintain your urologic health.

You Don't Have to Live with Cystitis

One of my major interests in recent years has been figuring out the many causes of cystitis. Contrary to what you, your mother, your grandmother, and all your family's doctors have been taught for generations, *cystitis is curable.* The prevailing notion that you are fated to develop a painful bladder infection at least once during your lifetime simply is not true. The fact that you may have already developed repeated infections is heartbreaking.

I have treated thousands of women for cystitis. Most infections could have been avoided had my patients known a few simple facts about female anatomy and how bladder infections arise. Indeed, cystitis is now an ailment most women can avoid. Urologists are learning more each day about the intricate mechanisms of bladder function and how the urinary tract works. New biochemical findings about this system are leading to better treatments and prevention of disease.

Tragically, American women continue to make more then 8.9 million visits a year to the doctor's office because of cystitis. It is the most common affliction prompting women to seek medical attention!

I am constantly surprised by how little my patients know about their urinary tracts and by the way they perpetuate myths about cystitis. But the patients are not entirely to blame.

To this day, urologists are taught that women may never be cured of cystitis. Women get cystitis again and again, we are told, because women are "built funny."

You should never get a bladder infection unless there is some anatomic or functional reason underlying the disorder. But if you are like most cystitis sufferers, your anatomy is perfectly normal. Your infection can be traced to a functional cause—that is, it is something you can easily prevent if armed with commonsense knowledge.

Commonsense Urology

The medical specialty of urology appealed to me for several reasons. I love puzzle solving, and urology is a field with few hard-and-fast answers. There is no single formula for any particular disease that makes everyone well. The urologic system is particularly complicated, and many parts of it can go awry in an infinite number of ways. Every patient is unique and needs to be assessed individually.

Working with patients has taught me how to be a keen observer. My medical school preceptor and I used to play a game. As we went on rounds, he would suddenly point to a patient and say, "What is wrong with that one?" I had to focus immediately on anything I could pick up about the subject at hand. It was like the game we played as children in which we looked at a picture for fifteen seconds, looked away, and then wrote down everything we could remember about it. Medicine is similar. You observe each person and focus on what he or she is saying. Today, I can often figure out what is bothering a patient just by looking at the way she sits, walks, or holds her body.

Throughout my residency training at UCLA, I was always the "but" person; I'd say, "But . . . what about this observation? But . . . what the book says doesn't make sense. But . . . this can't be right." When things didn't work, I wanted to know why not. I wondered aloud if something might be wrong with the logic being applied. Have we reached only part of the answer? Should we be content with "This is the way it is?"

It was this unwillingness to accept edicts, as passed down in some medical textbooks and by some professors, that led me to put more trust in my innate common sense on matters of female urologic function and health than in all those edicts. Everything you will read in this book is based on my practice of urology and urogynecology for the past fifteen years. The information does not necessarily reflect the opinions and training of the UCLA urology residency program, those of the American Urological Association, or for that matter other urologists or gynecologists. Rather, this book distills for women my own distinct approach to women's health.

As a urologist, I treat men, women, and children. A few years ago one male colleague told me, "I always knew it would take a woman to figure out women's problems. Put a woman into urology and things will change." He was right, but the change didn't come easily.

Women in Urology: A Splash in the Pan?

At the time I was chosen as the first woman ever to be accepted into UCLA's urology program, I did not realize it was unusual for a woman to choose this specialty. I presumed, in my naïveté, that women were involved in all fields of medicine. It was only upon applying for a residency position that I was informed by other (male) urologists that no woman, to their knowledge, had ever been trained in urology in the entire United States!

As it turned out, this was not true. In 1986 there were seventy-four women urologists in this country, but there has been little growth since. I believe, however, that as the surgical treatment of common urologic disorders—such as kidney stones, prostatic enlargement, cancer, and impotence—give way to newer noninvasive medical management, urologists will renew their interest in women's problems and with that will come the opportunity for women to influence the curriculum taught to urological residents.

I chose urology because I believed a woman could offer special insights into this fascinating field of medicine that affects so many other women. After all, at least half of all urologists' patients are women.

A few years ago, I presented a paper, "Women in Urology: A Splash in the Pan," about the history of women in the field. Everyone laughed at me, saying the talk would last but two minutes. Instead, I could hardly contain my lecture within the allotted twenty minutes.

Although over the centuries very few women have practiced urology, it turns out that one of the earliest specialists was a woman. Her name was Trotula, and she practiced in Salerno, Italy, during the eleventh century. Historians tell us she was a very attractive, feminine woman who treated both male and female patients. Her prescriptions for urinary tract infections and stone disease were numerous. Her teachings include twenty-nine observations she made on urine, and she is credited with the first description of the skin manifestations of the disease we now call syphilis.

During the late tenth century in Egypt, the demand for women in urology was great. Kidney stone disease was very common, yet male physicians were not allowed to touch women. Abou'l-Quâsim, a noted surgeon in the court of the Caliph of Cordova, stated that "one must find a woman well versed in urology but they were few and far between."

One of my colleagues recently noted that "overwhelmingly, the gynecological literature of medieval Europe was written for a male medical audience and was a product of the way men understood women's bodies, functions, illnesses, needs and desires."

It seems that for hundreds of years, right up to the late 1800s, when the Industrial Revolution brought women back into professional roles, women urologists were virtually nonexistent. It was a struggle for women back at the turn of the century to become recognized as full-fledged surgeons with medical degrees hung neatly on the wall. Many male medical school professors believed that women did not require and were not fit to receive the scientific education needed to become a first-rate physician. As one professor said, "For their own sake, it is not desirable that they should pursue some of the studies necessary such as anatomy." It was thought that the study of natural science would injure a woman's character. In the medical schools of those days, male students were assigned a dissecting laboratory separate from the female, or "hen," medics. Women were not allowed to dissect male genitalia. Instead they were given a castrated papier-mâché model of the male body.

But some women rebelled. Sophia Jexs-Blake, founder of the Royal Free Hospital for Women's Education in London, stated at the turn of the century, "If a woman's womanliness is not deep enough in her nature to bear the brunt of any needful education, it is not worth guarding."

I found a trail of many women who had practiced urology, some of whom developed innovative surgical and medical treatments. Unfortunately, none survived in the field. They were forced to treat only women and children or to turn to gynecology. The work they did was credited, as was then customary, to their male mentors.

In recent decades, many excellent women physicians fared no better in attaining what they really wanted out of medicine. Virginia Apgar, who developed the Apgar scale used worldwide to assess the health status of newborn infants, always wanted to be a surgeon. Yet her male colleagues told her that she did not stand a chance. She regretted to her death that she allowed them to talk her out of a surgical career.

* * *

By the early 1970s, when I was receiving my medical training, myriad social factors had changed for the better a woman's chances of entering surgery, urology, or other specialties formerly practiced almost exclusively by men.

Women have been allowed into these fields and are beginning to make unique contributions to the practice and study of medicine. Women physicians, however, must learn to rely on their unique experiences *as women* if they want to make a difference in how diseases of the female urinary tract are viewed and treated.

When you think about it, the way the medical community divided up female anatomy long ago made no sense. The gynecologists got the reproductive tract and the urologists got the urinary tract (except for bladder hernias, which only gynecologists were then taught how to repair). As a result, when a woman feels burning when she urinates caused by a vaginal infection she is punted to the gynecologist. When she feels burning when she urinates caused by a bladder infection she is turfed back to the urologist. This is the famous punt-and-turf game of specialized medicine.

As medical consumers, women are beginning to ask that the rules of the game be changed. A new field, urogynecology, has been established, in which the female reproductive and urinary tracts, like those of men, are treated by a single practitioner. Unfortunately, these urogynecologists can treat only the lower urinary tract, that is, the bladder and urethra, leaving problems with the ureters and kidneys "out of reach." Ideally, urology and gynecology should be wholly integrated into one field, with obstetrics/infertility/pediatrics as the other, complementary field. The idea is not new: This unification of fields was almost accomplished at Johns Hopkins at the turn of the century, but sadly, men made the decision to split the fields as we know them today. I strongly believe that physicians who treat women ought to understand the complexities of both systems, and I have found my own expansion into gynecology invaluable in treating my patients.

Grasshoppers and Ants

Private practitioners do not, as a rule, conduct basic research. But when a practitioner is confronted with a fundamental paucity of understanding about women's urologic health, a doctor must investigate these problems scientifically. As a result, I have published numerous original articles about cystitis and other urologic problems that tend to affect women. Much of this book is based on those scientific inquiries and results.

Someone once told me that scientific inquiry is conducted by two types of researchers, grasshoppers and ants. The grasshoppers are the mavericks, the bold leapers, the ones who propose new, possible answers to tough questions. The ants are the establishment, the detail gatherers, the phalanx of workers who ultimately follow many of the insights made by grass-hoppers. Both ants and grasshoppers are necessary for the advancement of science.

But if I had a choice, I would be like the grasshopper. Not all the leaps win gold medals. But they do stimulate awareness of medical issues and help promote research into long-ignored women's problems. Some of my leaps may prove wrong and some will prove right. Some treatments and therapies I use today may seem crude in twenty years, but if they stimulate scientific thinking in the right direction, they are worthwhile. Forward progress is extremely important, and I feel I have contributions to make.

The work I do is ongoing. As you'll see in this book, at no time do I claim that we understand each problem completely and here is the exact answer to each question. Rather, you will see that we are following simple logic in analyzing each question. We look at how problems evolve and how individuals can have many interconnected factors that lead to their cystitis, incontinence, or other urologic health problems.

The book is not meant to take the place of an office visit with your doctor. It is not a substitute for medical care. Rather, it is a guide to help you achieve a better working relationship with your own physician through knowledge.

I suspect that as you read the book, you may be struck at how simple and obvious some of the discoveries appear to be. I can hear you saying, "Of course! Why didn't they think of that ages ago?" But the solution to many of these puzzles about cystitis, incontinence, and other problems appear simpler than they really are. They remind me, to use a show busi-ness analogy, of Fred Astaire's dancing. He made his performances look simple. Yet his motion picture frames were timed to the second. It was hard work that gave the illusion of simplicity, but we mustn't forget that Ginger Rogers did everything Fred did backward and in heels! It is hard work, too, that is leading to a new understanding of female urologic health.

You Have Common Sense Too

I tell patients to use their common sense with regard to bladder infec-tions. Women are intelligent. If something makes sense, it must have some basis in fact. But if you can't understand a treatment or technique and it doesn't make sense to you, it can't be the right approach to your problem. For example, a woman given antibiotics for a bladder infection when none exists might ask, "Why am I taking these pills?" The answer, "To prevent you from getting an infection," doesn't make a lot of sense. The faulty logic of this common practice—some women are routinely given antibiotics to prevent bladder infections when they have no infection—is immediately apparent to anyone who thinks about it. But if you are intimidated by physicians and you want to get better, you don't necessarily think logically.

This book will teach you how to work with your physicians so you get the best value for your medical dollars. You want to understand what is being done to your body. If it doesn't make sense, you might be seeing the wrong physician. Don't be afraid to keep changing physicians. Find the one who can help you unravel your mystery. This book may help serve as your validation—that you are right to keep looking for answers to your problem—until you find that practitioner.

When you go to a new physician, you may find little opportunity to ask the kinds of questions that would help you figure out why you are getting cystitis or having other problems. Being in private practice, I sympathize with how little time most physicians have. With the demands of surgeries, emergencies with patients, and difficult diagnostic problems, we find ourselves hurrying through each day with never enough office hours.

On the other hand, I firmly believe that patients should spend far more time with their doctors. They should be equal partners in diagnosing and treating any medical problem. Of course, the only way to establish such a relationship is for the physician to spend more time with each patient. Patients need to be given more information about their bodies, reasons for problems, why treatments are tried, and what to expect from any course of action.

Time is precious in a healing situation. Knowledge is imperative. This book is an attempt to combine the two and help you regain and maintain your health. When you understand what is happening to your body, you can tackle any problem with far greater strength.

By educating yourself, you will also be helping your doctor. Urology is a fast-moving field. Physicians who left school twenty years ago may not, for example, have been exposed to some of the latest information about cystitis. Please understand that because medicine is so vast an enterprise, and none of us can be an expert in everything, most doctors choose to specialize in one small area; thus we tend, as physicians, to choose an area of personal interest.

Why You and Not Me?

When I began private practice, I became uncomfortable not knowing what caused cystitis in my patients. I didn't like giving medication without knowing why the patient got the infection in the first place and how we could stop it from happening again.

I am a healthy, sexually active woman. Yet I have never had a problem with my urinary tract. I have never had a bladder infection. As women continually seek my help for urinary tract infections and other problems, I always ask myself, "Why? Why is she different from me?" By asking this basic question, I have been able to shed light on several aspects of disease affecting women's lower urinary tracts.

No one, for example, had scientifically studied the effect of birth control methods, particularly the diaphragm, on cystitis. No one, for example, had stressed to patients the close link between lower back problems and cystitis. *Yet the bladder is one of the most sensitive indicators of lower back problems,* and many women with recurrent urinary tract infections can trace their problems to simple but nagging lower back injuries. In addition, a fundamental misunderstanding of female anatomy led thousands of women into having unnecessary surgery of the urinary tract.

And then there is the guilt. Many patients tell me that they feel it is all their fault they are having urinary problems. After all, if they hadn't had too much sex, they wouldn't have an infection. Some tell me that they are terrified to have sex, fearing they are doomed to repeated infections. Some have told me that they think a bladder infection is the way they have to "pay" for an emotionally satisfying experience.

Most women go to their gynecologists for treatment of their first and second urinary tract infections. But when they have had three or more bouts, they may be referred to a urologist to find out why they have the problem.

As many women came to see me with the symptoms of cystitis, I became unsettled on learning that many had rarely had their urine cultured. It was assumed they had bacterial infections of the bladder and they were prescribed antibiotics over the telephone. This practice, as I discuss in Chapter Two, may lead to a failure to diagnose a chronic pelvic pain syndrome called *interstitial cystitis.* It is, in my opinion, the orphan disease of men, women, and children.

It has now been twelve years since I established the Women's Clinic for Interstitial Cystitis in Beverly Hills, and I have seen over four thousand patients with this painful syndrome. I will discuss in Chapter Three my new understanding of the causes for this problem and how knowledge of neurology, neurosurgery, gynecology, gastroenterology, and endocrinology are necessary to unravel this complicated response of the bladder and pelvic floor. Finally, you will learn how treating the cause of the pain may result in your bladder returning to normal function. This chapter will discuss the importance of loving yourself if you are to find the inner strength to heal your body. During my work with pelvic pain, I have seen women who view themselves only as victims, blaming every failure in life on their pain. You will discover why "support groups" may hinder rather than assist you in regaining your self-esteem, especially if they are not led by health-care professionals.

In Chapter Four you will find guidelines on how to be a patient. In my experience, women are often unprepared for their doctor's appointment and speak from emotion rather than from an orientation to the facts. If you have a chronic health problem, you do not want to be dismissed as "another hysterical female" by doctor after doctor. By preparing for your next visit to a physician, you can overcome that bias.

The next Chapter, Five, walks you further through the anatomy and function of each component of the female urinary tract. I explain in detail why women are urologically different from men, which may help you better understand your body. I will tell you why your urethra cannot be in the "wrong place"—that is, too high or too low—thus causing urinary tract infection.

In the beginning of my practice, I did what I had been trained to do in medical school. I would look first for an anatomic explanation for the problem. This stems from the still widely held belief that female bladder function is affected by our "peculiar" female anatomy—that the urethra is "too close" to the anus and "too short" to keep bacteria out of the bladder. The perineum, the skin bridge between the anus and the vagina, is said to be a "breeding ground" for bacteria that get into the bladder.

Let me assure you, there is nothing wrong with the design of the female perineum! The perineum wouldn't have survived the trial of human evolution if it were such a handicap. The female urethra is not a shortened, amputated version of the male urethra but a separate, integrated unit with different functions. Therefore, other factors must be involved in the causes of cystitis.

After finding most of my patients to be anatomically normal, I began to suspect that what I had been taught about anatomy and cystitis in residency didn't answer all the questions. It became a very frustrating experience for both me and my patients to have them undergo expensive, invasive tests only to find no good reason for their infections.

Indeed, anatomic abnormalities are rarely discovered in mature women; such abnormalities almost always show up in childhood. Fortunately, pediatric care in the United States is so excellent that very few children with anatomic problems are missed. They reach adulthood without chronic urinary tract infections.

Some women have their urethras repeatedly dilated—that is, forced open with instruments—to prevent further infections. Efforts to stop cystitis in women with treatments like dilation are based on a male understanding of female urinary anatomy and function. In fact, dilation does little to prevent infections and harms the patient. It is what some urologists call "the rape of the female urethra."

Chapter Six is devoted to urinary incontinence, a rarely discussed topic. Yet some 10 million Americans suffer from incontinence—that is, they leak urine! You will learn about the different kinds of incontinence and how to treat each one. For example, a treatment available for one type of incontinence can be done in the office. You walk in wet and you walk out dry. Also, you will learn how to perform simple exercises that can reduce the symptoms of incontinence, called "vaginetics." I will discuss the value of saving the uterus to help support the pelvic floor instead of removing it during operations meant to alleviate incontinence. Newer surgeries that preserve the pelvic floor will be discussed in addition to minimally invasive techniques that are done through a microscopic lens system.

In the next chapter, Seven, I discuss women's urologic problems that arise during menopause. Three out of every five postmenopausal women in the United States have had a hysterectomy, sadly as a result of "fear of cancer" rather than necessity. This operation can have profound effects on a woman's urinary tract. In seeking to relieve lower pelvic pain, many well-intentioned gynecologists have performed hysterectomies, only to find that the operation did not correct the problem and take away the pain. Thanks to advances in microinstrumentation, fibroids can now be removed through tiny incisions, saving the uterus. I'll explain hysteroscopy, the technique of looking inside the uterus, and how it can stop excessive bleeding, preventing the need for a hysterectomy.

Hormone replacement therapy is very controversial. Deciding whether or not to use it can have profound effects on a woman's urinary system. You need to understand the trade-offs involved in such therapies to maintain a healthy bladder. You will also learn about PMS and how hormone problems can be improved through diet, exercise, and specialized nutritional supplements.

Chapter Eight delves into the effects of pregnancy on the urinary tract. For example, many women void differently when pregnant and some are misdiagnosed as having bacteria in their urine. Thus, they may be put on antibiotics even though they are perfectly healthy. You can avoid this problem through a simple technique that I will describe.

Chapter Nine is about children. After explaining some common anatomic problems, I describe causes for bed-wetting and how to stop it. A concept described in Chapter Two—the leaky cell membrane phenomenon—applies to bed-wetting. I'll show you how diet and a simple medical treatment can stop bed-wetting and give children control over their bladders.

Chapter Ten discusses bladder cancer, giving you an idea of what treatments are available. I believe patient attitude toward this disease is an important factor in treatment. You will learn how to deal with the emotional stress of cancer and how to look at trade-offs involved in different treatments. You will learn how the incidence of bladder cancer in women has risen in direct response to smoking, and how the daily intake of a simple over-the-counter medication may help prevent its occurrence.

Finally, Chapter Eleven discusses how nutrition affects the way cells function in your urinary tract and reveals dietary guidelines that improve the symptoms of interstitial cystitis, bed-wetting, migraines, and colitis. You will learn how to protect your bladder through a wise choice of foods and vitamin supplements.

The Appendixes include information about Healthy Life Publications, a resource for keeping you up-to-date on my work and other sources of information; nutritional formulations that may be helpful to you; a guide to the medications most commonly prescribed for urologic problems and which medications should be avoided by interstitial cystitis patients; a description of the tests and procedures used by urologists and gynecologists.

Throughout this book, you will read the stories of my patients and how they were helped. Every story is true, based on real people with real problems. To protect their privacy, only first names have been used, with one exception: Actress Pamela Sue Martin, who was known for her television roles as Fallon on *Dynasty* and in the title role of the *Nancy Drew Mysteries,* asked that her name be used to draw national awareness to the disorder of interstitial cystitis.

My Goals

This book has several goals.

First, I want to give you knowledge because with knowledge comes power, in this case the power to stay well.

Second, I want to help you learn how to be a successful health-care client. As women, we often have great difficulty relating facts to our physicians unless we are secure in that relationship. My goal is to give you the confidence to know that you can share personal observations with your doctor and not be accused of making emotional, irrelevant remarks. At the same time, I want you to learn how to take responsibility for your own health. Patients who get better do so through tremendous personal effort, or as one woman recently said, ''I think that each of us has within the power to heal.'' I take this to mean that you are responsible for your own wellness and road to recovery.

Third, I want to teach you about your body. It has become very clear to me from my own office practice that as a first step to permanent well-being, most women need to know more about how their urogenital system really works. As a rule, a woman who comes to my office for the first time does not know where her urethra is located. Men get that knowledge simply because they can look at each other.

Another of my goals is to better understand the cellular physiology of disease. On the level of molecules and cells, what factors contribute to problems of the female urogenital tract?

This book will give you the answers to this and many other questions about your urinary system's health. And it will help you find out why you are getting cystitis and how to avoid ever having it again.

ONE

Why You Have Cystitis

Any woman who has had cystitis cringes from the viewpoint held by many doctors that three or four bladder infections a year is no big deal. The pain of these episodic infections is excruciating. For hours and perhaps days, she can think of nothing else as her bladder controls her life. And while these common bacterial infections are not life-threatening, they are temporarily life-shattering. Cystitis won't kill you, but it does make life miserable.

Cystitis can occur at any time in males and females of any age. Children, grandmothers, husbands, and sisters can develop it, for various reasons. It is most common, however, in sexually active women. So to begin explaining how bladder infections develop in healthy people, we'll start with Tricia's story.

It was Monday morning. Tricia woke up and stretched, remembering the delightful evening before. It had started with a dinner date and wonderful conversation and ended with Tricia in the arms of her favorite man.

But now, as she sipped a first cup of coffee before work, she noticed something was not right. She had a strange need to urinate. There was a tingling sensation in her urethra and a feeling of pressure in her lower abdomen.

She had the feeling that she needed to go to the bathroom and needed to go now. First, while on the toilet, she removed her diaphragm. It had been in place about eight hours now, and she felt assured that it had worked correctly.

Moments later, Tricia's feeling of well-being was shattered. When she urinated, it hurt horribly. There was a searing, burning sensation as warm urine trickled out of her bladder. It felt as if someone were pouring acid on an open wound. She squeezed out everything she could and went back into the other room.

She thought, What am I going to do? At work, she had a report to finish before a 2:00 P.M. committee meeting and at least a dozen telephone calls to make. This felt like a bladder infection coming on. She knew from experience that it could knock her out of action for several days. She gulped down three glasses of water and went to work.

At the office, Tricia's symptoms grew worse. When she went to the bathroom, she noticed her urine was a smoky color. Later, there was a bit of blood on the tissue.

A colleague gave her cranberry juice and a vitamin C tablet. Another told her to wash her vagina with copious amounts of cool water. But Tricia developed a gnawing pain around her pubic bone and it seemed every time she urinated, the pain was more intense.

By 4:00 P.M., Tricia was in agony. She desperately wanted medical help. All the water, cranberry juice, and vitamin C had not helped. She couldn't stand the discomfort any longer. What went wrong? Why did this happen now?

Cystitis and Your Anatomy

Women who develop bladder infections constantly ask these questions. Why me? Why now? To understand what went wrong, you need to understand how your urinary tract is supposed to work and to know which parts of your body are affected by cystitis. (For more details on the anatomy and function of the urinary tract, see Chapter Five.)

Amazingly, most women do not know where their urethra is located. Many of my patients are embarrassed to tell me they don't know this simple fact. Others think they know where the urethra is located but are way off track.

Look at the illustrations on page 16 of the female lower urinary tract. Notice that the urethra is located just above the opening of the vagina. In fact, the vagina and urethra share a common tissue plane. The urethra is a specialized tube that connects the bladder to the outside. It transports urine out of the bladder.

Your bladder is located in the lower part of your pelvis, in front of your uterus. It is very much like a collapsible balloon in that it expands as it fills and contracts as it empties. It stretches slowly to make a reservoir for the urine that your kidneys are constantly making.

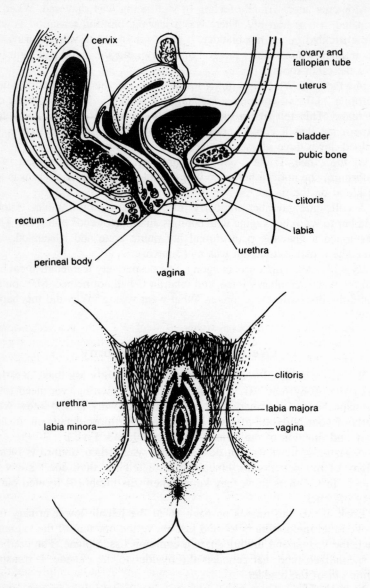

Figures 1-1, 1-2, Anatomy of the Female Pelvis

Frequency, Burning, Pressure

When bacteria multiply in your bladder, they cause you to feel sensations of burning, pressure, and frequency. Each symptom is correlated with how bacteria affect the tissue that lines your bladder.

The bacteria actually adhere to your bladder lining by secreting an enzyme called *urease*. They then split the urea in urine, which results in the production of ammonium salts and produces that burning sensation and special urine odor. As the protective lining is weakened by bacteria, urine crosses over to the cells and tiny capillaries that make up the bladder wall.

When urine comes into contact with these cells, it stimulates special chemical receptors that make you feel the need to urinate. These receptors are overly and improperly stimulated by the urine, giving rise to the sensation of frequency. Some women with cystitis may feel the need to urinate as often as every ten minutes.

When urine gains access to the nerves that lie between cells lining the bladder, the nerves fire. Smooth muscle within the bladder contracts, giving you the feeling of pressure.

The female urinary tract is highly efficient and—this is a very important point to remember—it is designed to perform differently from the male urinary tract. Many physicians, even urologists, mistakenly believe that the male and female urinary tracts are anatomically equivalent and that the female urinary tract is a shortened version of the male urinary tract. This is not so. The female urinary tract serves very different functions and women have different urologic problems from men.

When women void, the urethra is placed so that urine streams down over the labia, the vagina, the perineum (the skin bridge between the vagina and rectum), and then exits over the anal sphincter. We are built like French bidets; we thoroughly cleanse ourselves as we urinate. Because urine is sterile, any bacteria adhering to surrounding tissues is continually washed away. The next time you urinate, pay attention to how this works. Notice how the urine washes you off.

However, if something prevents the bladder from emptying efficiently, bacteria can be left behind—either in the bladder or on surrounding tissue, where they may find an ideal environment in which to multiply and thrive.

It is clear that one bladder infection means that things are not working according to nature's design. *Something*—and there are many possibilities—is compromising your natural system.

Let's Get Rid of the Old Wives' Tales About Bladder Infections

Before exploring the causes of cystitis, I want you to consider five basic concepts carefully that should dispel some of the misinformation or myths that you may think are true. These are commonsense concepts that will help you understand why you have contracted one or many bladder infections.

• *Bacteria often get into the bladder during sexual intercourse.* This is natural, normal, and nothing to worry about. The urethra is next to the vagina. During foreplay, bacteria that thrive on the perineum are easily mixed with vaginal fluids and massaged into the urethra by your partner's fingers. During the repeated thrusting motion of intercourse, the bacteria may work their way into the bladder. This is nothing unusual or threatening. It is normal!

• *The bacteria are your own.* They can come from your perineum, vagina, or anus. They *do not* come from your partner. In other words, he is not infecting you with his germs.

• *Your body has natural cleansing mechanisms.* Most of us don't get bladder infections because bacteria are washed away when we urinate after intercourse. Urine cleanses the bladder, the bladder neck, the urethra, and the vaginal area as well. Moreover, the bladder lining has intrinsic bacterial defenses in its tissue. Even when bacteria stay in there for several hours after intercourse, infections don't normally occur.

In 1961 doctors demonstrated this fact by placing stool directly into the bladders of medical students. After the students urinated a few times, the stool and the bacteria it carried were completely washed away. There were no infections. (This study was very critical to our understanding of cystitis, but it also gives you an idea of the regard doctors have for medical students.)

• *A urinary tract infection is not a problem of bacteria getting into the bladder.* It is a problem of bacteria *not* getting *out.* This is a mechanical or functional issue. When what goes in cannot get out, there is a setup of conditions for an infection to occur.

• *There is more than one way for bacteria to get trapped.* One way is for something to obstruct your normal flow rate. A second is a neurologic problem, such as damage to the nerves in your lower back that are associated with bladder function. In such cases, there is residual urine in the bladder that can feed the growth of bacteria. This leaves you susceptible to a bacterial infection.

Always Get a Urine Culture

If, like Tricia, you wake up one morning with what you think might be a bladder infection, you need to do one thing right away: Get a urine culture done. Many things can cause the symptoms of cystitis, and you *do not* want to take antibiotics if you do not have a bacterial infection.

After work, Tricia went to a nearby walk-in health clinic and left a urine sample. As her urine was "cooking"—left in a warm place overnight so that any bacteria present would colonize and show up the next day growing on the culture dish—Tricia began a course of treatment to knock out what we were pretty sure was a bacterial bladder infection. At this point neither she nor I knew what had caused her infection, but her discomfort was so great that we decided to treat her while awaiting results of the urine culture.

How to Give a Urine Sample

When you give a urine sample, the nurse will give you a sterile container and ask you to catch urine in midstream. Lean way forward so urine does not have a chance to flow up into the vaginal opening and back out again (this happens easily if you lean back against the toilet seat). Some of my patients call this the "skier's position." Be sure the urine does not come in contact with any pubic hair. Your goal is to catch a bit of urine that has come directly from the bladder and is not contaminated with any bacteria that might be residing outside the bladder. Urinate for a moment, to wash away bacteria around the urethral opening, and then place the cup under your stream of urine. Another way to catch a clean urine sample begins with doing what the men in your life have done since they were toilet trained: start facing the toilet with the seat raised. Now sit facing the back of the toilet, straddling the ceramic commode (this position is not recommended if you are wearing panty hose; however, it has been accomplished by several *very* determined women!). This changes the tilt of your pelvis so your urethra now faces straight forward. Begin urinating and you will have no difficulty catching your sample in the little container. As an extra bonus your hands will remain dry! If you do not have a bladder infection, this urine sample will be sterile. If you do have bacteria in your bladder, the urine sample should test positive for bacteria. Moreover, the culture test will indicate which bacteria are causing the infection and how significant the bacterial invasion and growth may be. The bacteria that most commonly cause cystitis are *E. coli, enterococcus,* and *strept fecalis.* Your physician will prescribe a different medication for the different types of bacteria.

The number of bacteria in both your bladder and in the laboratory doubles every few hours. The severity of an infection can depend on what is called the *inoculum*—how many bacteria get into your bladder initially. If you have vaginitis at the time of intercourse, more bacteria might be introduced into your bladder than otherwise. If your inoculum was 50,000 "bugs," it would increase to 100,000 in a short time. But if the inoculum was 5,000 bugs, it would increase to 10,000, then 20,000, then 40,000, and so on. The smaller the inoculum, the longer it takes for the infection to increase.

In my practice, I recommend patients take three pills of a cephalosporin (Keflex, Ceclor, Duricef) or sulfonamide trimethoprim combination (Bactrim, Septra) all at once to knock out an infection. Unlike many doctors, I do not prescribe a ten-day course of antibiotics for uncomplicated urinary tract infections because I do not think such a condition warrants long-term treatment. As long as the bladder is capable of normal function and empties properly, you should feel better in a few hours.

My attitude about antibiotics is different from that of many of my colleagues. In fact, when I began my practice I had a problem with some patients referred to me by other doctors. I have steadfastly refused to prescribe antibiotics for long periods except in rare cases. I also require that patients return in a few days to give a urine sample for a repeat culture.

Some patients reacted to my treatment as if I were asking for the moon. Some women were insecure with my approach because "no one else did it." I explained my reasoning: The bladder is a reservoir. The antibiotic quickly reaches the site where it is needed. A large single dose works to knock out infection rapidly and effectively. Why expose your entire body as well as sensitive bladder tissue to ten days of antibiotic therapy? To me, that didn't make sense.

Some patients, however, finding they couldn't talk me into giving them the drug for ten days, would call their old physicians to get a two-week supply of an antibiotic. The doctors would comply, thinking I must have made a mistake.

However, several infectious disease studies have shown that a single dose of antibiotics eradicates uncomplicated infections with complete safety. This approach, which makes a lot of sense to me, also eliminates the complications of yeast infections and diarrhea that some women develop when taking antibiotics for ten days.

Recently, one of my patients, Pat, confronted her gynecologist. She told me, "I asked him why he insisted on giving me a ten-day course of medication for each bladder infection. Why couldn't I take one or two days of medicine and then come back for a repeat culture to see if bacteria were still in my bladder? He said he couldn't do that because patients would not want to return to his office and pay fifty dollars for a second culture. I was furious," Pat said. "I told him he was not giving women a choice."

After a while, I managed to persuade most of my patients to adopt this commonsense approach to treating bacterial infections of the bladder. They have come to learn that antibiotics are not a safe panacea. Antibiotics are miraculous drugs that have a central role in medicine. But they should not be abused by patient or physician alike.

As all my patients do, Tricia came to my office three days after taking the antibiotic—recovered and rested, but with her recent activities still fresh in her mind—so that we could figure out together what caused her problem. Her first urine culture had grown one organism, confirming that it was a genuine bacterial infection. (If it had been sterile, we would have had to figure out other causes of her symptoms.) When she came back, we took a second urine sample to make sure her urine was normal and free of infection.

Some patients continue to feel the symptoms of burning and frequency several days after the medication is finished, even though the bacteria are gone. This is because the bladder lining needs time to recuperate after bacterial attack. You should not take a second course of antibiotics just because you still feel symptoms. Get a second culture and prove there are living bacteria in your urine before you expose yourself to more drugs. Symptoms of irritation will often be relieved by taking Pyridium (a prescription bladder analgesic) or ¼ teaspoon of baking soda in water.

Just one bladder infection is a sign that something is wrong with your "voiding unit." There are certainly many ways this unit can fail. If your food processor has ever broken you know there could be something wrong with the blade, pusher, chopper, switch, wiring, or other components. Similarly, there are numerous things that can go wrong with your urinary tract. Figuring out the reason is an exercise in problem solving. We need to examine all the possibilities and eliminate the ones that don't make sense for your situation.

A Visit to My Office: Six Questions for Tracking Down the Cause of an Infection

When Tricia came into my office, she filled out a questionnaire to help us decipher what caused her infection. I wanted to know everything that she had ever observed about her urologic history. Each of the questions that follows relates to a different aspect of my theories about the causes of cystitis. All my patients are given this questionnaire when they first visit my office, and the answers to these questions provide valuable clues in the search for the cause of bouts with cystitis.

1. Do you have a history of urinary tract infections dating back to your childhood?
2. When did your first infection develop?
3. What methods of birth control have you used and when?
4. When did you last have intercourse?
5. Do you have frequent vaginal infections?
6. Do you have a good stream when you void, particularly after intercourse?

Question 1: Do You Have a History of Urinary Tract Infections?

If you have a history of urinary tract infections, something is chronically causing your bladder and pelvic floor to malfunction. If you had infections as a child, it tells me you may have a true anatomic problem. Since anatomic causes are so rare, however, I would want to eliminate other possible factors before putting you through tests that examine your anatomy.

Question 2: When Did Your First Infection Develop?

The timing of your first infection gives me clues about the cause of your present one.

For example, for many women, their first urinary tract infections occurred with the onset of sexual activity. This can be a problem for teenage girls who develop cystitis but who don't want their mothers to know they are sexually active. Girls who don't seek help for their symptoms right away can damage sensitive bladder tissue and cause themselves even more grief. Cystitis, in fact, is often called ''honeymoon cystitis'' because it often appeared in young women who were just married and sexually active for the first time. Today, of course, mores have changed and many young women have sexual relations before they have a honeymoon. The woman who develops cystitis upon her first exposure to intercourse may have something wrong with the way her bladder functions. Or there may be some problem traceable to how she is performing intercourse.

On the other hand, there are women who have intercourse for years and never develop a bladder infection, then suddenly get one. This situation points to a change in the system and makes functional problems more suspect, for we know their systems worked fine right up to a certain point. Then we investigate what happened to make the change occur.

This question of whether you were able to have intercourse without getting infections or whether the infections began the moment you started having intercourse is important because it helps me determine whether the symptoms are related to a functional or an anatomic cause or some combination of both.

Question 3: What Methods of Birth Control Have You Used and When?

I ask this question because I have found that some women who use diaphragms are susceptible to urinary tract infections.

It was a very observant patient who first said to me, "You know, I think it's my diaphragm that's causing me to get these infections." This immediately piqued my interest. Here was one distinct difference between me (who has never had a urinary tract infection) and this patient: I had never used a diaphragm.

Could this widely used birth-control method be an accomplice in recurrent urinary tract infections? This connection had not been studied, and I decided to find out. I designed a study that would confirm or deny my suspicions.

THE DIAPHRAGM STUDY: THE DIAPHRAGM-CYSTITIS LINK

The first step in the study was the selection of patients. One hundred fifty women who had recurrent urinary tract infections agreed to participate. They were otherwise healthy and had no history of urinary tract infections in childhood and had never had vaginal or bladder surgery.

I asked them the same questions about their sexual activity and use of birth control. Ninety-four percent said they thought their infections were related to sexual intercourse, and 87 percent said their infections began only after they had become sexually active. A quarter of them had had recurrent vaginal infections with their bladder infections. And two out of three reported they had a poor urine stream after intercourse but a strong forceful one at all other times.

Of the 150 women in the study, 102 used a diaphragm. Each of these 102 came back to the office wearing her diaphragm and had the uroflow and residual urine check redone.

Interestingly, I found that when they wore their diaphragms, their urine flow rates changed dramatically. The pressure of their urine flow was lower and their bladders took longer to empty.

To make this a proper scientific study, I had to find out if one factor—the fitting of the diaphragm—was consistent. If the devices were fitted very differently, it would make other correlations less credible.

So, in the tradition of medical experimentation, I participated in my own study. I learned the names of all the specialists who had fitted the diaphragm wearers in my study. There were fourteen of them, gynecologists and nurse practitioners, all in the Los Angeles area. I called each one and made an appointment to have myself fitted with a diaphragm.

When visiting their offices, I did not tell them the purpose of my study. I knew confidentiality would be maintained and that they would not find out I had visited each one as part of an experiment.

Diaphragm sizes are measured in millimeters. An 80-millimeter diaphragm is large and a 65-millimeter diaphragm is considered small. At the fourteen fittings, I received thirteen 80-millimeter diaphragms and one 75-millimeter diaphragm.

Unfortunately, all fourteen were far too big for my small frame.

Back in the office, I compared my urine flow rate with and without the diaphragms. My normal average flow rate is 18 cubic centimeters of urine per second. With an 80-millimeter diaphragm it dropped to 12 to 13 cubic centimeters per second. This drop suggested that obstruction was occurring.

What does this finding mean? As shown in my patients, the diaphragms as fitted by most health specialists tend to reduce normal flow rates (see illustration page 25). The devices were obstructing normal urine flow by putting pressure on the bladder neck. In some patients, the diaphragm restricted urine flow by as much as 40 percent by altering the angle of the bladder neck. This means that urine could easily be left in the bladder along with bacteria from recent sexual intercourse. Since most women keep the diaphragm in place up to eight hours after intercourse, you can see how easy it might be for an infection to arise.

My patients found they had to squeeze very hard to empty their bladders fully when wearing their diaphragms. Without the diaphragms, their flow rates were perfectly normal; no urine was left in their bladders.

For example, one patient's normal flow left 2 cubic centimeters of residual urine in her bladder after voiding—essentially nothing. With an 80-millimeter flat-spring diaphragm, 40 cubic centimeters (about ⅙ cup) was left over, and with a 75-millimeter flat-spring diaphragm, 34 cubic centimeters were left in her bladder.

Now all these diaphragms were "properly fitted" by competent gynecologists and nurse practitioners. But after seeing the bladder neck obstruction produced in so many of my patients, I began to question the notion of what is considered "proper fit."

One popular book on women's health care written by a doctor asserts that using the largest possible correctly fitting size ensures that the dia-

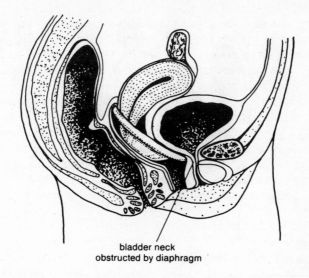

bladder neck
obstructed by diaphragm

Figure 1-3, Bladder Neck Obstructed by a Diaphragm

phragm will not be displaced during intercourse. But what is "correctly fitting"?

In essence you should not be able to feel the diaphragm once it is in place. Doctors and nurses are taught to fit diaphragm users with the "largest comfortable size." But for many women, this means that inside the vagina the coil-spring rim that gives the diaphragm its shape presses snugly against the pubic bone. When the diaphragm fits that tightly, it presses on the bladder neck. During intercourse, the diaphragm rim rubs and may irritate the bladder neck.

Many physicians will tell you that a diaphragm is a barrier method of birth control. That is, that the device itself blocks the entry of sperm into the cervix. I do not subscribe to this idea. Sperm are minuscule; we need a microscope even to see one. It simply is not possible to bar them completely from entering the cervix with a rubber disc. I tell patients, "They'll pole vault over the thing if they want to." So it does no good to make diaphragms fit tightly. It would take a diaphragm the size of a newborn baby's head to make a completely occlusive barrier.

Rather, I believe the diaphragm should be viewed as a receptacle for spermicide. In fact, Masters and Johnson have shown in their studies of sexuality that during intercourse the vagina expands and contracts. During intercourse, every diaphragm floats around somewhat, even the ones that fit tightly when the vagina is in a resting state. (Since the male penis

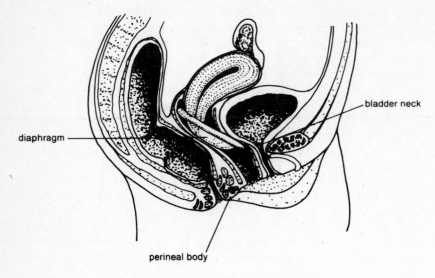

diaphragm

bladder neck

perineal body

Figure 1-4, A Properly Fitted Diaphragm

comes in all sizes and most women can accommodate the differences, it seems logical that a diaphragm of a smaller size would also be snugly held in place by good vaginal tone.)

Since the diaphragm is meant only to hold spermicide in place so that any sperm will be less likely to get by, a properly fitted diaphragm does not have to be as ''large as can be accommodated'' (see illustration).

It is critically important, however, that you put your diaphragm in correctly. The spermicide goes inside the cup and the cup rests against the cervix. As each thrust of the penis against the diaphragm pushes more spermicide into the cervical opening, the cervix becomes coated with the sperm-killing substance. This is what makes the device so effective.

My diaphragm-wearing patients continued the experiment for another year. I fitted most of them with a smaller diaphragm, the largest one that did not cause obstruction to the bladder neck but still covered the cervix. This usually turned out to be a 65-millimeter one. When inserted, the practitioner should be able to fit a portion of his or her finger between the spring and the vagina.

How can you tell if your diaphragm is the correct size? Very simply: You should *never* be able to feel the diaphragm once it is in place. If you do, it is too big. It should not obstruct the bladder neck.

How do you feel for your bladder neck? Put your forefinger inside your vagina. Press up against the pubic bone and roll your finger back and forth. You will feel a tube. That is your urethra. Follow the tube further up your vagina until you feel a V shape. That is your bladder neck.

After one year, all but one whose diaphragms were refitted were free of infection. Six women did not follow my recommendation to change diaphragm size and they still had infections. Others switched birth control methods and were infection free. Three followed recommendations but continued to experience infections for other reasons.

The startling discovery from this study was that, for diaphragm wearers, simply alleviating obstruction caused by too large a diaphragm or switching the method of birth control stopped recurrent urinary tract infections.

Thus, if you are trying to track down the cause of your infection and you use a diaphragm, the first thing I would advise you to do is to be certain your diaphragm is not obstructing the easy flow of urine. You don't have to give up the diaphragm; just get a smaller size. As my study shows, your risk of pregnancy is not likely to increase, and your risk of repeated cystitis may be eliminated. Studies have shown that the failure of the diaphragm to be an effective contraceptive method is based more on the "diaphragm in the drawer" syndrome than on improper fit.

I don't want to frighten you from using the diaphragm. In fact, just in the last year I switched to this method of birth control because I have reached the age when the pill is no longer recommended. I have not had a bladder infection. Rest assured, the diaphragm is an excellent method of birth control. It is safe and effective and has fewer side effects than any other method.

A good way to prevent infections is to void before you insert the diaphragm and have intercourse. Do not void again until you have to, so that you generate a good, efficient stream. If six hours have passed since intercourse, remove the diaphragm and then void. By removing the obstruction, you allow your bladder to function as nature intended.

Many doctors today advise cystitis patients to void right before and right after intercourse to prevent infection. This is not correct. You should not urinate after intercourse until you feel the need. You should wait until you can void with a forceful stream, for a few drops of urine dribbling out after intercourse is no protection at all. Your bladder should be at least half full. You can influence this cleansing mechanism by drinking fluids just before or after intercourse, thus assuring that you will have to urinate within a few hours. Remember, it's not simply the fact that you void after intercourse that counts. You have to void with some force to cleanse your urinary tract of any bacteria that might have been introduced during intercourse.

If you continue having problems with your diaphragm, you might consider alternate methods of birth control. Aside from the pill and IUD,

---

Four Steps for a Healthy Bladder

To keep your bladder healthy, you must empty it efficiently. This "mechanical" function is dependent on four factors:

- The amount of residual urine left in the bladder after voiding.
- The rate of urinary flow—that is, how forceful your stream is.
- The frequency of voiding; the less often you void, the longer urine stays in your bladder.
- The rate of bacterial multiplication, which depends on how large the initial introduction of bacteria into the bladder was.

These factors are implicated in cystitis. For example, the diaphragm can affect each one. It can increase residual urine by obstructing the bladder neck and decrease the rate of urinary flow. If you jump up after intercourse to void, your bladder may not be half full and capable of generating a good, forceful stream. Your stream should be capable of moving dirt on a sidewalk. If it can't move dirt, it's not forceful enough. Finally, if the diaphragm stays in for a long time, bacteria can stay in the bladder long enough to multiply into hazardous numbers.

---

which some women avoid because of side effects, other methods are available. Cervical caps and sponges are gaining popularity but must be used according to directions to avoid vaginal infections. If you have had all the children you want and find birth control methods problematic, consider a tubal ligation for you or a vasectomy for your spouse.

It is still news to many people that the diaphragm has been implicated in urinary tract infections. When I first began my study, I didn't think it was so unusual. One day I was driving a friend, who is a professor of pediatric surgery, along with his family and my daughter, to Disneyland. When I mentioned the link between cystitis and diaphragms he turned to me, surprised, and said, "My God, that's an interesting concept. Maybe that's what I'm seeing in my teenage patients." That was the first time I began to think that what I was doing was different.

At that point, I entered my scientific study in an essay competition sponsored by the Western region of the American Urological Association. I won honorable mention in the contest, beaten out only by a study on penile implants and another on prostate cancer.

My scientific article on the diaphragm was not published until a full two years after I had assembled the data and made the conclusions. In the world of research, this is a normal delay. It takes time to design a study, carry it out, write it, submit it, and then wait for other experts to referee it. If those experts find fault with a study, the author must convincingly counter those criticisms before the study is published. My study sailed through this process, but it still took two years to get published.

After I put together the scientific study, I wrote a popular article for a well-known woman's magazine. But the magazine refused to run it without making major changes—recommended by other doctors—that would have completely changed my conclusions. The magazine editors believed the article was too controversial because, in the minds of the doctors they consulted, the link was not yet "proven" and "wasn't true."

I demanded the article back and then submitted it to *Ms.* magazine, which published it without changing a word. The editors stood behind every point. *Ms.,* which considers itself on the cutting edge of women's problems, had the courage to take something that made sense and put it forth as a major health finding.

After the *Ms.* article appeared, I was called by editors of other magazines and by television producers who were excited about the new findings. By appearing on television, I found that I could get my message to a wide audience in a short time.

The response was very positive. At television studios, while sitting in the so-called green room before going on the air, women always approached me to discuss in private their urinary tract problems. They poured out their stories and were starved for information about cystitis, incontinence, and other urologic problems.

As I listened, I realized women were not getting information about urology. They had painful bladder infections and didn't know what to do about them. They leaked urine when they sneezed and didn't know why. But no one was talking about such problems.

On one show, there was a great debate before airtime over whether or not I should use the word *vagina*. Evidently, no one had ever used this word on the program. The staff had agreed that "vagina" would not be mentioned on the air. But I simply refused to talk to the audience as if they were children. There is no reason not to use correct terminology in discussing female health problems.

When I did use the word "vagina," I saw smiles cross the faces of the cameraperson and sound technician, both of whom were women, as this forbidden word was finally spoken.

On another show, I discussed diaphragms. This word was also taboo, but I ignored the rules and even showed an illustration of a diaphragm. The reaction of the studio audience was not one of shock, dismay, or disgust. Rather, after my segment on the show, they kept asking for more information. They commended the television producers for discussing—at last—issues that needed to be aired. Vaginas and diaphragms, the television producers realized, are not dark secrets. They are normal parts of life. These shows led to other appearances during which I talked about incontinence. It seems once we got past diaphragms, we could go on to that taboo.

Meanwhile, my study has been replicated and corroborated by other researchers. Doctors at the University of Washington recently found that women who use diaphragms have a rate of bladder infections four times greater than that of women who use other methods of birth control. Both the scientific article and the *Ms.* article on the diaphragm-cystitis link are often cited by other researchers because of their early significance.

What might be done to make diaphragms more compatible with a woman's body? Aside from using smaller diaphragms, the device might be designed differently. I have suggested one possibility, a diaphragm that uses a soft wire at the point where the device encounters the bladder neck (see Figure 1-5). It is a simple change because such a diaphragm would not put undue pressure on the bladder neck, and it would fit in just one way. A wearer would always know it was properly and securely in place. Unfortunately, the companies that make diaphragms still consult gynecologists who think the diaphragm should be a "snug" barrier method. It seems we still have a long way to go in persuading others to improve women's urologic health.

Question 4: When Did You Last Have Intercourse?

Of course, not all women who use diaphragms get bladder infections and not everyone who gets cystitis uses a diaphragm. What about my other patients?

Clues can be taken from answers to the fourth question on my questionnaire, for certain aspects of intercourse can lead to a urinary tract infection.

A little-regarded fact is the impact of sexual positions on urethral trauma and bladder infections. Many men, it seems, receive their sexual education from magazines like *Penthouse* and *Playboy*. Their photographs often depict men in a very dominant position for intercourse. The man is raised at arm's length above the woman, apparently ready to conquer all.

Unfortunately for women, men are not built to make this a satisfactory position. The penis is normally suspended at a 45-degree angle from the man's abdominal wall. When he enters from on high, in what we might

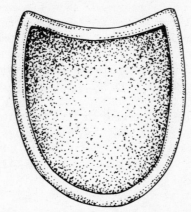

Figure 1-5, Improved Diaphragm Design

call the dominating missionary position, his anatomy forces him to thrust with a corkscrew up-and-down motion. This motion drags the urethra up and down in the vagina and the urethra quickly becomes sore and swollen. Abrasions can make bacteria adhere more easily.

This dominant position is extremely unhealthy and unsatisfying (see illustration page 32). The vagina has a G spot, or erogenous zone, along its top wall. The other erogenous spot, the clitoris, is outside the vagina. If the male enters at a lower angle, the natural alignment is such that the clitoris is compressed and the G spot is massaged. He performs a rocking motion which is more stimulating for both partners and the female urethra is spared unnecessary stress.

No sexual position is inherently dangerous. Rather it is alignment—the angle of the penis against the vagina—that counts. No position will damage the urethra if this alignment is correct.

Using spermicides for intercourse may be to blame for your infection. While they may be helpful in killing harmful bacteria (such as gonorrhea) in the vagina, excess amounts of chemicals can harm vaginal or urethral tissues. This is especially true of the foaming spermicides that are inserted as tablets into the vaginal opening. The foam can chemically burn the vagina or urethra, making it red, swollen, and tender to the touch. In some instances it can even cause ulcers, which can be mistaken for a breakout of vaginal herpes. Other spermicides come in a cream base that is gentler than foams. When inserted with applicators, the spermicide is right up on the cervix where it is expected to work.

A single contraceptive sponge contains 1,000 milligrams of nonoxy-

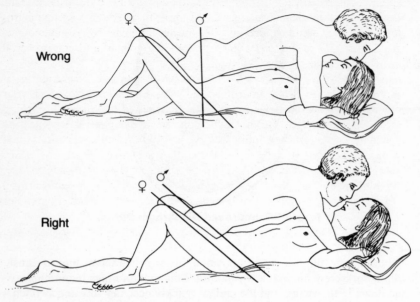

Figure 1-6, Right and Wrong Positions for Intercourse

nol 9, a chemical detergent that destroys sperm as well as the AIDS virus. However, because a chemical called peroxide (it's the same agent used to bleach hair white) is formed when the spermicide is exposed to oxygen, normal, protective bacteria, such as *Lactobacillus,* may be destroyed, allowing *E. coli* to set up shop or colonize the vagina. This results in a vaginal infection. Yeast infections can also occur with the use of spermicides, especially if you use sponges. However, newer contraceptive films have been found to decrease this type of infection, and I recommend them to my patients, especially if they use a condom.

One spermicide, Semecid, comes as a small corrugated shape, making it easy to insert into the urethral opening instead of the vagina by mistake. This results in a severe chemical urethritis and cystitis. If this should happen to you, immediately drink ¼ teaspoon of baking soda in water. The bladder analgesic, Pyridium, should also be used for the next three days. Elimination of the foods listed in Chapter Twelve should be done as this will also help decrease the pain. No permanent harm will come from this, but I guarantee you will never make that mistake again!

In any case, don't use too much spermicide. Excess cream or foam will spread outside the vagina and become a potential carrier for bacteria. This is also true of lubricants such as K-Y Lubricating Jelly or Vaseline petroleum jelly that some couples use to moisten the penis before intercourse. If you use gobs of lubricant, you are providing gobs of a viscous material on which bacteria can hitch a ride and grow.

A safer way to use K-Y Jelly is to put it on sparingly, where you need it. Put some on the tip of your index finger and open your labia with your other hand. Place the jelly on the back portion of the vagina's opening (see illustration page 34). This is the point where the penis creates friction and drag. If you are not lubricated by your own natural secretions or if your tissue is dry because of lack of estrogen, you can experience lacerations and tears to the vagina at this point, called the *posterior forchette*. By lubricating this place with a dab of jelly, you will prevent harmful friction and will minimize the amount of jelly that can spread beyond your vaginal canal and into the urethra.

Infrequent sex is *not* a factor in cystitis, as some doctors may have you believe. Rather, the problem lies in the lack of lubrication. If you are relaxed and your naturally lubricating vaginal fluids are secreted during foreplay, intercourse should not cause friction and damage your vagina or urethra. There are several products available that substitute for normal vaginal fluid. These moisturizers contain elements that mimic natural vaginal lubrication and can help restore the sensitive vaginal acid/base balance that is so necessary to prevent infection. Gyne-Moistrin, Replens, and Astroglide (not to be mistaken for an amusement park ride) are all available without a prescription.

As more women practice abstinence from intercourse in today's risky world, vibrators are seeing more action. However, you should remember to clean the vibrator with alcohol or bleach, as organisms that grow on plastic materials can be massaged into the urethra, causing an infection. Contrary to popular belief, oral sex is not a cause of cystitis either. Your partner's germs have nothing to do with your cystitis. In my fifteen years of practice, I've never found a strange throat organism in the urine being tested for bacteria. There is simply no basis for the old wives' tale that oral sex causes bladder infections.

Nor is there any basis for the belief that venereal disease is a precursor to cystitis. The two are not related. This old wives' tale may stem from a subtle male orientation that promiscuous women must get bladder infections. Not so.

Sexually transmitted bacterial infections such as trichomonas and chlamydia can cause symptoms of irritation leading to vaginitis and urethritis, however. Chlamydia is now thought to be present in the cervix of about

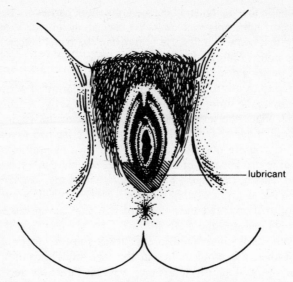

lubricant

Figure 1-7, Proper Lubricant Placement for Women

10 percent of sexually active women in America, especially those under twenty-two who have had herpes or other genital infections. Often, a woman infected with chlamydia has no symptoms. Her gynecologist may notice a mucus discharge on her cervix and that is all. When cultured, the mucus is shown to carry a cervical chlamydia infection.

Trichomonas is easily detected by looking at a smear of vaginal fluid under a microscope. The organism has a characteristic size and shape, including little tails, or *flagelli*. Gonorrhea and syphilis are long-recognized venereal diseases that require treatment for both partners.

If you have these symptoms and your urine culture is negative for showing bacteria in your bladder, you should probably be screened for these sexually transmitted bacteria because they are increasingly common. One woman was told by her physician that she had a "scaly urethra" when no bacteria were found in her urine culture. In actuality, she had urethritis induced by chlamydia.

Unlike nonspecific urethritis and urinary tract infection, which cannot be sexually transmitted, trichomonas, chlamydia, gonorrhea, and syphilis require that both partners take an antibiotic.

What if you have a normal flow rate, don't use a diaphragm, and still get infections? We will continue to look for reasons with help from the fifth question.

Question 5: Do You Have Frequent Vaginal Infections?

Vaginitis arises when the protective layer of tissue found on the vagina and urethra becomes decreased or absent for any reason. Normally, the layer protects sensitive tissue from bacteria. But when it is rubbed away, bacteria can invade the urethra. There is itching, discharge, burning inside the vagina, and burning on the outside of the urethra when you urinate. There may also be a mild feeling of frequency and urgency.

Since vaginitis is essentially increased bacterial growth in the vagina, it can lead to cystitis.

Using a diaphragm can lead to a vaginal infection. Since it is a foreign body, it can irritate the vagina. If left in the vagina longer than the recommended six to eight hours, the risk of vaginitis increases. If you forget and leave your diaphragm in for a day, I recommend that you douche with a mild vinegar-and-water solution (1 tablespoon to 1 quart water) to restore the normal acid-alkaline balance in the vagina.

With the growing awareness of sexually transmitted diseases, such as AIDS, it is imperative that women use condoms with spermicide for extra protection. But in following this necessary practice, some women are developing bladder infections for the first time. Maya came to my office in obvious distress. She had treated herself to a holiday cruise in Mexico, where she had a shipboard romance. For three glorious days she and her new love enjoyed the romance of the sea, but on the fourth day she woke up with terrible pain. Her vagina felt swollen and raw, and when she urinated, she found blood in the toilet. Suddenly her vacation had turned into her worst nightmare. When I asked her how frequently she had had intercourse, she smiled and said, "A lot!" But she couldn't understand how this could happen, as she didn't use a diaphragm and she was careful to urinate each time after sex once her bladder was full.

Maya had used a spermicide containing nonoxynol-9, a chemical found to protect against the AIDS virus. Each time she had intercourse, she inserted the proper amount and made sure not to douche for at least eight hours. However, she rarely went more than eight hours without sex. Researchers have now shown that this chemical changes the vaginal pH, creating a friendly atmosphere for bacterial replication. It's no surprise that Maya developed a vaginal infection that led to a bladder infection. Armed with this knowledge, Maya was reassured that she could prevent cystitis.

A seemingly ridiculous but common cause of vaginitis and urethritis is designer jeans or pants that are too tight for the build of your body. The center seam rubs your perineal skin and abrades the tissue so that bacteria can adhere. Irritation follows. I do not have one of those elite designer jean bodies, but I would caution you about trying to maintain that image. If the center seam pulls up on your labia when you sit and you have that tight, drawn-up feeling between the labia, the urethra, and the rectum, those are not the kinds of jeans you should be wearing.

Women who are prone to vaginal yeast infections often get the symptoms of cystitis. Such women tend to have abnormal sugar metabolism—either too much, as in diabetes, or too little, as in hypoglycemia. If you binge on sugar, you may set yourself up for yeast infections, and yeast in the urethra is very irritating. When this happens, you may feel that you have a bladder infection when in fact you don't. This is another example of why urine cultures are so important. If you frequently take antibiotics in the absence of infection, you are setting yourself up for potentially chronic bladder problems. In fact, antibiotics may actually damage your bladder and exacerbate the symptoms of cystitis. Many antibiotics cause upset stomachs, alter normal bowel metabolism, and make you even more susceptible to vaginal yeast infections. One truly distressing cause for chronic vaginitis is AIDS. As the immune system breaks down, repeated vaginal infections can be the first sign of this disease. Women who are at risk because of unprotected intercourse with more than one partner should be regularly tested for the virus.

Another source of infection in the vagina and the urethra is an allergy to the materials used in commercially available tampons and pads. Women with this allergy tend to get symptoms in the third day after their menstrual period begins. These women may make their own pads out of cloth rather than fiber, but then the problem is that cotton cloth does not carry blood away from the inner part of the pad, which is the part near the vagina. Bacteria grow in blood and are kept next to the urethra, and this easily irritates the urethra and causes urethritis, or inflammation of the urethra. I know one woman who solves this dilemma by making her own cotton pads and wrapping them in Handiwipes. Handiwipes are similar to the wrappings on menstrual pads that carry blood from the outside to the cotton inside. If you have to make your own pads for any reason, such as an allergy or because you are too large to wear commercially made pads, use Handiwipes to help protect you from infection.

I once had a patient come to me because she was developing a culture-proven bladder infection every month. This woman, who was a high-powered executive, did not wear a diaphragm, and had had intercourse for many years without ever getting infections. Her infections were in no way related to intercourse. We could not figure out what caused them until one day she said, "You know, the infection always happens by the third to fourth day of my period." I instantly realized how she could solve her problem. She was getting infections because she had switched to superabsorbent tampons, which tended, as they expanded, to obstruct her bladder neck. She would void two or three times before removing the high-capacity tampon. As soon as she started pulling the tampon out every time she urinated, she was infection-free and no longer had cystitis.

Once a nurse told me that her sister had chronic bladder infections that arose on the third day of her period each month. The infections had invaded the sister's kidneys on several occasions so that doctors had prescribed chronic antibiotic suppressive therapy. I told the nurse to tell her sister to pull out her tampons every time she voided. The infections stopped.

Again, this is a commonsense "cure" to cystitis that you could figure out by yourself. You've got to observe your habits and environment. Focus on everything you can. You are a partner in mystery solving every time you visit a physician.

If you wear tampons, I recommend that you make it a habit to pull one out each time you void. They are not expensive and the practice will keep your bladder neck and urethra free from obstruction. Next time you wear a tampon, listen to your flow and hear how it slows your urine stream as you void.

Question 6: Do You Have a Good Stream When You Void?

If your recent bladder infection did not come about after sexual activity or as a result of a vaginal infection, we have to look for other causes. The answer to the last question on my questionnaire can shed light on the matter: Do you have a good stream when you void?

Put another way, when you are in a public ladies' room, does your urinary flow rate sound as good as that of the woman in the next stall? Do you empty your bladder as quickly as your girlfriend does?

By paying attention, you may save yourself considerable trouble in the future. When Sarah came to see me last year, she was doubly perturbed. In recent years, she was having to urinate more and more frequently. "It built up gradually," she explained. "Eventually I couldn't wait an hour before having to go again. I found myself preoccupied with bathrooms. I chose dark clothing so that if I had an accident, no one would notice. Finally I got fed up and decided to get help."

Sarah went to her gynecologist, a woman physician, and explained her problem. The physician, recalling her training, said Sarah needed an operation to tighten the ligaments under her bladder and to remove her uterus. The reasoning: The ligaments had been stretched, and even if they were tightened, the uterus would make them fall again. This, the doctor said, was why Sarah had to urinate frequently.

A Uroflow Exam

A uroflow is simply a graph of how you void. As you urinate, it charts out—on paper—a graph of your flow rate. Actually, your perception of what is normal may be limited. A uroflow pictures your voiding pattern and eliminates misconceptions. It allows me to compare my flow rate, which is normal, with yours. If your flow rate is abnormal, the uroflow chart will show you the difference.

If you have an abnormal uroflow, it is likely that you will get bladder infections whether or not you have intercourse.

Sarah said she was appalled at this news. "I don't know the long-term consequences of a hysterectomy. Major surgery is risky. I was in a real dilemma. I felt my doctor was wiser than me. But the urinary problem was unbearable. My girlfriend was a patient of Dr. Gillespie's, so I called for an appointment to see if something else could be done."

When Sarah came to see me for a second opinion, we tested her flow rate. Sure enough, it was sluggish. Her stream was not forceful and her bladder never emptied itself fully. She kept having to urinate sooner and more often. Many women with this problem develop recurrent urinary tract infections. But Sarah was luckier. Her major symptom was frequency.

The cause could be traced to the nerves in her lower back. Without realizing it, Sarah had damaged a disk, which compressed the nerves that signaled her bladder to void. Her nerves were "shorted out."

"I was really surprised," Sarah said. "I felt only minimal back pain. Otherwise I was fine. I didn't exercise and I do wear high heels. Something had thrown my back out."

Sarah took a medication that stimulated these nerves to fire properly. "Within forty-eight hours," she said, "I felt relief. Gradually, I have been taking less and less medicine because I've been taking care of my back with proper exercises. I watch how I sit and lift, and I threw away my spike heels. I'm almost off medication now and my flow rate is normal. The thing that astonishes me is that I almost let someone take out my uterus, when all I needed was physical therapy and a few pills temporarily."

I often hear from patients that their streams are intermittent and tend to flow in spurts instead of in a smooth pattern. There is considerable straining to get all the urine out.

If this sounds like you, a uroflow exam could identify that you have a primary bladder problem. It will tell us if your bladder is unable to empty efficiently. Remember, it takes a good flow to cleanse bacteria from the bladder and to wash off the perineum and vagina. Residual urine is susceptible to bacterial invasion from your own body even if you are celibate.

BACK PAIN AND UROLOGIC PROBLEMS

There are numerous reasons why your bladder might not empty efficiently. One of the most common is lower back stress. You may be going to a gymnasium or exercising at home without proper supervision. If you lift weights you may injure your lower back without knowing it. You may use a rowing machine that puts stress on the lower back muscles.

You may wear heels that are too high for your hip and leg structure. This will cause you to have a swayback and increase pressure on your lower spine. The medical term for this swaying of the back to compensate for high heels, pregnancy, or other imbalances is *lordosis*. It is just one reason why many women suffer bladder dysfunction.

A recent study indicated that from 70 to 90 percent of the U.S. population will have low back pain at some point in their lives. Lower back pain is the number-one cause of disability in people under forty-five and the number-three cause in those over forty-five, according to orthopedic surgeons.

Lower back pain is also a leading cause of urinary tract infections in women. This fact is rarely addressed at urology meetings and few physicians have taken the trouble of studying the relationship in detail. Nevertheless, the fact that lower back damage can cause bladder infections has long been known by urologists everywhere.

Why is it so often overlooked? I can only guess that subtle biases may be at work. Gone are the days when lower back pain in a woman was automatically attributed to a "tipped uterus" (such a condition is extremely rare), but many doctors fail to look for other causes of lower back pain in women. Some seem to believe that women have a lower incidence of lower back injury because women tend to lift fewer heavy objects than men. But this is not the case. Women strain their backs just as often as men.

Some physicians are trained to look for overt injury to major nerves in the lower back before making a diagnosis of back injury. But there are many fine nerves in this network that can become strained and then contribute to bladder problems. Indeed, in studying patients orthopedists have found that a certain percentage of people who complain of minor backaches tend to go on to develop ruptured disks. It appears that vague back pains can be indicative of changes in disk support, presaging more serious trouble.

The point is that the bladder can pick up signs of back trouble long before there is more obvious damage to the nerves and disks.

When Irene came to see me, she had been having repeated bladder infections for three years. They came upon her at any time with or without intercourse. Irene constantly took antibiotics. Whenever she stopped, she got another infection. A culture was not taken every time, but when it was, it showed that her problem was with genuine bacterial infections.

I asked her to give me a uroflow, the first she had ever had done. It showed a severe abdominal straining pattern. Her bladder muscle was not working properly. Upon probing, I found she had an achy lower back. To Irene, it was a minor discomfort, but I convinced her to have X rays taken of her spine. They showed a major instability of the fifth lumbar vertebra. It was the kind of problem that usually requires surgery.

Then it hit her. Her bladder infections began at the same time, three years ago, that she had had a sledding accident. She came down the hill, fell, and landed hard on her tailbone. Her lower back was injured, creating her bladder problem. If someone had given her a uroflow when her infections first began, she could have avoided years of taking antibiotics and having recurrent infections.

Indeed, the bladder is the most sensitive indicator of lower back problems. Helen, a forty-five-year-old accountant, had bladder problems for three weeks. Her uroflow showed abdominal straining. I told her that I suspected it was her back. She laughed, saying her back felt fine. Then one day she called to say she was in traction. She had a slowly moving disk that did not hurt until it had slipped a certain amount. But it had caused bladder problems immediately and was a sure sign of impending back trouble.

Nina is an artist who makes silk screens at a nearby university. As she leaned over her table to reach for supplies, she strained her back and began developing bladder infections. Once she learned to stand straight, her bladder got better. Studies have shown that when you sit, the pressure on your lower disks is 40 percent greater than when you stand. Thus people who have sedentary jobs—artists, secretaries, writers—have a higher incidence of disk rupture than do people who stand and walk around on their jobs.

Virginia, an avid gardener, gets cystitis every spring. "It's because I sit on the cold ground," she said. "It weakens my bladder." But Virginia also has a lower back problem. Every spring when she goes out to start her garden, she strains her back and initiates cystitis. It has nothing to do with sitting on cold ground.

Joyce took stock of her lifestyle at the age of forty-two and decided she needed to get more exercise. She joined a health club and focused on the Stairmaster, working up to as much as thirty minutes a day. At the same time, she developed her first bladder infection. When I asked her about her exercise program, she proudly informed me of her stepping time and the free weights she could now lift, as well as any of the younger women. Imagine her surprise when nerve conduction testing showed she stretched the sensory nerves in her back, especially at the fifth lumbar–first sacral level. An X ray showed subtle changes of alignment in her spine, suggesting instability. When I suggested that she quit her routine, she wailed, "But I'll get fat!" Life is full of choices, so I recommended that she try walking in the mall on flat ground rather than face repeated bladder infections. She wasn't thrilled with this suggestion, but she agreed to try it for two weeks. When she returned to my office, not only was her uroflow normal but she was wearing a new outfit—something she spotted on her daily mall walk.

I frequently find that exercise programs can be detrimental to a woman's back health, in part because few women have professional trainers to ensure they use the proper technique during their program. As you tire, your body recruits other muscles to perform the task at hand—in some cases the wrong ones. The net effect can be to weaken rather than strengthen back support. Even exercising with free weights can be fraught with danger, because perfect form is essential. If stair climbing is your favorite exercise, I recommend you use the stairs at work or at home, which give you a natural fluid motion. Learn how to weight train properly by using the resistance methods, such as Nautilus or other isolated muscle techniques. Be careful about the use of back-loading exercise, such as the cross-country ski machines. Women with scoliosis and a swayback should not use this type of equipment as it increases the force on the lower back, putting a strain on the sensitive nerves to the bladder.

I belong to the school of thought that believes if God had wanted women to exercise He would have strewn the floor with diamonds! But I am concerned about the kinds of exercise women are choosing today. Little has been done to study the difference these exercises may have on women's pelvic floor musculature as opposed to men's. I raise this concern because of a discovery I made while studying healthy women I recruited from a health spa. I will discuss in the chapters on interstitial cystitis changes in the nerves of the pelvic floor that can be detected through a simple nerve-conduction test, which measures how long it takes to receive an electronic signal sent along a nerve pathway. Women from the spa who had never had a vaginal delivery (which stretches these nerves normally) or any history of cystitis volunteered to serve as my normal controls. But when I examined this group, all of them showed a delay in transmission of the signal to the nerves in their pelvis. The one activity they all had in common was *prolonged jogging.*

The design of the male pelvic outlet (the space between the pubic bone and the rectum) is quite narrow for obvious reasons: They don't have to "birth no babies." During jogging, the up-and-down motion of the pelvic floor is restricted, as there is not much space for the contents of the abdomen to bounce against. However, the female pelvic outlet is wide, allowing for necessary stretching during childbirth. It would seem that prolonged jogging may be similar to continual straining during delivery, which has been shown to result in damage to the pudendal nerves—the ones that send signals to the pelvic floor musculature.

A large group of nerves to the bladder originate in your lower spine between two vertebrae (see illustration page 43). The point is called the *lumbar fourth and fifth interspace.* Compression of the disk or bending backward in this area may short out the transmission of one of your body's chemical messengers that helps your bladder function. You can think of the bladder as a battery. The nerves leading to the battery from your lower back are like battery cables. And the chemical *acetylcholine* is like the battery acid. If the cable cannot transmit enough current, the charge in the battery does not build up enough to start the car—in this case to generate a normal, efficient bladder contraction.

Injury or damage to the nerves of your lower back may impair the transmission of "current" to your bladder. Like a weak battery, the bladder does not function well. It does not empty efficiently and may leave residual urine, which can lead to infections. This type of infection is best treated with a longer course of antibiotics. Depending on the individual, the drug may be needed for five to seven days.

The condition can be corrected in two ways. One is to give you bethanecol chloride (a synthetic acetylcholine) on a daily basis. The extra chemical, commonly used in your body as a neurotransmitter to help nerves "fire," aids in restoring normal bladder function. A second approach is to resolve your lower back stress. Many of my patients stop having bladder infections once they discover how they are straining their backs. I have found the use of a specialized chiropractic technique, called flexion/distraction therapy, very useful for these problems. This is a nonadjusting therapy. That is, there is no bone cracking or popping. Instead, gentle flexion of the back in a prone position coupled with massage helps to improve spinal alignment. My patients have felt the results within two weeks of therapy when this approach is helpful. If you cannot find a chiropractor with an electronic flexion table, locate a licensed deep muscle massage therapist. Several patients have discovered massage not only helps their bladders, but relieves emotional stress at the same time.

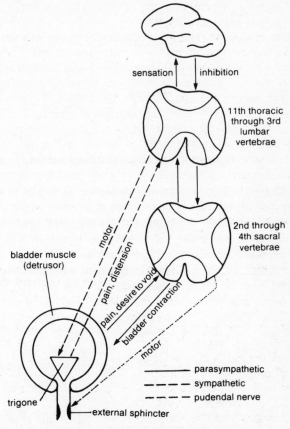

Figure 1-8, Nerve Network to the Bladder

Compare in the diagram on page 44 my uroflow with the uroflow of a patient with lower back injury. Mine is a smooth bell-shaped curve, like a smoothly accelerating and decelerating automobile. Hers is a zigzag shape, like a car that is lugging with loss of power.

If this appears to be your problem we can help resolve it by giving you a single X ray. If we see a narrowing between the disks where these nerves to the bladder originate, or any evidence of instability, we know you have a physical problem that will benefit by intense physical therapy or orthopedic manipulation. Oral doses of bethanechol chloride can help support neural transmission until the primary problem is resolved.

If you show no damage, we can treat your ''silent disk'' with stretching exercises such as yoga. Swimming is another excellent exercise that

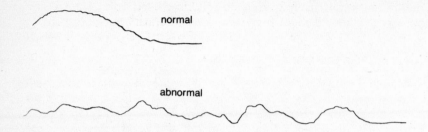

Figure 1-9, Normal and Abnormal Uroflows

strengthens the back and stomach muscles. In fact, it is perhaps the best therapy of all, but I must caution you to perform only the backstroke and the Australian crawl. Swimming styles that arch your back, such as the butterfly, will only make your symptoms worse, as will swimming with your head above the water. If you have access to a gymnasium, lie face-down across the piece of equipment called the horse. Support your stomach and hips and let your legs and toes touch the floor. Then bring your legs up so that your body is horizontal, over the horse. Pull your legs apart and then together before dropping them to the floor. If you do this ten times, you will work the muscles of your lower back in proper alignment. You can also lie on the floor on your back. Bring both knees up to your chest and hold them, while rolling gently from left to right.

If these exercises work, you may not need continuous medication. You can watch your progress when new uroflows are taken. It is truly rewarding to watch the smile on a patient's face when she looks at a successful comparison of her first uroflow and, after some hard work on her part, a later uroflow. The payoff is there, graphically displayed.

Yet another factor in lower back injury is being overweight. If you are carrying ten pounds of extra weight on your stomach, the weight is centered about 10 inches in front of your spine. Your back muscles are located 2 inches behind your spine. To balance this weight, your back muscles must exert a force of 50 pounds to counterbalance the 10 pounds on your belly. You can see that just a few pounds extra weight exerts a strain on your back.

Unfortunately, many urologists do not bother to evaluate lower back strain by asking their cystitis patients to take a uroflow exam. Rather, they assume the infection must be sexually related. The lower back simply is not considered. They assume that minor back problems are irrelevant and that only major problems, requiring surgery, could be related to urologic health. As a result, many women are prescribed unnecessary chronic suppressive antibiotic therapy to prevent recurrent urinary tract infections.

HAVE A UROFLOW DONE

A uroflow is useful for making sense of another common misdiagnosis of cystitis patients, that of "the narrow urethra." Almost weekly I see new patients, like Jenny, who tell the same sad story: "My doctor told me I have the urethra of a child," Jenny said. "It was too narrow and too tight so that my urine didn't flow as it should. I needed dilations every six weeks to stretch out and help mature my urethra."

Although the dilations were terribly painful, Jenny said she found she voided better for a few days afterward. "I didn't dare not go back," she said. "He said I would keep getting infections if I didn't come in regularly. I took antibiotics for several days after every dilation. Finally he said I could avoid the inconvenience of regular dilation simply by having surgery that would make it wider."

Is there such a thing as a narrow urethra? The answer is, emphatically, *no*. Incredibly often the poor urethra is blamed for the problem caused by a lazy bladder muscle, which can be traced to lower back problems.

Does it make sense to have your urethra snipped? The answer, again, is no.

When Jenny gave a uroflow, her problem was immediately apparent. She showed a marked inability to achieve a normal flow rate. Her infections could be traced to a bladder that did not contract, not one that could not drain.

Upon examination, her urethra was perfectly normal. For a discussion of why urethral dilations came into vogue and why they have no place in modern urology, please see Chapter Five, Anatomy Is *Not* Destiny.

Jenny asked why she seemed to void better for a few days after the dilations. The reason is simple: The procedure would paralyze her urethra, which contains muscles to hold in urine. When the muscles are knocked out of action, gravity would drain her lazy bladder and she felt better. The proper treatment for Jenny was exercise to correct her lower back problem and medication to stimulate the muscle to contract fully. She never had another dilation.

A woman recently came to me with bladder infections caused by a highly unusual set of circumstances, and the diagnosis was aided by an examination of her uroflow, which was very odd. The uroflow showed a high ascent curve with straining and then it got sporadic. It appeared that she could generate pressure well enough in the beginning by pushing with her abdominal muscles, but then there were stops and starts that did not seem to reflect that she was straining to urinate. I suspected that she was not relaxing her pelvic floor when she voided.

When I pointed this out to her, she said that her doctor told her that voiding and defecating at the same time was proof that she had a neurologically damaged bladder. He made her practice controlling her anal sphincter by squeezing it when she voided so as to gain control. This would be like doing Kegel vaginal exercises when you need to have a bowel movement. This, of course, is nonsense. But the woman tried so hard to hold back her stool if she was voiding that she never fully emptied her bladder.

We solved her problem with reeducation. She temporarily took medication to increase her bladder contractions and also enrolled in a yoga class to strengthen her lower back. She also practiced a self-regulatory mechanism. As she sat on the toilet, she completely relaxed her buttocks until she felt her vagina drop down. She felt herself relaxing more and more as she subconsciously pictured urine flowing out. After several weeks of practice, her bladder tone improved and she broke her spastic habit. Her cystitis was cured.

This relaxation exercise can be very helpful to women who have experienced chronic urinary tract infections. With an infection, it is extremely painful to urinate. Thus, you hold back, trying to stall off the inevitable pain. Once your infections are arrested, however, you might continue this learned response and hold back when you start to void, thus disrupting your normal pattern. Relaxation exercises, practiced at home, can help overcome this fear and restore normal function.

Mysterious Conditions That Can Cause Infection

Finally, what if you don't fit any of these categories? Do you get infections whether or not you have intercourse? Is your back fine, your uroflow normal, your birth control method nonobstructing?

You may have an acquired anatomic reason for your infections. That is, an explanation lies in some change your body has undergone since childhood. For example, there are glands in the urethra, called *Skene's glands,* which produce wetting agents. They help protect your urethra from urine. Skene's glands, however, can become clogged and infected with bacteria. During intercourse the bacteria are ''milked out'' of the glands. A urine culture may raise the clinical suspicion that this is your problem if you grow bacteria but have no cystitis symptoms, and a test called the *Tratner urethrogram* can confirm the diagnosis. The glands can be excised to stop the condition.

Similarly, a different gland further up on the urethra can become enlarged, causing what is called a *urethral diverticulum.* These glands can become traumatized during childbirth, enlarging and filling with pus. They hold bacteria that constantly seep into the urine. Women with this problem may be prescribed long-term antibiotic therapy. Every time they stop medication, however, the same bacterial organisms reappear in the urine. This condition can be diagnosed with the same test, the Tratner urethrogram, and surgically removed as well.

Another rare acquired condition is *chronic pyelonephritis.* The kidney may serve as a breeding ground for bacteria because of its spongelike nature. It may be difficult to knock out such infections and, in this instance, longer term antibiotic therapy is called for. To test if bacteria are stemming from the kidney and not the bladder, a catheter is put up each ureter to draw urine directly from the kidneys. If the bladder urine is positive on culture but the kidney ones are not, the problem is a lower tract infection.

Consider the case of Marion, whose infection turned out to be quite dangerous.

Infections Can Be Dangerous

At thirty-two, Marion decided it was time to interrupt her career and have a baby. She consulted her gynecologist, who told her it was a good idea to get off the pill and use a diaphragm for a few months before getting pregnant. This would give Marion's body time to adapt to its normal hormonal balance before embarking on pregnancy.

However, the first time Marion used her new diaphragm, she got a bladder infection. A second infection soon followed and, suspecting it to be the culprit, Marion put the diaphragm in the drawer. At that point, she and her husband decided to buy a house. She resumed taking birth control pills for another year and then saw a new gynecologist for advice on when to get pregnant.

The second doctor, who was a woman, gave Marion the same advice about waiting a few months before getting pregnant. She said to Marion, "Doctors have the habit of fitting diaphragms too small. Here's a different size for you that should work fine."

"The new one felt uncomfortable the moment I put it in," Marion said recently. "But I was determined to use it."

During intercourse with the new diaphragm, Marion felt pain in her side. But she simply ignored it.

The following week, she said, "I felt run down and irritable. By Saturday I was achy all over and grumpy. We made love again but used a condom. I just couldn't put the diaphragm in again."

On Saturday afternoon, Marion and her husband went shopping for a new piano. "When we got back, I should have felt elated," she said, "but I felt awful. I began to feel like I was getting a bladder infection. I thought, 'Oh, no! Not on a Saturday.' I went to the bathroom and sure enough there was blood and pain. I knew I had an infection, my third one."

Marion said her husband was sympathetic and suggested they cancel plans to join friends that evening to see a film. "I blew up and screamed at him," she said. "I told him, 'You don't understand women! I'm not sick! It's just a bladder infection!' I was really acting irrationally."

Marion telephoned her doctor and explained the symptoms. "She was extremely reluctant to prescribe an antibiotic over the phone," Marion recalled. "She made me go through my symptoms carefully—the achiness, blood, and pain. Finally, she said it sounded like a true infection and phoned in a prescription. I got the pills and took one at three o'clock. But I still didn't feel any better."

At 5:00 P.M. Marion and her husband met their friends at the theater. "I sat on the aisle because I had to keep getting up to go to the bathroom," Marion said. "I felt worse and worse. Finally, in the bathroom I began to vomit. My head was hot. I thought I was allergic to the medicine. I was so weak I could hardly stand up.

"By the time we got home, I went to bed and heaped covers over myself. I kept shaking. My fever was one hundred two and I thought it must be the flu. My body hurt so bad I couldn't sleep.

"At seven the next morning," Marion continued, "I knew I needed help. I called the doctor and woke her up. She said, 'It might be a kidney infection. To play it safe, meet me at the hospital in one hour.' I could hardly walk. Everything hurt."

At the hospital on Sunday morning, Marion was given immediate treatment for pyelonephritis. The bacteria in her bladder had worked their way into her kidneys—quietly. She received medication intravenously for a full-blown kidney infection. This is not usually life-threatening, but it can require hospitalization.

Marion said she felt better by the following Friday morning. Yet in the following days and months, her urine still tested as positive for having bacteria. This is because the kidney is very much like a sponge. Tiny abscesses throughout the organ can harbor bacteria long after an acute infection is brought under control. Thus bacteria from Marion's kidneys continued to work their way out of her body for months after her infection.

Another diagnosis you could possibly hear, but one you should beware of, is that your urinary tract infections are caused by polyps of the bladder neck. The polyps are said to act like baffles in that they impede the flow of urine. The polyps are said to create turbulence in the area of the bladder neck and to prevent bacteria from getting out of the bladder. Furthermore, many women are told that these polyps must be cauterized to restore normal bladder function.

Women come to my office after having had these "polyps" surgically removed, with still-persisting bladder infections. The reason is simple. The polyps are not the cause of bladder infections but rather the result. When you have a nose cold, your nose secretes mucus. When there is inflammation of the bladder (which may or may not be caused by a bacterial infection), these polyps—more accurately called *pseudo polyps*—may form.

Having these polyps removed makes as much sense as having your nose cauterized every time you have a cold. In other words, the so-called polyps are a reaction to an inflammation, not the cause. They are temporarily caused by swelling of the mucous glands and soon go away naturally.

What if you continue to have symptoms in the absence of bacterial infection; that is, you are told there are no bacteria in your urine. Is there nothing wrong with you? Or could you have another disease? Perhaps you've been told you have urethritis, trigonitis, or an "angry bladder." There is inflammation, you are told, but no infection.

If this sounds like your problem, you may have interstitial cystitis, the topic of the next chapter.

Self-Help Do's and Don'ts for Fighting Cystitis

There are many things you can do for yourself to figure out why you have cystitis. Your doctor can help you but you need to think about your lifestyle and how it might contribute to your infections.

• Whenever you develop symptoms of cystitis—burning, frequency of urination, pressure—get a urine culture as soon as possible. It is extremely important to differentiate between true bacterial infections and symptoms produced by other problems. Leave a urine sample for culturing before starting an antibiotic.

• Vitamin C will increase the burn you feel with cystitis. Cranberry juice contains hippuronic acid, an antiseptic that prevents adherence of *E. coli* to the bladder lining. This acid is also found in blueberries. However, once you have an infection, cranberry or blueberry juice cannot eradicate the bacteria. So drinking cranberry juice may be helpful in preventing an infection, but not in treating an existing one. Cranberry juice is simply not acidic enough to kill bacteria in urine, and the extra calories are not worth it. It is a good idea, however, to drink plenty of water when you have cystitis to help cleanse your system.

• Drink ¼ teaspoon (no more) of baking soda in a glass of water to help ease symptoms

• Look at different methods of birth control. Consider changing diaphragm sizes if you wear one and can feel it when it's in place.

• You can buy urine sticks from a pharmacist to test your urine for bacteria at home. The sticks are color coded and will show you several measures of urine contents.

• Know how to put your diaphragm in properly to prevent additional bacteria from growing on your urethra. The amount of sexual activity is not the culprit in your infections. You could hang from a chandelier and not get an infection. If you use a diaphragm properly, it does not matter how many times you have intercourse.

• Think about voiding properly and completely after intercourse. The bladder needs to be half full to generate a good contraction. You can drink fluids before or after intercourse. A good stream of urine will cleanse away any bacteria that may have reached your bladder.

• Do not squeeze out a few drops after intercourse and consider that you have reduced your chances of getting a bladder infection.

• Remove any obstructing foreign body, such as a tampon, before voiding.

• Be kind to your urethra. Avoid sexual positions that compromise your urethra.

• Think very seriously about avoiding repeated urethral dilations, particularly if your lower back and bladder functions have not been evaluated.

• And don't let anyone give you a ten-day course of antibiotics if you have an uncomplicated infection. In general, if your infection can be traced to intercourse, you probably have an uncomplicated infection and can take fewer antibiotics. But if you suffer nerve damage and your bladder is functioning poorly, you may need a longer course of drugs.

• Never take an antibiotic without leaving urine for a culture before you start the drug. Do it at home, do it at a clinic, just do it. You must determine if bacteria are present or not.

• Learn how to give a urine sample. A urinalysis is not enough, by itself, to reveal a bladder infection in women. You can contaminate your urine sample by improper collection.

• If you have back problems, consider avoiding the use of a diaphragm.

Start all exercise regimens under proper supervision to strengthen your muscles and help prevent bladder problems.

If you follow these simple guidelines, you should not get cystitis. Use your common sense in figuring out what functional or mechanical thing you are doing that encourages bacteria to stay in your bladder.

TWO

Interstitial Cystitis: The Real Story

O N the television saga *Dynasty,* the character Fallon Carrington Colby endured dramatic pain and suffering dreamed up weekly by imaginative scriptwriters. Little could those writers imagine, however, the real-life pain and suffering experienced daily by the actress who played Fallon, Pamela Sue Martin.

Pamela suffered from interstitial cystitis throughout the years she played Fallon on *Dynasty.* There were hours on the set when her bladder burned with "electric shocks." As Pamela now recalls, "I was continually plagued by it the last year on the show. Like any health problem, it was exacerbated by pressure. I ignored it as much as I could. But I was in terrible pain."

Today Pamela is no longer controlled by this crippling disease. Her own story, unlike Fallon's, has had a happy ending. She underwent treatments with me in 1984, and has since been free of interstitial cystitis symptoms. "Once the disease was explained to me," she said, "I understood why everything done to me previously didn't work. I knew what my body had been through and I could now understand why other treatments were ineffectual. Dr. Gillespie's therapy worked. I've been fine ever since and I feel cured."

Pamela's story is like that of many interstitial cystitis patients:

"I was about eighteen years old when I had my first attack. I remember it very well. I was working in New York City as a model, when I suddenly had to go to the bathroom. It was just uncontrollable. I managed to get to a ladies' room, and when I finally went, there was a lot of blood in the urine. Accordingly, I was treated for a bladder infection.

"But after that, the problem continued. I would go through bouts of increased urinary problems. I'd feel great urgency to urinate but very little would come out. There was a lot of pain involved. For the next twelve years, no matter what my symptoms were, I was treated for recurrent bladder infections. Many times urine cultures were not taken. It was always explained to me that I had a bladder infection that just repeatedly came back. And I was always prescribed pretty much the same medicine. They were large red pills that would relieve the pain and supposedly stop the infection.

"Some years were better than others. I'd have a month of pain and then many months pain free. But then it would always come back. I found different things would set it off. If I had no sexual contact for a long time and then resumed it, the problem would recur. If I was under pressure, the symptoms would worsen. But one thing was consistent: No infection was ever found.

"Over the years I saw about ten doctors. Usually I was given antibiotics. Sometimes they changed their approach. One gynecologist performed a D and C [dilation and curettage] operation that scraped my uterus 'clean.' He said I had 'excessive infection with a lot of buildup.' It didn't make sense to me why he'd operate on my uterus to fix my bladder. But the funny thing is that I did feel better for a while. I'd believe in these aggressive treatments for a while. Then the pain would come back.

"Finally, one of my gynecologists sent me to a urologist. I'll never forget it. First thing, he wanted a urine sample. But instead of asking for it, he stuck a catheter up into my bladder. Now I was there because I had horrible pain. And he just went ahead and catheterized me. Of course, my urine turned out to be sterile. It was the most excrutiating thing anybody had ever done to me. Except he then proceeded to give me these so-called urethral dilation treatments to widen and stretch open the urethra. After he did that, the urine would just pour out of me for a while and I did seem to get better. Then the pain would come back.

"I had maybe three or four dilations, always accompanied by another dose of antibiotics. By this time, I was really getting scared. The last dilation gave me a genuine infection. I was worse off after going through more excrutiating pain. I got to the point that I knew something more serious was wrong with me. I knew I wasn't being cured. I was uncomfortable so much of the time. One morning I looked into my medicine cabinet and saw rows of pills that I had been taking for years and I really felt very desperate."

You Are Not Alone

If you identify with Pamela Sue Martin, you are not alone. After her successful response to therapy in 1984, she and I appeared together on *Hour Magazine,* a television talk show hosted by Gary Collins. My office received more than twenty thousand letters from women around the country who said they had the same problem. One wrote, "I was ironing and listening to you talk when all of a sudden I realized you were talking about me!"

If you pay close attention, you will probably notice some hallmarks of this disease. The pain in your bladder feels worse after you urinate. It hurts both before and after you go to the bathroom. In fact, the only time you get relief is during those few moments when you are voiding.

You also have probably noticed that some foods make your symptoms worse. Perhaps you have eliminated coffee, tea, and orange juice from your diet, but you continue to have unexplainable bouts of pain.

Moreover, your doctor is as baffled as you are. She or he knows you're in pain but can't find anything to explain it. When your doctor looks into your bladder in the office with a cystoscope, an instrument that illuminates the inside of the bladder, everything appears normal. Your urine cultures turn up negative. You do not have a bacterial infection.

Finally, your doctor may tell you that the only way to cope with this chronic pain is through psychiatric help. He or she argues convincingly: It is a well-established tenet of urology that chronic, nonbacterial cystitis may be caused by emotional distress. *Campbell's Urology* (fourth edition, 1979, by J. Hartwell Harrison, M.D.; Ruben F. Gittes, M.D.; Alan D. Perlmutter, M.D.; Thomas A. Stamey, M.D.; and Patrick C. Walsh, M.D.), a textbook memorized by every resident in training, included the following assessment in its fourth edition.

"Interstitial cystitis—a disease that is taunting in its evasion of being understood—may represent the end stage of a bladder that has been made irritable by emotional disturbance."

The text then goes on to tell the story of a twenty-nine-year-old woman whose "bladder had come to serve as a pathway for the discharge of unconscious hatreds." This hatred, it said, "combined with a bladder infection during puberty to set up a vicious sequence of hate, repression of this hostile emotion, enuresis [bed-wetting] as an expression of the hatred, superimposed infection, and inflammation, all of which apparently culminated in chronic interstitial cystitis." Thankfully in the most recent edition this chapter has been replaced with more logical thoughts!

This was the first disease I had ever heard about in which the mind could cause an organ to burn, ulcerate, and shrink. It was the first psychiatric disease that could mysteriously cause tissue to scar. So I raised one of my "buts": But you must be telling us that women have incredibly powerful minds if we can cause our bladders to shrink. Are you giving us all that credit?

Don't Let Them Tell You It's All in Your Head

As an openminded woman, you feel perhaps there may be some emotional problem at the root of your bladder pain. After all, you do seem to cry easily in recent months. The constant pain has had an effect on your personality. No one has a perfect childhood or nontraumatized life. So you go into therapy.

After six months, however, it becomes clear that while you do have some problems to work through, the problems are not causing the real and genuine pain you feel before and after you urinate. Your therapist, too, agrees that you are a victim of real and not imaginary pain. But she can't help you eliminate the pain. She can only help you cope with it.

If you, as a reader, recognize this as the story of your life, then I would like to assure you that *you don't have a psychiatric disorder. You are not crazy. Your childhood mishaps have nothing to do with the constant pain you are coping with every day of your life.*

Rather, you have the devastating disease called interstitial cystitis. It is one of the least understood and most under-diagnosed diseases in modern urology. Most practitioners are under the impression that interstitial cystitis is rare. But in actuality, the failure to suspect interstitial cystitis is why so many of you are not diagnosed as having this disease.

Twigs in the Bladder

Interstitial cystitis is not new. The problem was first described by a French physician in 1836. He saw so-called ulcers on the floor of the bladder that would rupture.

The disease was again described and popularized in 1914 by Guy Hunner, a Baltimore gynecologist. He reported that he was finding a rare type of bladder ulcer in women. The back wall of the bladder was congested with blood vessels, he said, that appeared to mingle and then split up into "numerous twigs." An ulcer was frequently noted. This condition became known as *Hunner's ulcer.* Hunner did not know what caused the "twigs" but he did note that many of his patients had had scarlet fever, an association which, as we'll see later, turned out to be important.

Other physicians found these "ulcers" and, in listening to their patients agonize about the pain, developed various treatments. One urologist, for example, put sandalwood oil directly into women's bladders in an attempt to keep urine from burning the tissue. Other palliatives were devised and tried but interstitial cystitis was deemed incurable. In worse cases, women had their bladders surgically removed.

Interstitial Cystitis Defined

Over the years, physicians began to refer to Hunner's ulcer as interstitial cystitis, a more general name. "Hunner's ulcer," meanwhile, turned out to be a somewhat misleading term. Hunner saw true ulcers because his patients were suffering from an advanced stage of disease brought on most likely, we can speculate in hindsight, by streptococcal bacteria. After the advent of antibiotics in the 1940s, strep infections were largely arrested before they could damage bladder tissue and lead to interstitial cystitis. Unfortunately, physicians were taught to look for an ulcer in making a diagnosis. When they examined the bladders of women with the symptoms described by Pamela Sue Martin and others, they could not see any ulcers. Thus they failed to make the diagnosis of interstitial cystitis.

But it was also not clear that interstitial cystitis is a progressive disease, going from microscopic ulceration to a shrunken, scarred bladder. It has a continuum of stages. It has not one but many clinical manifestations. Thus today you do not have to have an end-stage bladder that holds only a half cup of urine to be finally diagnosed as having this disease. Your symptoms do not have to be so obvious that even an elevator operator could diagnose your case.

First, it is important for you to know that interstitial cystitis is not the same disease as common cystitis. There is a world of difference.

Common cystitis is an episodic inflammation of the urinary bladder caused by bacterial infection. When bacteria get into the bladder and cannot get out, they multiply and thrive in wet, warm urine. Pain is caused when bacteria attack your bladder lining, causing superficial erosion of the lining. Urine then comes into contact with sensitive tissues, setting up sensations of burning, frequency of urination, and pressure. It hurts when you urinate.

Such bacterial infections respond to short-term antibiotic therapy. Antibiotics work by different mechanisms. Some are like detergents—they lower the surface tension on bacteria, causing the organisms to rupture and die. Others inhibit protein synthesis in the bacteria, which prevents them from multiplying rapidly.

Interstitial cystitis, on the other hand, has nothing directly to do with bacteria. It is a chronic condition caused by an inflammation of the space (called the *interstice* or *interstitium*) between the bladder lining and the bladder muscle. It is induced by a variety of agents, but bacteria generally are not present in the bladders of its victims.

However, and this is an important point, earlier in their lives the majority of people who get interstitial cystitis have had bouts with bacterially induced cystitis. The bacteria seem to presensitize the bladder before the numerous agents we call *promoters* start the ulcerative process.

And what are those agents? We're only just beginning to find out. In my research, published in the *British Journal of Urology,* with more than four hundred interstitial cystitis patients—the largest group of such patients ever studied—I identified several factors and cofactors that promote the disease. These include certain drugs, hormones, back problems, and a virus. I am certain there are others we have not yet identified.

The agents are different, creating different damage to cells, until they funnel into a common process: interstitial cystitis. In other words, interstitial cystitis does not have a single cause, and no single treatment can help everyone who suffers from it.

In working with interstitial cystitis, I have become convinced that environmental causes can play an important role in disease formation. When presensitized people come into contact with one or more environmental factors, the disease process can begin. It involves, as we shall see later on, a slow destruction of bladder tissue by urine. The immune system may try to cope with this destruction by making adaptations to bladder tissue. It is as if the body is trying to heal itself but is thwarted by a constant attack—that of urine on injured tissue.

Interstitial cystitis is not necessarily progressive and it exhibits a wide range of symptoms. In its earliest stages, frequency of urination without bacterial infection may be all that is noted. It usually starts out as a mild condition, in which the bladder's protective inner lining becomes inactivated.

In severe cases, the bladder rapidly becomes ulcerated and scarred. It literally shrinks and may hold only 1 to 2 ounces of urine. In every case of interstitial cystitis, sensitive tissue is continuously exposed to an acid burn from urine. As a result, it is painful to hold urine.

In fact, as noted, the only time an interstitial cystitis patient feels relief is when she voids. During those moments, the capillaries that filter the contents of urine have no blood flow. Filtration therefore stops. But when she finishes voiding, the vessels quickly refill, causing increased filtration of acid and other elements in urine. Pain resumes.

Interstitial Cystitis Around the World

As time went on, many physicians from around the world began to notice that interstitial cystitis does not occur with the same incidence in every country. In England, for example, it has been found in 1 of every 660 outpatients with cystitis. In Scandinavia, it has been identified in 1 in 350 such patients. In the United States, some physicians believe that 1 in 20 cystitis sufferers is a victim of interstitial cystitis.

However, with increased awareness of this disease over the past decade, the reported figures have risen rapidly. Today, statisticians believe that there are between twenty thousand and fifty thousand men, women, and children in the United States alone with this problem. Is there some explanation for the higher incidence?

One reason has to do with underdiagnosis. In England, for example, women are not thought to have the disease until their bladders shrink to half of normal capacity. In fact, physicians in that country prefer to think of this problem as one caused by a "hypersensitive bladder" and not "interstitial cystitis" if the patient's bladder can hold a normal amount of urine.

If interstitial cystitis is an environmental disease, such variations in incidence are to be expected. Women in Europe are exposed to different drugs, pollution factors, and diets from American women. These differences, I believe, explain the different rates of interstitial cystitis occurrence around the world.

Why Are So Many Cases Misdiagnosed?

Why are so many cases (perhaps yours) of interstitial cystitis overlooked or misdiagnosed? Why do some physicians believe it is a very rare disease? The answer is complex and reflects the dynamic nature of medical knowledge itself.

Interstitial cystitis is a particularly enigmatic disease. Because it was first described in detail by a gynecologist, many physicians to this day are under the false impression that only women can develop interstitial cystitis. But men get it, too. They tend to be diagnosed as having a bacterial prostatitis or nonspecific urethritis, vague-sounding conditions about which very little is known. In my experience, many men thus diagnosed actually have interstitial cystitis. If you think it is difficult to get properly diagnosed when you are female, you should consider what it is like for men with this disease. Many are given unnecessary prostatectomies (as their female counterparts are given unnecessary hysterectomies) as a way of treating the symptoms of lower pelvic pain.

Because different causes for interstitial cystitis share the same symptoms in both men and women, medical investigators have been confounded in their attempts to explain the disease. Also, much of the medical detective work today that is leading to treatments for interstitial cystitis is based on very recent medical findings. The biochemical aspects of this disease are on the forefront of the field of biochemistry itself.

Many doctors have seen only one "classic" case in their medical careers and are simply unaware that the disease exists widely. By looking for Hunner's ulcer, they miss other signs that would lead to a diagnosis. Some physicians are aware of interstitial cystitis but think it is a hopeless problem. Some, in fact, regard interstitial cystitis as a disease worse than cancer. At least there are well-established approaches and methods for treating cancer; the doctor knows what to do. But there are not yet widely agreed upon treatments for interstitial cystitis among the nation's urologists. Underdiagnosis has made it a rare, orphan disease.

Hence some physicians, when they suspect you have interstitial cystitis, might opt not to tell you. They believe they can't do anything; they don't know of any treatment that works. They think that you have an incurable disease, and that if you knew, you'd get more upset than you already are.

Here is where the importance of knowing how to be a patient comes in (see Chapter Four). If you have this chronic disease, you know how much pain there is. You know how easy it is for you to cry and become emotional about the disease. You know that the pain sometimes really does drive you crazy. To many doctors this is proof that you are suffering from a psychiatric disorder. You act unbalanced. Your fixation on your bladder, they say, is causing it to shrink so that it may ultimately have to be removed.

You may be blubbering all over his desk, and he is a caring physician and feels helpless. So he does what any gallant gentleman does to help a lady in distress. He offers the best help he can, which is psychological counseling. He wants to help you learn to cope with the pain and look into your soul for the reason you hurt. You are referred to a psychiatrist.

Barbara's Story

In recent years, the research that several others and I have done has confirmed my suspicions that interstitial cystitis is not psychiatric. I began to suspect that the emperor had no clothes. It just did not make sense.

This became apparent when Barbara came to see me in 1980, the first year of my private practice. Her arrival marked for me the beginning of a great adventure in urology. Together we embarked on an investigation that was to be full of mysteries and surprises.

It is my habit to open the door to my waiting room and personally invite each patient into my office. It is my environment and I like to invite people in just the way I invite them into my home after opening the front door of the house.

I was immediately struck by the way Barbara walked. I still like to exercise my observational skills when meeting patients. She was dressed in a loose empire waist dress and flats and her hair seemed rigid, as if she had pushed it stiffly into place. Her face was drawn.

Before standing up, she looked at me with a quick, almost furtive glance that seemed to say, "I'm scared and suspicious of you. You probably won't believe what I say."

She stood up painfully and began to walk. Her legs were apart and she took small, slow, careful steps to avoid jarring her body. It was what I have come to call the "classic interstitial cystitis walk." In my office, she gripped the arms of the chair and lowered herself, again slowly, into the seat. Then she shifted her weight off her pelvis.

I asked her what I could do to help. Barbara did not, could not, look me in the face. This was a pattern I was to see many times in people with this disease. She refused to meet my eyes out of a fear that I would not believe her story. Like many interstitial cystitis patients, Barbara had been told there was nothing wrong with her.

The facts of her story were tragic. She recounted them recently, going over some of the things she told me when we met: "I began having urinary problems six years ago, when I was twenty-eight years old. It began with urine retention for no reason anyone could figure out. I was dilated two or three times a week. They couldn't find a cause for my problem. Although I started out with bladder infections, later they could not find infections. It was just bladder pain that continued for four to five years.

"I reached the point where the pain was so great I began to go to other doctors. I was told I had kidney problems. I was told I'd be on dialysis by the time I was forty. The pain increased and I was given antibiotics. I was maintained on antibiotics for years. The sulfa drugs made me shaky and the other antibiotics made me tired all the time. No one warned me of the side effects. My energy was draining and draining. I was working as a literary agent in New York and was always exhausted.

"Then I developed lower back problems. They seemed to be related to the urinary retention. I went in and out of emergency wards for dilation, back traction, and new regimes of antibiotics.

"I knew I could not maintain my life the way it was. At thirty-three, I left New York for California, believing inside of me that I would not live long. Every day, every night I was frightened and no one could give me a reason for my pain and fear.

"The search for doctors who could help continued. My pain increased and my back problems worsened. I'd suddenly be unable to walk, spend two weeks in the hospital and six months recovering. I found urologists mostly to be plumbers. They described the machinery, how it worked, and told me everything in my body worked fine. One doctor scraped the inside of my bladder and trigone. It was called a curettage, supposedly kind of like a D and C of the bladder. It made me much worse.

"I was always left with the feeling that I had somehow done something wrong to my body. I was somehow responsible for creating the mysterious pain. This implication, that the pain was not there, is, for me, the hardest part. It eroded my spirit."

Imagine a woman in pain whom no one has ever believed! She was trying to cope but the pain was winning. Barbara had been to fifteen doctors (about average for women with this problem) complaining of unremitting lower pelvic pain. She was occasionally told she had pelvic inflammatory disease, or PID.

In reality, the pain of PID cannot match the pain of interstitial cystitis. I have had a child and occasionally experience menstrual cramps so I know what pelvic pain can feel like. But with interstitial cystitis, there is a continuous acid burn of the tissue on top of the cramping.

As Barbara told her story that day in my office, she began to weep. Her emotional pain predominated her physical pain. And as she spoke, I realized why other physicians probably had had a hard time listening to her: Hardly any facts were being related; it was all emotion.

After she finished, I said, "I think I know what's wrong with you." Barbara looked stunned. It was the first time any physician had said that. As she calmed down, I asked her questions.

Does it hurt before, during, or after you urinate? She had not thought to pay attention before but, yes, it only stopped hurting when she voided.

Are you very meticulous and obsessive about neatness? Do you make lists? This question was prompted by my then recent medical training, which taught me that interstitial cystitis patients are so-called Type A personalities. Today I think these personality traits are irrelevant to the disease. Anyway, Barbara's answer was affirmative; she was Type A.

Have cultures been done on your urine? She answered, "Very few." Nevertheless, Barbara was repeatedly prescribed antibiotics to combat infections. I found this interesting. I never give antibiotics without first getting a urine sample for culturing. As time went on, Barbara said, she began to notice that the antibiotics made her symptoms worse. She had to urinate more and more often.

Did you try psychotherapy? Yes, and after several years, she found she could handle the pain better. But the pain did not lessen.

The GAG Layer

To understand what happened to Barbara's bladder and perhaps to yours, you need to visualize how a healthy bladder works. On the bladder surface there is a protective layer that is secreted, like mucus, from the cells that make up the bladder lining. Scientifically speaking, this secretion is made of sulfated glycosaminoglycans, but from now on we'll simply call it your GAG layer.

The GAG layer, a fouling barrier, is your first line of protection against anything that enters your bladder. Urine contains many toxic elements that your body has excreted. The GAG layer repels them. It is like a moisturizer that keeps harmful elements from interacting with tissue.

Perhaps most important, the GAG layer is impervious to acids and toxins found in urine. It is believed that by binding to underlying cells, the GAG layer creates an electrically neutral barrier to urine. Specifically, the GAG layer is designed to prevent protons—electrically positive-charged elements in urine—from binding to the surface of the underlying tissue. Without a GAG layer, the underlying bladder tissue cells would readily interact with electrically charged chemicals in your urine. A tiny electric current would be established across the cellular membranes—protons would flow from urine into the unprotected cells and you would feel "electric shocks."

Furthermore, your GAG layer is the primary antibacterial defense mechanism of the bladder. When bacteria enter a normal bladder under normal circumstances, the layer prevents them from adhering to the interior tissue. The bacteria are soon washed away and no harm is done. But if bacteria remain in the bladder, they begin to colonize. Growing bacteria secrete enzymes that help them adhere to tissue. The more bacteria, the more enzymes. Eventually, the GAG layer is eroded. Bacteria begin to adhere to underlying bladder cells.

When this protective layer is damaged, urine gains access to tissue below. This can have several effects. Cell membranes begin to leak. Capillaries are exposed to urine. And nerve networks in the bladder are inappropriately triggered. Between epithelial cells (the cells of the bladder lining) there are branches of sensory nerves that are connected to the sympathetic nervous system. When a normal bladder is half full, the GAG layer is slightly stretched, which allows ions or chemicals in urine to leak across the barrier and tickle or excite these nerves below. This gives rise to the signal to void. But in a damaged bladder, ions in much smaller volumes of urine get through the barrier. You feel burning, pressure, cramping, frequency, and pain—the hallmarks of cystitis.

In a study of 300 patients with interstitial cystitis, I found that more than 95 percent of them had a history of at least one bacteria-proven bladder infection. This led me to speculate that when a healthy GAG layer is damaged—particularly by recurrent bacterial infection—it may change, or mutate. The affected bladder may later be more susceptible to other chemicals and be ineffective at deflecting them from the tissue. Once your GAG layer is compromised, your chances of developing abnormal tissue reactions in response to urinary toxins are higher than if your bladder was never modified.

As previously stated, there are many agents, certain drugs, hormones, pesticides, a virus, and so on that may serve as promoters of interstitial cystitis. In Hunner's day, scarlet fever was such an agent. If you have interstitial cystitis, you have probably been exposed to something that has compromised your GAG layer. Thus it is important to recall any circumstances surrounding the onset of your disease.

The onset of interstitial cystitis can be insidious and slow, but it can also be sudden and traumatic. Diane, for example, went to a friend's wedding and began the two-hour drive home with a full bladder. She had to urinate but decided to hold it in since she was "almost home." She had had a few bladder infections in her life but noticed nothing unusual. Once home, she ran to the bathroom and sat down to void. At that moment, she developed tremendous pain. And from that moment forward, she never voided normally again. Her onset was related to the way she overdistended her bladder by holding in urine for so long. Upon questioning, it became clear that her bladder was not normal, as she came to realize she had been having symptoms of frequency and mild burning for quite some time. But she had paid them no heed until the wedding episode precipitated her problem and made her look into it.

Symptoms and Concepts

As I listened to Diane and then to hundreds of other women with interstitial cystitis, I slowly pieced together different aspects of this enigmatic disease. Each patient's story contained clues about what causes interstitial cystitis and clues to developing treatments that work. Deciphering the meaning of various symptoms has led to developing fundamental concepts of the disease.

Symptom: *Acid Foods Make Me Feel Worse*

One of the first things I asked patients in those early days of my practice was simply, "What makes you feel better or worse?" Frequently, one answer was, "Acid foods make me feel terrible."

"I discovered I couldn't drink orange juice, grapefruit juice, or other acid drinks without increasing the burning and pain," said Paula, an Orange County housewife who was immobilized for several years with interstitial cystitis. "Wine was the worst. My bladder would start to hurt almost instantly."

Esther said she had been taking vitamin C by the handfuls. "Before I'd have breakfast I'd feel better. An hour later I'd be uncomfortable. I also lived on grapefruit and toast for breakfast and drank cranberry juice all day long. I thought I was doing my body all sorts of good."

So in looking for a common element, I decided to look at how acids might be involved with bladder pain. The simplest way to do this involved testing the pH of urine voided by my patients.

The symbol *pH* is used to describe the acidity or alkalinity of a solution. Acid solutions have a pH measuring from 0 to 7. Alkaline solutions have a pH of 7 to 14. A neutral solution, which is neither acid nor alkaline, has a pH of 7. Acids, by definition, are solutions that donate positively charged hydrogen ions (called protons). Alkaline bases, by definition, are solutions that accept protons.

At first, I suspected I would find that my patients would have very acid urine. After all, they complained of acidlike burns in the bladder. When they ate acid foods, their symptoms worsened. Was acid urine to blame?

Surprisingly, I found the opposite: My patients all had very alkaline urine! Now I had been taught that alkaline urine is not abnormal. They were merely called "alkaline tides" and were supposedly related to dietary influence.

But this didn't make sense. I was measuring alkaline urine in patients who hadn't eaten for twelve hours. When you don't eat for that long, your urine becomes acid. These patients should have been, to use the medical term, acidotic. I tested urines at different times of the day and consistently saw alkaline urine in association with severe pain, burning, and frequency. It became clear to me that the high pH of their urine was not related to diet.

To prove it, I had patients' husbands eat exactly the same diet as their wives and then I recorded their urinary pH. The husbands' pH hardly ever went above 5.5, which is normal for most urine samples. Yet the wives, with the same diet and fluid intake, showed pHs of 7.5, with marked symptoms of pain and burning.

I then asked myself: Is the urine in their kidneys alkaline or is it just urine in the bladder that has an elevated pH? Logically, if alkaline urine correlated with what you ate, the urine in the kidneys should show it.

I ran a very simple experiment in the operating room. While patients were anesthetized, I ran catheters up their ureters to get urine samples from the kidneys. Sure enough, the urinary pH in the kidneys was in the normal pH range of 5.5. Urine in the bladder was somehow undergoing significant pH changes. Since the bladder serves as a reservoir for fluids, there would be plenty of time for a chemical change to occur there.

Concept: How Leaky Cell Membranes Contribute to Pain

This discovery of pH changes was the first breakthrough in solving the mystery. It pinpointed that interstitial cystitis involved the chemistry of the bladder lining. The pH changes were not irrelevant. Rather they were a clue to explaining the disease process.

I reasoned there must be an ion exchange occurring on the bladder surface. Positive charges found in normally acid urine were disappearing! Instead, the urine was showing excess negative charges, resulting in an alkaline urine. What could account for this basic chemical change?

I began to think about cells. Cells are fundamentally alkaline. They contain high levels of bicarbonate, which gives them an alkaline pH (see illustration page 67).

If cells were leaking, two things could happen. First, the cells would lose bicarbonate as negative charges in the cells flow out toward the positive charges in the urine (positive and negative charges attract one another). That would explain how the urine became alkaline. Second, positive charges in urine would start flowing toward negative charges in the cells. Urine would enter the leaking cells. And it would burn.

At that point, I remembered what I had been taught about burn patients. They lose massive amounts of bicarbonate, an alkaline salt. In fact, one of the most critical aspects of treating burn patients is to give them lots of sodium bicarbonate (a sodium alkaline salt) to arrest the cellular leakage of bicarbonate.

It occurred to me that my patients were describing the identical problem. If you drip acid on your arm, you will get a burn and a loss of bicarbonate. If you keep acid urine on your injured bladder, you will experience burning and loss of bicarbonate. The pH readings proved it.

Suddenly I knew the direction to take. By postulating interstitial cystitis as a "leaky cell membrane" disease, I could look for factors that would cause the leak to occur. And I could try to find ways to stop the leak.

Clearly, healthy bladders with intact GAG layers do not leak. Urine, with all its toxic substances and high acidity, does not burn or injure a normal bladder. But if you constantly put urine directly on skin that has no protective GAG layer, you will get a burn. Men and women who are incontinent develop terrible burns on the skin in their genital area; their skin takes on the texture of nonpliable leather.

I developed a model of a leaky urothelial cell, that is one that has lost its GAG layer protection (see illustration). When the GAG layer is lost, the charges from urine can affect the exposed bladder membrane. The cells, in turn, exchange negative charges for the positive ones in urine. A balance is achieved.

As I developed this model, a patient one day told me she was taking baking soda for her symptoms and found it helpful. Instead of dismissing this as irrelevant, I wondered how that could possibly help.

Baking soda is alkaline. It would make the urine in the kidney less acid, I reasoned. In turn, urine reaching the bladder would be less acid and therefore less highly charged.

This turns out to be beneficial for the person with leaky cell membranes. When cells leak, they lose sodium and gain hydrogen. It is as if the cell pumps one element in and another out. When urine pH is altered with baking soda, the pump mechanism is reversed. The cells begin to regain sodium bicarbonate and to lose hydrogen ions (protons). This restores the normal alkaline balance of the cells.

Another patient said her symptoms were relieved by Pyridium but not by Urised, both bladder anesthetic agents. I looked up Urised and discovered it would only work in an acid medium. Since my patients' urine was not acid, the medication Urised naturally did not work, and neither did it turn their urine blue, as it does for people whose urine is acid. Pyridium, on the other hand, is not related to pH. It, by the way, turns urine orange by releasing mahogany dye. One patient said she felt like an Easter bunny: She dyed all her underwear red or blue depending on which medicine she was taking.

Symptom: Urinary Frequency

About this time I started asking patients to describe their pain in more detail. What kind of pressure feeling is it? Many then said it felt like spasms.

"You don't sleep at night," said Pam. "You lie there looking at the ceiling and say, 'Why me?' The pain is constant. You feel like you've swallowed a strep throat and it's lodged in your bladder."

This was puzzling. Urologic investigations had shown that the smooth bladder muscle, the detrusor, does not actually spasm. But there was no denying that patients were describing real cramps, even to the extent of comparing them to the cramps of childbirth.

It made me think. If you keep putting acid on a wound, it eats away at tissue and gets right down to the bone. If the urine is burning bladder tissue, the bladder would "want" to rid itself of urine as quickly as possible. It makes sense that bladder spasms are a protective response of the body, to keep its surface from being burned further. If you keep washing

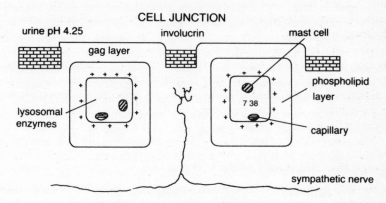

Figure 2-1, Leaky Urothelial Cell

the acid away, you may contain the burn to a lesser level. Thus the symptom of urinary frequency became one of the earliest indicators that the process of interstitial cystitis had begun.

I also reexamined what I'd been taught about diagnosing this disease. One of the hallmarks of the disease is a shrunken, shriveled bladder. Thinking again of burns, I realized that when the skin forms a scar, the skin contracts—plastic reconstructive surgery is based on concepts of how to release scar tissue and regain mobility and flexibility.

A bladder with end-stage interstitial cystitis would shrink as if with scar tissue. As the burning continued, the bladder would no longer expand and contract normally. I remembered Hunner's ulcers. Now it was clear to me why the disease had been classified as ulcerative. Urine is indeed ulcerating and could burn away the very lining of the bladder.

Concept: Urethritis as an Early Sign

I realized that the ability to diagnose their disease only at this very late, ulcerative, stage was little help to my patients. I needed to find the earliest sign of the disease. I pulled charts on patients I had diagnosed as having "urethritis." The term *urethritis,* defined as inflammation of the urethra, has no real meaning, but it was the term available at the time.

I called some of those patients months after having seen them to ask, "How are you doing? Do you still have your symptoms?" They were surprised to hear from me but, yes, the symptoms were continuing. "I have to urinate every hour," said Cindy. "It feels like pressure in my urethra, a kind of irritation down there. It isn't getting any better."

I began to suspect that urethritis could be the beginnings of interstitial cystitis. Upon reexamination, these women had nothing wrong with their urethras. There was no inflammation and no redness. I wondered if something could be happening in the bladder that was causing the external sphincter in the urethra to go into spasm. This would make their symptom a referral pain; that is, pain that originates in one place but is felt in another. Was the urethra being blamed for a problem in the bladder? At the time, there was no known nerve pathway that could account for this kind of referral pain. (The pathway was later found. See page 97.)

Symptoms: Antibiotics Make It Worse

By asking patients, "What makes you feel worse?" another pattern emerged.

"I had dozens of attacks," said Linda. "My doctor was great about it. I'd just call him and tell him I had another infection and he'd renew my prescription for an antibiotic. We didn't bother to do urine cultures because we knew I was just one of those women who got cystitis a lot.

"But after a while, I noticed that the antibiotics weren't working. My symptoms wouldn't go away in a couple of days. In fact, sometimes they got worse. We tried several antibiotics but I kept getting worse."

Before long, more than thirty patients told me, separately and without any coaching, that their symptoms got worse when they took antibiotics. But not just any antibiotics but three particular drugs: nitrofurantoin, tetracycline, and erythromycin.

These patients' past urinalysis reports showed marked elevation of urinary pH but no bacterial growth in the urine culture. There seemed to be no explanation for their urinary symptoms.

But a pattern seemed to be emerging.

When one patient informed me that her urine smelled like "a dead mouse" just before a bad attack, I pulled the charts on past patients and realized that the patients who were coming back to me because of chronic urethritis were the very ones for whom I had prescribed nitrofurantoin. These were patients I may have chastised for wearing tight jeans, saying, "You're bringing the urethritis on yourself by causing irritation to your urethra."

But maybe they were telling me something else, something significant. I had given them antibiotics three or four months at a time, but the treatment I had been taught to give in residency training was not working for these patients. They were not responding; in fact, the patients' symptoms had changed for the worse: Now they felt pain and burning all the time, except when urinating. Their stories were sounding exactly like interstitial cystitis. It suddenly felt more like a murder mystery than a simple medical mystery. Were doctors doing in their own patients?

Concept: Antibiotic-Related Interstitial Cystitis

Like other urologists, I had been taught that so-called chronic antibiotic suppressive therapy was the proper way to treat women complaining of repeated urinary tract infections. In this therapy, the patient takes antibiotics every day for three to four months. The rationale? Something is chronically inducing her infections, so you should simply knock out the bacteria before they take hold.

There are several problems with this concept. As discussed in Chapter One, there is usually a commonsense cause for repeated urinary infections. When something obstructs the normal flow of urine, bacteria have greater opportunity to grow in the bladder. Lower back problems are also often a reason for cystitis, as will be discussed. In my opinion, the only time it makes sense to take antibiotics for long periods is when conditions such as a chronic kidney infection or bladder paralysis are present.

Another question was whether or not bacteria were present when these medications were taken. Many patients told me they did not give urine cultures before taking long cycles of antibiotics.

What if they had not had bacteria in their urine? What if they were taking antibiotics in the absence of infection? What if their symptoms—urinary frequency, burning, pain—were *not* caused by bacteria?

I began to think about how antibiotics work. There are two main mechanisms. Bacteriocidal drugs—ampicillin, penicillin, and sulfa drugs—work by killing bacteria outright. Other antibiotics attack the bacterial membrane. They invade the outer membranes of bacteria and cause them to "leak to death." These bacteriostatic drugs include nitrofurantoin, tetracycline, and erythromycin.

Now there was a key to the mystery. Could it be that antibiotics—in the absence of bacteria—end up attacking what's available, namely bladder tissue? Could it be that tissue, which had already been sensitized by certain bacteria, could become "leaky" too? Remember: The bladder is a reservoir. An antibiotic excreted in urine that is not put to work killing bacteria would remain biologically active in the bladder. In addition, some patients could have metabolic difficulties in digesting or breaking down the drug normally. As a result, *a different or more toxic form of the antibiotic might be excreted in urine.*

There are scientific papers suggesting that this may be the case. When bacteria invade the bladder, they excrete an enzyme that yields a good supply of *ammonium ions,* a breakdown product of ammonia. Bacteria then use the ammonium ions to help them adhere to the bladder surface. An ammonium ion works by binding to a portion of the GAG molecule and impairing the molecule's ability to repel charges.

You can think of the GAG layer as being like a perimeter alarm. Its job is to keep out intruders, such as electrically charged chemicals in urine. By producing ammonium ions, bacteria inactivate the perimeter alarm. Intruders cross into unprotected cells of the bladder. The GAG layer is weakened by bacteria. It is simply inactivated.

The antibiotics tetracycline and erythromycin and nitrofurantoin (which is an antiseptic or detergent) work by inactivating the protective coat (which is much like a GAG layer) around individual bacteria. When the drugs reach a bladder that contains bacteria, they selectively target the bacteria and make them leak to death.

As it turns out, nitrofurantoin contains ammonium ions. If it were excreted into a bladder with no bacteria present, it could conceivably interact with a presensitized GAG layer and inactivate the perimeter alarm. Symptoms of burning and pain would thus accompany taking the drug.

Once a GAG perimeter is altered by bacteria (particularly by repeated infections), it may become easier for agents that are not as potent as bacteria to breach the perimeter. There are weak links in the fence.

Thus the perimeter alarm is presensitized. Although it functions, it no longer functions well. And, continuously assaulted, the perimeter eventually breaks down and loses resistance. Perhaps this is why chronic antibiotic therapy in the absence of infection seems to be a common link among patients with interstitial cystitis.

It might also explain why some patients noticed their urine smelled like a dead mouse. Something—perhaps a metabolic problem in breaking down proteins—could be producing excessive ammonium ions in urine. The result is a noxious smell, hence the graphic description.

The antibiotics associated with interstitial cystitis are not always prescribed for bladder infections. Many women take these drugs for acne or bronchitis. In cream form, they can be absorbed into the body in large amounts. Thus, some patients may later develop interstitial cystitis without ever having had cystitis. Antibiotic-related interstitial cystitis is largely an American version of the disease. In certain European countries, for example, nitrofurantoin, erythromycin, and tetracycline are not generally prescribed by physicians. This may help explain the relatively high incidence of interstitial cystitis in the United States, where these drugs are given routinely for the presumptive diagnosis of infection.

Please understand me: Antibiotics are not bad for you if you have a case of true bacterial cystitis. In that case, the antibiotic does what it is designed to do—inactivates the bacteria.

But if you insist that your doctor give you an antibiotic over the telephone without an exam every time your cystitis "flares up," or you get a cough or flu attack, you may be inviting more pain and suffering upon yourself. If the physician prescribes medication without taking a urine culture first to prove there is bacteria in your urine, you are asking for trouble.

Incidentally, to date there has never been a satisfactory animal model for interstitial cystitis. The complex of symptoms and the disease, however, are real. One difficulty with the studies that have been done is that they use animal bladders that have not been presensitized by a previous bacterial infection. In addition, one virus implicated in the disease cannot be introduced into rats, mice, or rabbits. Without laying this basis, as well as introducing important cofactors in the disease process, the results of research on animals have been confused and conflicting.

Finally, it is important that urologists discard the notion that women are "loaded" with bacteria and fated to get recurrent urinary tract infections. It is this bias, I believe, that leads to the improper use of antibiotics in treating the symptoms of cystitis.

More Symptoms

CHOCOLATE AND OTHER FOODS

While patients said acid foods worsened their symptoms, other foods were also singled out.

"I get really bad when I eat chocolate," said one.

"Champagne and red wine destroy me," said another.

"If I eat Mexican food, the burn really increases," said another. One Chinese woman told me ruefully that she could not tolerate soy sauce.

Soon I found myself sitting with a list of foods. What common element did they have? How could they be implicated with bladder function?

The list multiplied like rabbits. It soon included carbonated drinks, coffee, cheese, nuts, bananas, yogurt, avocado, and raisins.

THE ELECTRIC SHOCK SYNDROME

Meanwhile, many patients reported they felt a bizarre sensation in the bladder. "The pain is somewhat like a cramp," said Georgianne, "with a little electric shock in it. Zit! It keeps getting you every ten to fifteen seconds. It goes on all day long until you become debilitated and exhausted by the pain.''

These ''electric shocks'' were somewhat different from the chemical burn most patients felt. The sensations were sharp, tingling, as if they involved nerves.

Such symptoms, interestingly, were exacerbated by stress. ''I really notice it when I'm under pressure,'' said Nancy. ''The more stress at work or home, the more my bladder hurts.''

OTHER DRUGS INTENSIFYING DISCOMFORT

Other patients said certain medications made them much worse. These included several over-the-counter cold medicines and some long-lasting cough drops.

Louise was addicted to diet pills even though she had bladder attacks every time she took amphetamines. Like many compulsive dieters, she denied she might be hurting herself with so many diet pills. And for Louise, the correlation between the pills and her bladder was unmistakable. She chose to ignore it for a year and then checked herself into a drug therapy program. When free of the diet pills, her symptoms abated.

Mary asked me why her symptoms always flared up when she had dental work done. ''Are my teeth related to my bladder?'' she asked. I investigated the drugs used by dentists, Xylocaine (the trademark for lidocaine) with epinephrine. How might they fit the puzzle?

There were also some patients who found that the antidepressant Elavil (amitriptyline), prescribed by their psychiatrists, really helped quell their symptoms. ''The first time I took it,'' said Betty, ''it felt like the fire was stomped out. But it was too strong to take at the dosages given me so I cut my pills way down and used only a small amount every night.''

PAINFUL INTERCOURSE

A most debilitating symptom for many of my patients is painful intercourse. There are sharp pains in the vagina upon penetration which go away (temporarily) only if an orgasm is achieved.

''It is ruining my marriage,'' said Astrid. ''My husband thinks I'm making it up and just want an excuse not to sleep with him. But the pain is terrible. It hurts and it doesn't go away with time. I've tried relaxing, different lubricants, even aspirin before sex. It just plain hurts.''

Concept: How Nerve System Chemicals Can Trigger Bladder Pain

About the time I was trying to make sense of all these various symptoms, new scientific findings were published about an important chemical component of the nervous system. Very powerful chemicals previously identified in the brain (the neurotransmitters acetylcholine, norepinephrine, and serotonin) were found to exist—to everyone's surprise—in the gut and bladder.

Reports pointed out that these chemicals are carried along nerves that go from the brain, to the heart, to the gut, to the bladder and urethra, and finally to the tip of the penis or its feminine counterpart, the clitoris. It is an integrated system.

These nerves comprise a kind of network to be used in the body's "fight or flight" response. When an animal is stressed, these nerves "fire" their special chemicals more rapidly to help the animal escape (flight) or otherwise deal with the stressful stimulus (fight). The same is true in humans.

In bladder tissue, the nerves were found throughout the lamina propria, the bladder's very thin, smooth muscle layer in the interstitium. Previously, this layer was thought to have no function.

Since these nerves are there, I thought, what could affect their function? I had little training in nutrition but soon found that some foods contain these same powerful chemicals. These chemicals are later excreted in urine.

It was thus I discovered that foods on the list compiled by patients all contained tryptophan, tyramine, and tyrosine. In the body, these compounds stimulate the synthesis of serotonin and norepinephrine, both neurotransmitters used along this newly found system. In other words, when you eat chocolate or bananas or drink red wine, you promote the manufacture of serotonin, and a higher than usual amount of its metabolites are excreted in urine.

I searched for scientific articles on serotonin. In one study, a researcher reported cutting his finger and accidentally dropping serotonin on the wound. As a result, an enormous burn developed, and his finger swelled dramatically. There is a rare syndrome in which people produce too much serotonin. Some victims suffer itching under the arms, sore feet, hivelike sensations, and a needlelike tingling on their skins. Serotonin release destabilized cell membranes. If a woman had a leaky perimeter alarm, an influx of ions could flow across the membrane like an electric charge. Could this produce the "electric shocks" some patients were experiencing in their bladders?

Norepinephrine and acetylcholine, the other neurotransmitters found in this nerve system, fire more rapidly along nerves when the patient is under stress, and also give rise to the symptoms of burning and cramping.

But there was another key. These neurotransmitter-conducting nerves go from the bladder through the urethra and out to the clitoris. If there was a membrane leak in the bladder stimulating transmission along these nerve routes, pain could be referred along these nerves to the next system down the road—namely the external sphincter in the urethra and the clitoris. This sounded like the needling, shooting urethral pains described by some patients. Many women had told me they had a bruised, achy feeling in the clitoris. They also said they never dared tell this symptom to a male doctor for fear he would think they were crazy.

For example, one of my patients said she told her gynecologist many years ago that her clitoris felt bruised and achy, almost throbbing with a sensation of pressure. His response was, "If it hurts, don't touch it." She said she was so shocked at being made to feel guilty for describing this observation that she never dared volunteer the symptom to another physician.

Another patient—a young woman who had been sexually active for six years and married for more than one year—said that her physician, upon hearing the symptom of clitoral pain, told her, "Oh, don't worry. You're just a nervous bride!"

But now the reason behind painful intercourse is clear. These nerves travel a route between the vagina and the base of the bladder. On one side, nerves enter the bladder's sensory region, the trigone. On the other side, they enter the vagina's sensory region, the G spot. During intercourse, the normal focal point of stimulation in the vagina is at this G spot. Now imagine there is a burning sensation in the trigone as ions stimulate the nerves of this system. The stimulation of intercourse would be like someone rubbing your sunburned back. Instead of feeling warm and tender, you feel an intensified burn, almost as if you had a third-degree sunburn in the vagina.

An orgasm, however, eradicates the pain because the nerves are temporarily inhibited. Many physicians, as well as husbands and lovers, have thought that women use interstitial cystitis to avoid sex. But in my experience, patients are deeply disturbed about the loss of sexual pleasure. They mourn the loss of pleasurable sexual intercourse.

Carolyn broke down and cried one day in my office. "Sex has always been good between my husband and me," she said. "It's just a nice thing we do together. Now I see him and he looks so sad. We lost something we valued so much. I feel bad, not for me, but for him. I see that look in his eye and I want to cry. I know he's afraid of hurting me, even when I do feel better."

As a woman, I have been deeply moved by the sexual problems faced by Carolyn and other patients. Many women are frightened of losing their marriages. Others feel they could never commit to matrimony because the pain of intercourse would prevent such intimacy.

Husbands and lovers are also deeply affected by this disease. A lover does not want to cause pain. When he cannot give sexual pleasure to his partner, he feels inadequate; he loses self-esteem and feels sexually inadequate. Thus, interstitial cystitis can change the body image and sexuality of both men and women.

Sex is possible for interstitial cystitis patients who have not completed therapy, however, with some modifications. There are many ways to express intimacy. The idea is to prevent the angle of the penis from stimulating the base of the bladder. Only certain positions accomplish this. The woman on top can lower herself onto the penis and monitor the angle herself. Or she can rest on her hands and knees as her partner enters from behind. Or he can sit on the side of the bed with the woman sitting on top of him. In this position pelvic rocking motions should not overstimulate the bladder, for the penis is against the cervix rather than the bladder.

Pain management techniques, like those taught in natural childbirth classes, work well for many patients. Peggy, for example, has her husband stroke her stomach every night at bedtime. "He uses a feather-light touch," she said, "and traces circles over my abdomen. He can feel when my bladder is tight or in spasm." According to Peggy, the technique of light stroking (called *effleurage*) relaxes her bladder. "It gives my husband a sense of really helping me," she said, "and enables me to have intercourse without bladder pain."

Other strategies for controlling the pain also work. When I began to put my patients on a diet that restricted foods containing precursors to serotonin, their symptoms lessened. I then looked for drugs that might block serotonin's effect on membranes. I recalled the patient who told me that Elavil (amitriptyline) made her feel better. It is an antidepressant that works by blocking the uptake in membranes of serotonin, norepinephrine, and acetylcholine. This drug's blocking effect decreased the burning sensation. Only minute amounts, about 10 to 40 milligrams, eliminated most of the burn.

Other medications became suspect as agents that exacerbated symptoms, such as the over-the-counter pain-relief tablets. For reasons I will discuss later, medications that prevent the release of prostaglandins, such as ibuprofen, increased pelvic pain in my patients. This was apparent when Tanya complained that the only time her symptoms flared up was on the first day of her period. As most of my patients found relief from their symptoms at that time of the month, I asked her if she was taking any special medication for cramps. She replied "No, but I do take six tablets a day of Advil or Motrin like my gynecologist recommended." When I suggested that she use Tylenol her symptoms dramatically improved. However, for severe cramps, she was given a prescription for Percocet, a nonaspirin-containing pain reliever. This worked out well for her, but her response led me to consider how the stomach and digestion could affect pelvic pain.

We soon discovered why other medications increased pain. Many cold remedies contain ephedrine, a drug that increases the production of norepinephrine and its uptake by membranes. The dentist adds epinephrine to the Xylocaine (lidocaine) to make it last longer. And amphetamines also increase the effect of norepinephrine on membrane surfaces. This stimulates the norepinephrine-related nerves in the lamina propria, causing increased cramping.

All these symptoms now made sense in light of the brain-to-bladder chemical system of the body. With this knowledge, we could begin to treat symptoms by finding and using agents that blocked serotonin uptake and recommending that patients avoid substances that promote serotonin production.

Symptom: "Migraine" of the Bladder

Patients are very adept at describing their discomfort. The pain of interstitial cystitis has been likened to putting hot coals, Ben-Gay, or sandpaper in the bladder.

But one of the most enlightening descriptions for me was "You know, it feels like a migraine in my bladder. The pain throbs. It's as if there were a vice grip inside me and something is applying merciless pressure."

Serotonin is an agent that causes narrowing of the blood vessels. Migraine headaches are related to reduced blood flow through the small blood vessels in the brain. When there is increased serotonin available, the vessels go into spasm. This is the throbbing sensation of vascular congestion. I was struck by the fact that many patients said their migraine headaches also went away when they followed the interstitial cystitis diet restrictions! At the same time, I suspected that serotonin was not the only factor in this complex of symptoms. In examining the bladders of scores of patients, I was struck with how reddened the tissue appeared. The bladder walls were streaked with numerous blood vessels and spiraling capillaries. Normal bladders are clear and have just a few well-defined blood vessels.

I began photographing these abnormal bladders with special camera equipment (see photograph on page 77). A pattern emerged. Indeed, these were "angry" red bladders, always showing the "twigs" described by

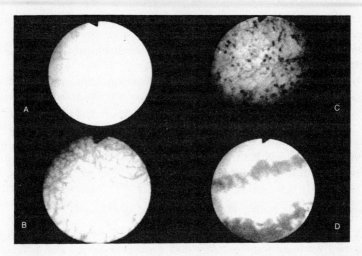

Figure 2-2, (A) A normal bladder. (B) The "angry" red bladder of interstitial cystitis. (C, D) Diverse manifestations of interstitial cystitis.

Hunner. The more I looked at them, the more they seemed to remind me of something familiar.

One day, sitting at my desk with pictures of bladders spread out in front of me, it hit me: These bladders looked like the back of the eyes of patients who have been blinded by diabetes. One of the complications of diabetes is massive capillary growth in the eye, and these bladders were marked by massive capillary growth. Some capillaries took the shape of dramatic spirals, something never seen in healthy bladders.

Other researchers had mentioned that there were vascular changes in the appearance of interstitial cystitis bladders. Yet no one had thought it amounted to much.

How Abnormal Capillary Growth Causes "Angry" Bladders Concept

By coincidence, at this time I read a paper on angiogenesis—a fancy word for capillary growth. Researchers at a major university had shown that capillary growth was involved in the growth of tumors. Cancerous tumors, they found, somehow encourage the proliferation of tiny capillaries, which connect the incipient tumor to nearby arteries and veins. The increased blood supply nourishes the tumor. They also found that cancer cells make a protein that promotes this capillary growth. Through special genetic engineering techniques, they are learning to make this protein in quantity for laboratory experiments.

This protein stimulates capillary growth. But if blocked, might it arrest capillary growth? I wondered.

I began to see a fuller picture of what is happening in the bladders of interstitial cystitis patients. When you cut or burn yourself, millions of tiny capillary loops are formed to seal the edges. A scab forms and later new skin grows there. But in the bladder, urine continually rips the scab from the healing site. New capillaries are continuously formed. The body is trying to heal itself, but the urine defeats it. Capillaries continue to grow unabatedly and to mature into larger vessels.

Symptoms: Joint Pains, Wheezing, Bowel Problems

As if patients with interstitial cystitis don't suffer enough, many report symptoms such as joint pains, bowel problems, fever, and asthmalike wheezing. Estelle's thumb always ached just before an attack of interstitial cystitis. She thought it was a sign of arthritis, even though the pain in her thumb correlated exactly with the pain in her bladder.

I began to wonder if perhaps the body's immune system was somehow involved. Many researchers over the years have suggested that interstitial cystitis may be an autoimmune disease. This means that the body has somehow made a disastrous mistake; it recognizes something in itself as being "foreign" and wages an immune system attack on its own tissue, in this case bladder tissue.

The immune system, in broad terms, involves the interplay of two agents—foreign invaders (*antigens*) and the body's own defense substances (*antibodies*), which immobilize invaders. An antigen can be a bacterium, a virus, or any number of agents from outside your body. Antibodies are proteins that recognize antigens with high specificity.

There is a highly significant test that can tell whether or not tissue from an organ has been attacked by antibodies. Called *immunofluorescence,* it literally tags the invading antigens with a fluorescent green dye. The antigens seek out antibodies (as heat-seeking missiles find a target) in tissue. If the antigen recognizes an antibody, a complex is formed and the dye fluoresces under a special light. It "sticks" to the tissue that has the antigen-antibody complex.

I wanted to know if the bladder tissue of my patients showed the presence of antibodies. Their presence would indicate that the immune system had somehow been activated. I presumed (and later proved) that normal bladder tissue does not show such activity; when tagged with the glow in the dark dye, it doesn't light up.

I sent some tissue samples from the bladders of my patients to an immunopathologist who specialized in this technique. He questioned why he should run the tests. "This is a waste of your patients' money," he said. "The bladder is not an immunologically active organ."

I insisted he run the tests on just five patients. If no activity was evident, so be it. But if antibodies showed up in the tissue, he would agree to perform this test on the biopsies of all my patients.

The tissue samples of all five patients were strikingly positive, lighting up like the glow-in-the-dark wands used by kids on Halloween. He concurred, "There's something here all right. All other bladder tissue we've seen has been totally negative." He agreed to keep investigating more patients with me.

We did 100 more tissue samples, and a pattern emerged. There were distinct categories of antibody reactions in these patients. It looked as if this was not one disease, but many. There were at least five different immunofluorescent patterns that kept repeating. In addition, virtually every patient showed fibrinogen (a scablike material) in her lamina propria (that smooth muscle in the interstitium). This was the first definitive hallmark of interstitial cystitis.

At first, we thought these results could have been caused by bacterial infections. Maybe bacteria were causing the antigen-antibody reaction. But urine cultures done at the same time as the biopsy all turned up negative. Cultures for the bacterial venereal disease chlamydia were also negative. Moreover, none of the patients at biopsy was taking suppressive antibiotic therapy; therefore the response was not likely to be a direct result of the antibiotics.

But something had activated the patients' immune systems. What was it? In an attempt to explain these observations, we returned to the patients' charts. And there we found some definite correlations. For example, the tissue of women who had taken only tetracycline therapy turned up with one pattern. Those women who had taken only nitrofurantoin showed another pattern. Women who had taken both antibiotics for a long period showed still another. A much smaller, rare group of women that had not necessarily taken many antibiotics at all showed a different antibody. Another group showed only fibrinogen in the interstitium.

But the question of what a truly normal bladder looks like remained. Virtually all bladder biopsies are taken from people who come to the doctor because something seems to be wrong. Thus no "normal normals" were available for comparison with the findings in my interstitial cystitis patients. I needed to make sure that the immune system is not activated in a healthy bladder by the biopsy technique alone.

I quickly cast my eye toward the operating room nurses at Century City

Hospital, where I perform surgery. These nurses were familiar with interstitial cystitis patients. At first they believed, as they had been taught, that this disease was psychosomatic. But as time went on, their attitude changed. Each of them peered through my cystoscope to see the bladder interiors directly. They saw the inflammation, the hemorrhages, the capillary growth, and the ulcerations. And they saw the incredible pain experienced by patients after their bladders had been distended as part of an operative procedure.

And so they volunteered to undergo cystoscopy and bladder biopsies in my office—without anesthesia. The actions of these truly generous and dedicated nurses indicated an enormous trust in me and empathy for the patients. As one of my patients said, "I cry every time I think these nurses did this."

The tissue samples taken from six nurses have served as the normal controls for my continuing studies. There was no fibrinogen in the interstitium of their bladders. Nor did they show signs of antigen-antibody activity.

In addition, we used their tissue to develop a brand-new staining technique that shows what normal and abnormal bladder tissue looks like. Normal tissue has a well-defined thin top layer which represents the GAG secretions that are believed to exist in the bladder (see photographs on p. 80). It came out pink in the staining technique. Underneath was a blue layer (consistent with urothelial cells). Next was a reddish layer (consistent with the interstitium that contained normal amounts of capillaries). The result resembled the NBC peacock.

Abnormal tissue obtained from patients with interstitial cystitis lacked the pink layer. This meant the GAG layer was gone. The blue layer was replaced by a brown material that represented an antibody. And the reddish area of the interstitium was infiltrated by a brown substance (fibrinogen) with huge, dilated, and ruptured capillaries. This staining technique helped to confirm the theory that interstitial cystitis is the result of the loss of the protective layer on the bladder surface.

With the results of this color-staining technique, we were able to see that interstitial cystitis is not one disease but many.

Patients with the disease can now be divided into three major categories. One group of patients has inflammation primarily on the surface of its bladder cells. A second group shows capillary growth and major involvement of its immune systems. A third, those who had fibrinogen only, has cell-mediated disease such as thyroid imbalance.

These results led to the first real diagnostic technique for the diseases that cause interstitial problems. They also led me to think about a new and different concept of autoimmune diseases. The findings indicated that

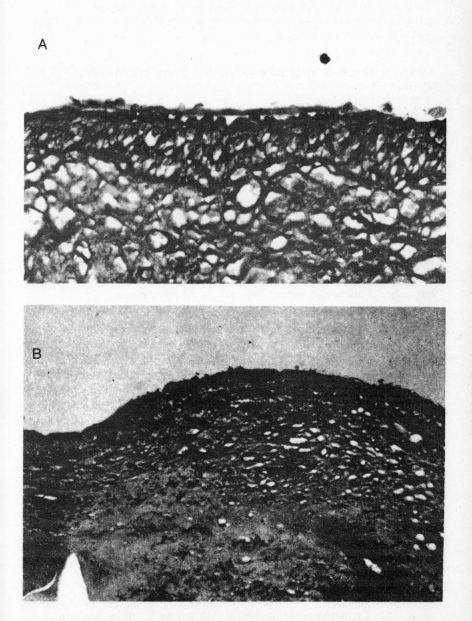

Figure 2-3, (A) Normal bladder. (B) Bladder with interstitial cystitis.

the bladder could be damaged in numerous ways, but they all resulted in a common process called interstitial cystitis, in which the immune system was definitely involved.

Concept: The Role Your Immune System Plays in Interstitial Cystitis

Why should the immune system become chronically activated in a disease such as interstitial cystitis? Granted, a bacterial invasion of the bladder could mount a brief antigen-antibody response, and once the infection was over, the reaction would disappear. However, interstitial cystitis patients do not have bacteria in their bladders.

Physicians have been taught that an autoimmune disease is one in which the immune system turns on itself. Instead of protecting the "self," the body recognizes something of itself as "foreign." Antibodies attack the tissue. Such diseases include arthritis, asthma, and lupus.

This has never made much sense to me. Why would the body destroy itself? I turned the question around: Maybe the body is trying to *protect* itself. Perhaps the immune system, in these diseases, has not gone haywire but rather is attempting some "logical" or adaptive repair.

In interstitial cystitis, the GAG layer is missing or damaged. Urine constantly burns tissue. Nerves are exposed to urine and fire randomly. Capillaries grow continuously. The bladder cramps as it tries to expel urine.

In this theory, the immune system is trying to substitute for the missing GAG layer. It is therefore to protect or adapt for the tissue's deficient components by placing fibrinogen as the next best impermeable barrier. Fibrinogen serves as the "scab" trying to keep the environment from getting into damaged tissues.

By extension, other autoimmune diseases might be viewed as immunologic adaptations of the body whenever GAGlike layers are damaged. There is a GAG layer in your joints and in your bowel. Could this be implicated in arthritis and colitis? Much more research will have to be done to explore this possibility. The bladder is an excellent organ in which to carry out research because, with instruments, it is readily accessible.

Symptom: Chronic Fatigue

At this point, I was pleased that so many pieces of the puzzle were falling into place. But some patients still didn't fit any of the categories. Many had never taken antibiotics for cystitis, although they may have taken them for acne or other conditions. In any case, antibiotics taken in the absence of infection could not have been a cause in Hunner's day; the drugs hadn't been invented yet. There had to be other factors in the disease that we had not unearthed.

Margaret had been my patient for a year. One day, she came to tell me that, at long last, she had been diagnosed as having chronic Epstein-Barr virus (EBV) infection. This is the virus that causes mononucleosis. It is very prevalent in our society and 90 percent of the U.S. population has antibodies to it.

But some people such as Margaret, for an unknown reason, have a chronic infection of the virus. The virus remains active in their bodies. Various agents in the environment seem to activate the virus and make it flare up in these unfortunate people, who are predominantly women.

"I'm exhausted all the time," Margaret said. "I have sore throats, headaches, swollen lymph glands, and a low-grade fever. I know that the virus is the cause of my interstitial cystitis. I know it."

I shook my head. "That's not possible, Margaret. I've never heard anything about Epstein-Barr virus except that it causes mono. You're telling me that it's not ordinary mono and that you're tired and weak from it?"

But what she said piqued my interest. Other patients had been describing symptoms that sounded like a viral infection. They had headaches, sore throats, and diarrhea. Yet plenty of research had been done trying to relate viruses to interstitial cystitis. All the results had been negative.

Except no one had ever looked at EBV.

"Okay, Margaret," I said. "Just to humor you, I'll test the next five people who walk through my office door for chronic EBV. You'll see. They won't have it."

But they did. They had massive infections.

Concept: Environmental Factors May Trigger Episodes

Very little is known about chronic EBV infections. The virus seems to lie quiescent in the lymph system or in damaged epithelium until something in the environment triggers it to multiply. An infection ensues. Such patients have chronic sore throats and are often given antibiotics for strep throats. Yet their throat tissue is rarely cultured to see if streptococcal bacteria are present.

I theorized that the virus could be responsible for initiating the changes in bladder tissues of interstitial cystitis patients. Such patients would feel fine for a while and then, boom! something would activate the virus and promote the disease we call interstitial cystitis.

Working with EBV authority Dr. Jim Jones, of the National Jewish Center for Immunology & Respiratory Medicine, we came upon one possible agent—phorbol esters. These chemicals are used in paints, lacquers, solvents, and a wide range of other industrial chemicals. For a list of agents containing these chemicals, see Appendix C.

More of my patients' symptoms began to make sense. Janie got sick every weekday evening after her husband came home but was fine when he was there on the weekends. The possible reason? He is an automobile mechanic and uses chemicals containing phorbol esters that cling to his clothes. He would bring the chemical into the house after work and Janie's bladder would hurt. On weekends he was free of the chemicals and Janie felt fine.

June got sick when exposed to household cleaners, particularly chlorine bleaches used to whiten sinks. After she hired a cleaning lady, her symptoms improved.

Lisa noticed her bladder hurt every time she went to the manicurist. Phorbol esters are in the glues and polishes used by beauticians to create that long-nail look. Nancy stopped having her nails done.

Leona was informed her office was going to be renovated. At the same time, she began to feel "like a Raggedy Ann with the stuffing knocked out of her." She developed headaches, fatigue, bladder pain, and constant coughing along with a sore throat. I informed Leona she had "Sick Building Syndrome." We discussed that it was possible that the glues used to lay down new carpeting and the cleaning products used in the building were causing her symptoms, and after she put an environmental air filter device into her office, her symptoms disappeared.

Chronic Fatigue Syndrome (CFS), or Fibromyalgia Syndrome (FMS) as it is now called, has been the focus of new research into the category of what I call "invisible diseases." Like interstitial cystitis, patients with this disorder have low serum serotonin, low cortisol production, low levels of tryptophan, low magnesium and growth hormone levels, and low blood pressure. In others words, these patients are running short on gas. In addition, these women seem to be more prone to premenstrual irritability.

As you will read in Chapter Eleven, I studied the metabolism and digestion of patients with interstitial cystitis and found several abnormal metabolites in urine that could cause bladder pain. These were all related to poor digestion in the stomach, especially of foods high in tryptophan, tyrosine, tyramine, and phenylalanine, essential amino acids necessary for hormone and nervous system function. Not surprisingly, CFS and FMS patients were also found to have poor digestion in a study done by Dr. Daniel Clauw at Georgetown University.

Interstitial cystitis patients also noted that many individuals had low blood pressure, a finding recently reported in CFS and FMS patients. The treatment of adding salt to their diet helped to correct this problem. I recommend if you suffer from hypotension, or low blood pressure, to try using natural sea salt, or kosher salt, as these salts are lower in sodium and contain numerous trace minerals important to the adrenal gland. The difference in taste is amazing. Just put a little of iodized table salt in your mouth. It has a bitter, metallic taste. Now try the sea salt. Notice how sweet it tastes? That's because the balance of trace minerals in sea salt does not cause the salivary glands to release zinc—which gives regular table salt its bitter, metallic taste.

Symptom: Menstruation, Menopause, and Pregnancy Coinciding with Flare-ups

Cathy's bladder began to hurt five days before her period and it kept hurting until twenty-four hours after she started to menstruate. It happened every month. "It's a dull aching toward the base of my bladder," she said.

Estelle's interstitial cystitis had responded well to treatment. She could travel again and her life was back to normal. Then, as she entered menopause, her gynecologist gave her a combination estrogen and progestin therapy. Her bladder pain returned with a vengeance.

Marlene had bladder problems since she was eighteen. When she was twenty-five, she got pregnant, and to her astonishment, her symptoms disappeared. She had a blissful pregnancy. Then, six weeks after the delivery, the bladder pain came back worse than it had ever been.

Concept: How Cycles Alter Bladder Behavior

Perhaps in this complicated disease, equally complicated hormonal factors come into play. Women develop interstitial cystitis far more frequently than men, at a ratio of one hundred to one. Men do not have monthly hormonal cycles. Maybe there are clues to be found in this fact.

It has been shown that estrogen increases the GAG layer and that progestins decrease it. Now don't confuse progestins with natural progesterone, which supports estrogen's effect on tissue. Many physicians misrepresent progestins such as Provera as a progesterone. It is not the same thing! Progestins are not natural, but are a synthetic product that blocks estrogen. Natural progesterone is much weaker and has fewer side effects. However, its delivery and absorption are not as controlled as the synthetic progestins. At the same time the body increases natural progesterone production, a chemical called angiotensin is released from the ovaries, which stimulates the rapid increase in blood vessels in the uterus, forming the lining for the egg. At the moment angiotensin production ceases, shedding of the uterine lining begins.

For two weeks before her period, as her progesterone and angiotensin levels rose, Cathy gradually developed urinary frequency. Her urinary pH rose to 7.5, indicating leaking cellular membranes. When her period came, she felt relief. Her pH fell back to normal range and she felt fine until the next time she ovulated. If this was the cause of some of my patient's symptoms, why not try a drug that blocks angiotensin?

As a senior medical student at UCLA, I wrote an article on treating renovascular hypertension with one of the first experimental angiotensin blockers, called saralasin. I realized that these drugs worked through competition for the same receptor site as the hormone, angiotensin. So it was important that I start Cathy on her medication when angiotensin was at its lowest level. As this medication may cause low blood pressure in normal people, I recommended that she take this medication at bedtime. She began taking Vasotec the first day of her period. She was amazed when she had few or no symptoms with her next period.

Estelle was fine until she took progestins at menopause. Repeatedly, she experienced excruciating bladder burning, pressure, and urinary frequency with each cycle. Unlike "normal" women who may tolerate progestins without a side effect, the blockade to bloodflow in the bladder of women with interstitial cystitis causes severe symptoms. In other words, most interstitial cystitis patients are "progestin intolerant." I encourage you to read Chapter Seven for a more detailed discussion of what this means for hormone replacement therapy.

Marlene's entire hormonal balance changed during pregnancy. Six weeks after she delivered, however, her bladder problems resumed. The protective effects of estrogen, oxytocin, and prolactin, pituitary hormones released by nursing, were gone. I have advised women to nurse as long as possible to continue the production of oxytocin and prolactin, which relaxes smooth muscle. Not only does your baby get the added immunological and psychological benefits of nursing, but your child could be giving you the gift of pain relief.

It may be that some women have naturally immature GAG layers. This would predispose them, from birth, to factors that alter bladder GAGs. I call them members of the teeny-weeny bladder club. Almost all of these women have hormonal abnormalities that affect receptors on the bladder surface, increasing their chance for a membrane "leak" to occur.

The complex effects of hormones and subhormones on bladder tissue during menstrual cycles is an area that needs much more investigation. However, until women can write their names in the snow, it will remain a low priority.

A New Understanding of What Causes Capillary Growth

As my interest in angiogenesis increased, I voraciously read research articles by scientists in fields considered far astray from urology. I have always believed that nothing in medicine is new; it's the application of the principle that is different. As a result, I began to subscribe to journals in gastroenterology, endocrinology, gynecology, neurology, neurosurgery, and basic science. Because I was not prejudiced by doctrines taught to others in their fields, I found it much easier to see the possible applications of others' work to urology.

When I came across research by David Knighton on the cell's response to injury, I made an important connection. In his article, he discussed the reasons behind rapid capillary growth, or angiogenesis. He found that it could be triggered by tissue losing oxygen as a result of acidosis, excess CO_2, low potassium, and low blood sugar. This caused blood vessels to go into spasm, which changed the blood flow to the cell. The capillary became "leaky" and the body responded by trying to bring more oxygen to the tissue through the birth of tiny new blood vessels or capillaries. Could this be the underlying reason for the changes in blood vessels in the bladder seen in patients with interstitial cystitis? Many of my patients complained of low blood pressure and hypoglycemia. This was not a case of reading "the handwriting on the wall"; this was skywriting by NASA!

I was now forced to think about this disease in a completely different manner, and in doing so I began to understand that interstitial cystitis may not be a disease after all, but a syndrome or collection of symptoms caused by tissue losing oxygen through changes in blood flow. There are many ways this oxygen loss could happen, which would explain why not everyone would respond to a single type of treatment.

So, out came all the charts again! This time, I began looking through the long stories written by patients about their own observations. Many described back problems before their symptoms began. Another group had a diagnosis of irritable bowel syndrome, and yet another crowd had distinctly hormonal problems, while others developed their bladder pain after pelvic surgery. No wonder there was so much dissension in the medical community about this problem. If you saw a gastroenterologist, he diagnosed you with his invisible syndrome, irritable bowel. The gynecologist thought you had pelvic inflammatory disease, while the urologist called you the unhappy owner of an "irritable bladder." Women were certainly being diagnosed as a "hole" in this case.

Back Problems and Pelvic Pain

Reatha always considered herself a calm, controlled woman. After all, she was a nurse and understood that doctors don't always have the answer.

She was calm, that is, until she was struck down by pain. While driving home, she was involved in a head-on collision, which threw her out the back window of her truck, causing her to land on her back and hip. Miraculously, she appeared to have no significant injuries. However, six months later she began to have urinary frequency, which worsened to the point where she couldn't even stand without terrible pain in her pelvis. Unless she rushed to the bathroom, she would leak urine down her legs. Gradually she developed mild aches down the backs of her legs, but she ignored this discomfort, as the pain from her bladder was far greater. She went to her urologist, who told her she needed to have a bladder "tuck." After all, she did have two children and, "every woman needed it sooner or later." He ignored her pain, telling her it was caused by the stress of being a single mother.

Not content with this explanation, she saw several doctors and detailed the circumstances of her accident and symptoms. She was given a myriad of diagnoses while her bladder began to shrink. Finally a doctor told her she had an incurable disease called interstitial cystitis. "He didn't seem to think there was much he could do about it, and it was a problem most women were going to have to learn to live with." So she tried exercising on the Stairmaster, jogging as much as she could without leaking, and taking pain medication as little as possible. She continued to ride her favorite horse, even though she had to wear pads because she leaked so much with every spasm. Over the next two years she lost more than half her bladder capacity and thought she would soon be losing her mind.

"It got to be so painful that it was just about impossible to take a trip. If I went out, a table near the restroom was essential so I could go as frequently as I needed. I went to urologists. I went to gynecologists, and I complained of pain in my back every time my bladder filled up, and they told me that the two things had nothing to do with each other. Then my bladder shut down—I couldn't urinate. They did a hysterectomy and nothing changed! They kept blaming it on my large children and saying there was nothing they could do. My doctor told me I could only hold two ounces and that in a few years I might not have a bladder at all."

When she came to see me, she filled out the special questionnaire in Appendix B. I developed this form so that patients could be free to express their thoughts in their own words. I have often reviewed records with patients only to discover that their intial complaint had been completely transformed, their words twisted to "fit the diagnosis." This questionnaire also helps people to concentrate on their complaints and put their observations together in an orderly, logical manner.

As you will read in Chapter Four, How to Talk So Your Doctor Will Listen, it is important to limit the emotional aspects of your presentation.

You will see I've included a long list of adjectives to help you accurately describe your pain. In this way, your choice of words can help me to work with you in discovering the cause of your problem.

Reatha made it clear that her pain began after her accident, yet no one had looked at her spine as a possible cause for her problem. *Spinal problems are the most frequent cause for bladder pain.*

We began by having Reatha do a uroflow test. This demonstrated that she was unable to relax her pelvic floor properly when she started to urinate. Urologists have called this problem "pelvic floor dyssynergic voiding," or a lack of coordination between the pelvic muscles and the bladder. Normally, your bladder sends signals to the brain that it is full and needs to empty. The brain sends signals back to the pelvic floor muscles telling them to relax. As this process begins, the external sphincter within the urethra stops all activity and the bladder muscle begins to contract. At the end of urination, the reverse happens. In Reatha's case, there was a "hitch in her gitalong." This was one of the first clues I had that interstitial cystitis could be the result of abnormal nerve signals to the bladder.

Today, many urologists perform complex urodynamics, or pressure/electrical studies of the bladder and pelvic floor. However, I have found that these studies never tell me why the bladder is acting up. So again, I wondered why we were not finding the cause, instead of looking at the result of a problem. This led me to the field of neuroconductive studies.

In the early 1970s, a neurologist by the name of Scott Haldeman, began to investigate the function of the male genitourinary tract by nerve conduction studies. He demonstrated that a test called the bulbocavernosus reflex response (BCR) could objectively measure the smallest delays in the sacral reflex arc. Instead of just reporting this reflex as merely absent or present, one could measure actual time for transmission of a stimulus through the arc. This test was easily performed in the male, as it required only the application of a stimulus to the dorsum, or top of the penis. The female equivalent, the clitoris, is more like a microprocessor in size. Nevertheless, a uniquely Frankensteinian torture method, which involved clips placed on the clitoral hood, was devised. Volunteers were few and far between. This changed with the invention of the bipolar sponge electrodes. Some readers may be disappointed to read that stimulation of the clitoris by this method will not cause you to have an orgasm—doctors do not sell a home unit!

Reatha's pelvic studies were within normal limits, so we proceeded to the next area of study, her spine. Blood supply to the spine flows from outside the spine into the spinal column, creating a unique situation for injury. If we look at Figure 2-4 of the spine, you can see there are three

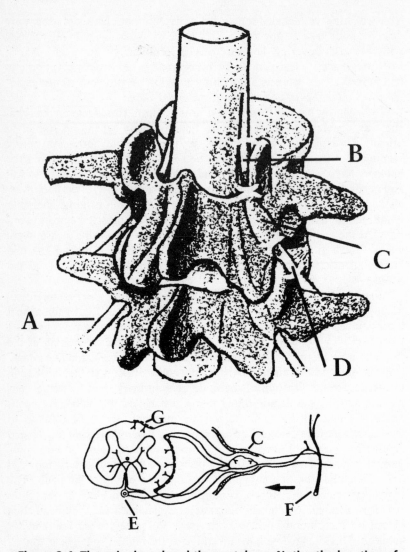

Figure 2-4, The spinal cord and the vertebrae. Notice the location of the nerve (A), which can be compressed at several levels as it exits from the spine (B, C, D). The dorsal ganglion is identified by the letter C in both pictures. The segmental artery (F) brings blood to the anterior spinal artery (E) and the dorsolateral artery (G).

zones in which the nerve exiting from the spine can be prone to injury. The first area is inside the backbone (called the *entrance zone*) and is where the nerve root is located (B); the second zone is underneath the bony bridge called the *pars articularis* (C), and the last site is where the nerve exits the bony skeleton at the facet joint (D). Even the slightest narrowing or compression at any of these points can result in oxygen loss to the nerve caused by decreased blood flow to the nerve root. (See illustration page 92.)

Most nerves have both a motor and sensory branch that travel in the same sheath, or tube. They have different functions: The motor branch controls muscle contraction while the sensory branch regulates blood flow, pressure, pain, and tactile responses. It was clear to me that interstitial cystitis could represent a sensory disorder. There had to be tests that could identify whether there was a sensory change to these nerves, especially as they exited the vertebrae.

Somatosensory evoked potentials (SEPs) have been used in neurology since 1973. However, the technique was not practical because it took a long time to study each nerve. A technique called dermatomal somatosensory evoked potentials (DSEPs) was later developed. I began to use it in my continuing search for an answer. A small, low-grade conduction signal is sent along the end of the fourth, fifth, and first sacral nerves, which are located on the foot and ankle. Small, surface electrodes are placed on the scalp to receive the signal. The time it takes from the moment of stimulation on the foot to the reception of the signal in the brain is called the *latency*. If a nerve is compressed, even a little bit, it will show an increased latency.

The Bladder as the Messenger in Interstitial Cystitis

Increased latency can be a red flag indicating nerve injury because blood flow in nerve roots is essential for normal function. You see, two basic requirements must be met if a peripheral nerve is to function normally: (1) its connection to the "mother cells" in the spine or central nervous system must remain undisturbed, and (2) it must receive a continuous and adequate supply of oxygen through the nerve's blood-supply system. If a nerve is severed from its blood supply, it loses its ability to excite its target area and the tissue dies or contracts. However, if blood flow is restored to the nerve, it can recover its function. Any temporary or permanent interference with the microcirculation or blood flow in a nerve may cause the nerve to function abnormally. To me, this sounded like the kind of event that could lead to the wide spectrum of changes in the bladder seen with interstitial cystitis. What was more exciting, however,

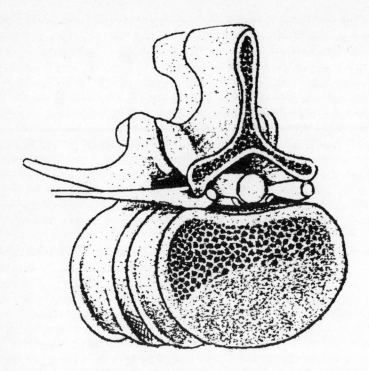

Figure 2-5, The dorsal ganglion is being compressed by a bony spur, or *osteophyte*, causing it to leak chemicals that can change the amount of blood flow to the nerve root.

was understanding that nerve injury could affect bladder function in the absence of damage *directly* to the bladder. It was the messenger that was malfunctioning, and we as urologists were "shooting" it with surgery and medications instead of finding the cause for its diminished response.

• Reatha underwent the DSEP studies along with another test called the H reflex (see Appendix E), which clearly showed her nerves were very "unhappy." In order to find out why, I ordered a magnetic imaging study (MRI) of the lumbar spine. This remarkable technique allows doctors to peer into the spine without invading the body with needles or scalpels. Soft tissue can easily be seen without the danger of X rays as the MRI machinery scans the targeted body parts.

Reatha was found to have a ruptured or shattered disk along with bony spurs that were stabbing into the dorsal ganglion, a warehouse of chemicals for the nerve. She underwent spinal surgery. "It's been two years since my surgery and I have a normal bladder. I even got married! I went back to my urologist and he apologized for not being able to treat my problem. For thirteen years I suffered greatly because nobody was willing to listen. I asked him at that time to just *listen* to what the patient has to say."

In 1991, I reported the association of far-lateral lumbar nerve root compression with the symptoms of interstitial cystitis; the association was especially strong in cases where the fifth lumbar nerve was compressed. My article, as published in the *British Journal of Urology,* reported the results of using microsurgery to decompress or relieve pressure on the excited nerve roots in patients with interstitial cystitis. The results were very encouraging. However, the spine is a very complex area and I was only just beginning to understand the mechanisms unique to that part of the body.

Instability: A Key to Intermittent Symptoms

Nancy felt like her insides were going to fall out. Rationally she knew that couldn't happen, but the pressure made her feel like she was about to deliver a 10-pound bladder at any moment. Sometimes it let up and she could go for days with hardly any symptoms, but other times, her bladder suddenly cramped so badly that she felt like she needed to squeeze every drop out, as if she was wringing a sponge dry. She never made a connection between her symptoms and her infrequent trips to the gym, during which she stayed especially long on the Stairmaster. She was proud of her flexibility, and delighted in showing anyone how she could not only touch the floor but contort herself like a human pretzel!

To understand how exercises that rock your spine back and forth can cause problems, look at Figure 2-6. Inside the spine there are ligaments that help to keep the spine stable, called the *ligamentum flavum.* It forms the roof over the nerve root as it travels down a passage to exit at the *foramen,* or opening. The intervertebral foramen is like a doorway to the end of the passage, its height being determined by the height of the corresponding disk space. If you rock side to side you intermittently narrow the doorway for your nerves, and the pinching causes edema or swelling. This does not happen to everyone, only those with chronic instability in their backs.

Nancy came to the office full of fear that she wouldn't have any symptoms that day. I assured her that with nerve conduction tests, we could pick up any damage that was being done to her nerves if this condition was indeed the cause for her bladder pain. Sure enough, the tests showed that she had an unstable back. She was started on back exercises and told to give up the Stairmaster and the "human pretzel" routine. After six weeks of therapy, she no longer had killer spasms. She followed the recommended course of exercises and diet and was no longer a victim of pain. Yet I had done nothing directly *to* her bladder. I had only changed the neural message it was receiving.

Endometriosis: The Silent Destroyer

Rebecca was really frightened by her pain for which she could get no diagnosis. She saw doctor after doctor, as each became frustrated by her confusing symptoms. She lost a bit of her self-esteem, as with every visit she was told she was neurotic and bladder obsessed. It took six physicians before she found one who became a partner willing to help her with her problem. "I needed to take control of this disease, my treatment, and my care and move forward with my life. I started to keep a journal of my symptoms and I became my own advocate. I put together my own support network and I started painting again. I couldn't let the pain define who I was anymore. I had to keep everything in perspective."

When she came to my office she shyly produced two paintings that represented her pain. I'm not an art therapist, but with one look I knew the cause for her problem. In the first, she had painted her bladder as a fiery, raging balloon, her ovaries and uterus barely visible in the background. In the second she painted what she imagined it would be like not to have pain. Surprisingly it did not show any reproductive organs at all. The answer to her problem, I told her, was within herself. Suddenly she gasped and said, "I have endometriosis."

Endometriosis is another of the "invisible" disorders. For unknown reasons, tissue similar to the lining of the uterus grows in other areas of the pelvis and sometimes in the lungs, spine, and brain. The tissue looks like caviar, or black fish eggs, sticking to the side walls of the pelvis, bladder, and bowel. When it covers the fallopian tubes or consumes an ovary, it can interfere with fertility.

The symptoms of endometriosis are as variable as those of interstitial cystitis. Typically endometriosis is associated with pelvic pain, abnormal menstrual cycles, and pain with menstruation. The most common area for endometriosis to occur is behind the uterus, between the rectum and vagina, making both intercourse painful and bowel movements painful. The

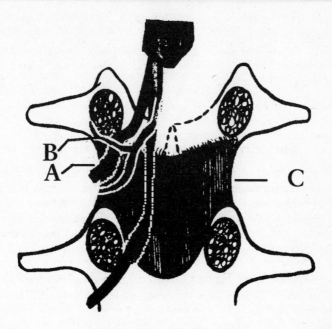

Figure 2-6, Two lumbar vertebrae viewed from within the spinal canal looking out. The L5 nerve root (A) is kinked forward by the thickened ligamentum flavum (C). The artery supplying the nerve and the facet is compressed (B).

amount of endometriosis in no way correlates with the degree of pain a woman may suffer. Unfortunately the diagnosis can only be made through surgery.

"I felt like I was having a period, but only on the *inside,*" said Rebecca. While her uroflow was abnormal, nerve conduction testing of the spine was within normal limits. When we did the next test, the BCR, her study was very delayed. An ultrasound of her pelvis failed to show any gross lesions considered hallmarks of this disease: chocolate cysts of the ovaries or fluid in the pelvis. This is not unusual, because many women with "clinical endometriosis" do not have easily identifiable markers. That's why so many women are underdiagnosed with this disorder. But if endometriosis was the cause for her interstitial cystitis, why don't *all* women with endometriosis have interstitial cystitis?

The answer is really very simple. It is the *location* of the endometriosis with respect to the sensory nerves that feed the bladder that makes the difference. This would also explain why many women are found to have "asymptomatic" endometriosis while undergoing pelvic surgery for another problem.

The Birth of Laparoscopy in Urology

As in other fields of medicine, advances in diagnosis and treatment of a problem may be dependent upon the available technology. Nowhere is this more evident than in the treatment of gallbladder disease. As instrument companies saw an opportunity to sell instrumentation to another specialty, they funneled more money into research and development that benefited everyone. As a result, the field of laparoscopy exploded around 1990.

I have never believed that all I needed to know about medicine I learned in medical school or during my residency, so I have frequently sought out other medical professionals who could enhance my ability to diagnose and treat patients. There was no country I wouldn't travel to if I could study at the hands of another expert who was thinking in new, innovative, unique ways.

I had long suspected that many of my patients with interstitial cystitis had other gynecologic problems, such as endometriosis or adhesions. But since I was not trained in laparoscopy, I needed to study with doctors who could teach me the necessary skills. I went to Germany to study with the "father" of laparoscopy, Dr. Kurt Semm.

Imagine his surprise when he learned a urologist wanted to learn gynecologic laparoscopic skills. What would I do with this training? Although he thought I would be wasting my time, his team of surgeons agreed to introduce me to new concepts in surgical technique. Eventually it helped me to both diagnose the cause of my patient's problems and minimize scarring and time spent in the hospital.

Upon my return to Los Angeles, I took several more courses, including one in which I learned how to remove gallbladders using this technique. After all, an ovarian cyst is very much like a gallbladder. The location was different, but the means of handling and removal were the same. Once I felt I had sufficient skills, I applied for and became the first urologist in my hospital to have laparoscopic privileges. With the help of the many gynecologists on staff, I began to explore the other side of my patient's bladders.

The Clue to a New Nerve Pathway

Breakthoughs in medicine are often 99 percent perspiration and 1 percent inspiration. However, in this instance, it was trusting a patient's observation that started me on one of the most exciting adventures of my medical career.

Mary Alice had a uterus that had served her well. It had held, nurtured, and delivered three wonderful children before losing its place in her pelvis. Gradually, she began to experience pressure and burning before and after she urinated. She was diagnosed as suffering from interstitial cystitis by an observant, compassionate gynecologist, and I concurred with his diagnosis. One day I received an excited phone call from the doctor who made this initial diagnosis. "I'm not sure what to make of this, but I went to block her cervix for a biopsy and she told me all her bladder pain went away." Instead of dismissing this observation as just another coincidence, I asked him how he performed the block and immediately tried the same procedure on my next patient. She felt the same relief! After ten more women found this procedure beneficial, I knew it was time to search the Biomed Library at UCLA again for answers to this unusual response.

The Ureterovesical Plexus: A Forgotten Pathway

I began a search of anatomy articles and found a French article by Laterjet in 1933 detailing the location of nerves—known as the *ureterovesical plexus*—that travel with the ureter to the base of the bladder, or trigone. Another network of nerves, called the *Frankenhauser ganglion,* sent fibers to the uterus and cervix. Political battles in medicine were evident even in Laterjet's time. He railed against those who taught and believed the Frankenhauser ganglion, which controls pain signals from the uterus, was located in a ligament supporting the uterus near the vagina. In reality, he wrote, this ganglion is over the rectum. He predicted problems with too much tension on the ureterovesical nerves by a falling uterus and warned surgeons not to take all the tissue "en masse" with the uterine artery when removing the uterus.

Laterjet's placement of the ganglion of Frankenhauser, or the *hypogastric plexus,* over the rectum could explain why several women complained of severe bladder pain *after* a bowel movement. The rapid contraction of the lower bowel would stimulate this pathway, sending increased signals to other parts of the system servicing other areas. If my medical textbooks had perpetrated the same mistaken anatomy that Laterjet condemned, it was time to do some new dissection work.

Dr. Mikel Snow, a professor of anatomy at USC (who fortunately didn't hold my collegiate affiliation against me) offered to reexplore the female pelvis, looking for the origin of the ureterovesical plexus. Luckily, he found a ninety-one-year-old female cadaver who still had her uterus! After weeks of dissection he confirmed the presence of a nerve bundle or plexus that ran underneath the ureter, alongside the uterus, and entered the base of the bladder. Laterjet had been right.

The LUVE Procedure

For several years, I had been blocking these nerves and asking women to observe if any *negative* symptoms developed. They assured me they still were aware when their bladders were appropriately full; they didn't lose control of their urine and the nerve block had no effect on their ability to have an orgasm. However, it had one significant *positive* effect: the pain was gone. The problem was figuring out how to make it last longer than a few hours.

Like Alan Shepherd, the first astronaut to risk his life by getting propelled into space on the back of a rocket, Sandra felt she had nothing to lose by being the first patient to have the ureterovesical nerves in her pelvis severed. Her bladder could hold no more than 50cc at a time, and her life revolved around the toilet and pain medications. She had an excellent response to the block, but as with all "firsts," you can't predict the unexpected. I chose to find these nerves through a vaginal rather than abdominal approach. An old gynecologic procedure that had "lost favor" as a technique for treating pelvic pain served as my map to finding these nerves. When she woke up, she gave me a very quizical look. I prepared myself for the worst. "One side of my bladder is perfectly fine, but it feels as if a line was drawn down the middle and you didn't touch the other side." Unbeknownst to me, the pathologist later confirmed that I had indeed removed the nerves from only one side, the very side on which she felt complete relief. I had created my own "control" for the procedure by mistake, but the response was unquestionable. When I developed this procedure laparoscopically, I called it "The *L*aser *U*retero *V*esical *E*xcision" or the *LUVE* procedure.

Rebecca had an excellent response to the block and underwent laparoscopy where I confirmed she had severe endometriosis. The lesions, which involved the ureterovesical plexus, were treated with laser therapy. After surgery, her bladder pain was significantly reduced. However, over the next year, her endometriosis recurred despite hormonal therapy and she elected to have a hysterectomy. Finally, she was free of both pelvic and bladder pain.

"I believe I will never learn as much about myself as I did confronting my pain. I asked myself, 'What's the gift; what am I supposed to learn from all this?' I found that by taking control of my disease and not letting myself become a victim of the disease, I really grew up. I've been more creative at this part of my life than I have at any other time. There is a sense of strength that I derived from this. Although endometriosis destroyed my reproductive organs, I feel more like a woman than ever before because of the sense of self and poise I have developed. I know what it is to heal from within. When it gets too dark inside, I can turn on the light and that light is my sense of self. I've come to respect the limitless potential and adaptability of the mind, the body, and the spirit. I grew up when I found my ability to take care of myself and heal from within, instead of thinking it all came from outside. It's a lesson we struggle with our whole lives, looking outside for all the answers when we have them inside all along."

Post-Hysterectomy Syndrome

Carole was diagnosed in 1986 as having severe endometriosis along with a "dropped uterus." She was advised to have a total hysterectomy because doctors predicted she would be pain free. That didn't happen. Carole went from doctor to doctor, still in pain, only to hear over and over again that it was all in her head.

"My life was a mess. I ended up in therapy, my family fell apart. After twenty years of marriage I lost my husband. He was resentful that pain had taken over my life, and my oldest son became impatient with me. I turned to counseling and that helped me to trust myself. I knew I wasn't a hypochondriac."

"I had had problems with my bladder since I was eighteen years old, and I had been taking medication off and on since then. I was tired, hurting, and without validation that my pain was real. Finally I was told I had interstitial cystitis but it was a disease I was just going to have to learn to live with. 'There are books in the library,' my doctor said. 'Go check it out.' When I found Dr. Gillespie's book it was like candy to a baby. Give me more information!"

Carole suffered from multiple problems, not unlike many of my patients. She had chronic fatigue syndrome from the stress of constant pain, and her uroflow and nerve conduction studies showed she had a problem both in her spine and inside her pelvis.

"I talked. She listened. She talked. I listened. She told me the steps I needed to take. I took those steps and I'm really proud that I did. Before I went into surgery, Dr. Gillespie promised me that I would have some kind of a life. I asked would I be able to play tennis again, and she said, yes you will. So I went out and bought a can of tennis balls and put them up in my closet. And that was my goal. I thought to myself, I'm going to get back out there and I'm going to play tennis. And on Easter Sunday I got to go out and play tennis. That was wonderful. That was great."

When she underwent laparoscopy, I found recurrent endometriosis in addition to adhesions involving the ureter and the vaginal cuff, the closed edge of the vagina formed after the cervix is removed. Carole had what is termed the Post-Hysterectomy Syndrome. Previously, women would complain of pain that began *after* a hysterectomy and caused them to have difficulty urinating. Now I understood one of the reasons for their pain. Just as Laterjet predicted, the problem was putting the nerves under the ureter on too much tension with the closure of the vagina. When I cut these nerves, the pelvic floor muscles could relax and function normally during intercourse and voiding.

"Today I'm much happier. It's been four years and I'm not in pain. I do regular exercising and I'm healthier. We worked together because we were a team. All those years the pain I had been going through, the aching in my back and down my legs I know today is from the bulging disk in my back. I know that certain foods I had been eating and should not have been eating caused spasms in my bladder. I have the energy to take long walks on the beach. I get to be physical. I'm considering going back to school, writing a book, becoming an interior designer. Today I have dreams, hopes, and desires that anything can happen for me. In 1986 I was griefstricken with pain and hopelessness. The transition I have been through, what I have learned about myself, I wouldn't give up. I'm alive. I'm happy. I get to live again! I wouldn't take away a day of the pain or the lessons I learned in life, because if I hadn't found Dr. Gillespie's book, truthfully, I don't know if I would be here."

I reported the results of my findings in the first 175 women who underwent this procedure in the *British Journal of Urology* in 1994. At the time of surgery, 55 percent of my patients had unsuspected endometriosis involving the inferior ureterovesical plexus. This study led to a guest appearance on *Good Morning America,* a nationally syndicated show, and an overwhelming response from viewers.

Bladder Pain *Without* a Bladder

Margaret woke up July 4, 1986, with terrible pain. Her bladder felt like "lakes of fire" and she couldn't stop going to the bathroom. Her back hurt and her legs felt as if they were dragging 50-pound weights for feet. Her vagina hurt to touch and she could barely sit down because of the pain. She immediately went to see her family doctor who diagnosed a bladder infection and gave her two weeks of antibiotics. When this didn't help, she saw another doctor, and another, until she was finally told she must be imagining her symptoms because all of her urine cultures were negative. After two months she was diagnosed with interstitial cystitis.

"I had no life. It just stopped. It was as if this disease had begun to steal it an inch at a time. It was like being locked in a room with some vicious predatorial invisible animal, not being able to fight the thing and knowing it was going to leap out and grab you at anytime. But I was powerless. There was nothing I could do."

Margaret continued having excruciating daily pain and going to see specialists around the country. Finally, she was told the only treatment was to have her bladder removed. "I began to give up parts of my body simply desperate to be rid of the pain and frequency. It seemed a fair trade—one body part for some relief." But when she woke up from surgery, she could still feel her bladder and the pain was the same. Researchers have reported this finding in other patients; however, they believed the problem was coming from within the brain and never considered the possibility that a spine problem could be causing all the trouble.

"I had no bladder but I still had all the symptoms. I gave it up for nothing. I thought of suicide on a daily basis. I planned solid ways of doing it, because my family and friends suffered as much as I did and nobody could seem to help." Gynecologists thought it was her uterus that was causing her pain, so she had a hysterectomy and the symptoms became much worse. "I gave up my bladder and all my female organs with no results other than I was down considerably more body parts."

Vulvodynia: Another Invisible Disorder

Another member of the Invisible Disorder Club is vulvodynia. This problem is much like interstitial cystitis, as it is characterized by burning, stinging, irritation, or rawness of the labia and posterior vaginal area, called the vulva. Like its sister disorder, it was long thought to be gynecology's psychiatric disease. It's amazing how unexplained female physical problems must be all "in our heads" when medicine doesn't have an easy answer. Research has focused on an infectious origin, such as herpes and yeast infections, yet when treatments for these causes fail to stop the problem, doctors are left with the same dilemma facing urologists: an unhappy, miserable woman who can't even wear underwear!

Like interstitial cystitis, vulvodynia has many potential causes, but those with "essential" vulvodynia may have compression of the first sacral nerve root, which connects to nerves outside of the spine that innervate the labia and vulva. Like endometriosis, not all patients with spine problems will develop this symptom complex. It is the type and location of the compression that may play a significant factor. If you look back at Figures 2-4 and 2-6, you can see some of the possible ways in which nerves can be compressed as they exit lateral to the spine. Compression in these areas is associated with bladder symptoms. However, if the spine slips forward, stretch is put on the sympathetic plexus, a group of nerves that regulate pressure and pain in the pelvis because they run down the front or anterior portion of the spine. People with swayback are more prone to anterior slippage. As you can see, the spine is a fascinating, dynamic organ. Just by stretching nerves, even slightly, you can change the signals sent to tissue far away from the spine.

Gradually, Margaret's condition worsened until she was unable to walk, sit, or lie down without pain down her legs and into her vagina. Finally, she forced her family doctor to investigate her spine. She had a myelogram, a test where dye is injected in the spinal canal in order to better see the nerve roots. Her test was positive. She had a herniated disk at the fifth lumbar area. "I thought, Hurray! I finally have an answer, but they told me it was just a minor anomaly, which in no way could be causing my pain."

When Margaret came to see me, she brought all her studies and records from the past eight years. From the questionnaire alone, it was obvious she had a spine problem. Margaret lived on a farm and her daily chores involved feeding her chickens, ducks, and geese. She carried heavy buckets of feed and cut her own wood. When she developed interstitial cystitis, her mother came to live with her because she could no longer care for herself or her farm. She had become entirely dependent, like a child again.

Margaret's nerve conduction studies were grossly abnormal. She recalled falling down some cement steps while carrying buckets of feed just before her pelvic pain began. I explained to her that the disk she had herniated was putting pressure on the nerves that help to regulate blood flow to her pelvis. You can think of a disk as a giant marshmallow between two crackers or vertebrae. If you push the crackers down on the right, the marshmallow pushes out on the left, and vice versa. If you move one cracker forward, the marshmallow pushes out the back and sides. The cause for her bladder pain was *not* in her bladder, as all her previous surgeries had unfortunately shown.

The instability of her spine was so pronounced that she underwent spinal fusion surgery, which involves fixing the lower part of the spine to the sacrum. In its fixed position the lower vertebrae won't pinch the nerves in the back or slip forward with movement. From her hospital bed Margaret tearfully announced that all her pelvic pain had disappeared. It's been three years since her surgery and she's never looked back.

"I kept going because I knew there had to be a logical explanation for this problem. I talked to many people with this disease and they were rational, intelligent people. It wasn't in their minds; they weren't crazy; they weren't neurotic. They needed physical help. There had to be a physical cause for this thing, I knew that. I'm not a stupid person. There had to be someone, somewhere looking for a reason for this disease. I read Dr. Gillespie's book and it helped me right away with the diet, but she was on a trail, like breadcrumbs, looking for the answer and she was only just beginning."

Environmental Issues

In my fifteen years of work on interstitial cystitis, my patients and I have uncovered many factors contributing to this painful bladder syndrome. We've seen how antibiotics, hormonal cycles, Epstein-Barr virus, scarlet fever, spine problems, endometriosis, vulvodynia, and food or drugs that increase serotonin production can affect the GAG layer.

But the mystery is not solved. The puzzle has many missing pieces. Why, for example, do cases of interstitial cystitis cluster in an Indiana neighborhood? Women from the same block have the disorder while women across town do not.

Why does a woman who moved next door to a landfill in New Jersey suddenly develop bladder pain and why do kids on her block suffer nosebleeds? What have they been exposed to?

Doctors working in California's Central Valley have reported clusters of interstitial cystitis patients in areas known for pesticide contamination of groundwater. Is there a link? Maybe. Maybe not.

Radon is an invisible gas that is released from rock containing radioactive elements. Such rocks are abundant in many parts of the United States and have been used in building the foundations of numerous homes. Epidemiologists have recently shown that exposure to radon gas correlates with lung cancer. We may find a similar but different agent that relates to interstitial cystitis.

How Antibiotics and Pesticides May Affect Your Hormone Balance

In 1962, Rachel Carson warned consumers about the dangers posed by manmade pesticides in her book "Silent Spring." It described in chilling terms how these chemicals were accumulating in our bodies. Foremost on her list were 209 compounds classified as hormone-disrupting synthetic chemicals: DDT, Dioxon, and the Furans. Unlike natural plant estrogens, man-made compounds such as this group of polychlorinated biphenyls (PCB), resist normal breakdown in the body, and accumulate in animal and human fat. The effect is low-level but potentially devastating long-term exposure. These compounds can mimic estrogen and interfere with thyroid and adrenal function. In addition, they can accelerate the breakdown and elimination of hormones, leaving the body short not just of estrogen but of the other steroid hormones mentioned above which are critical to normal human development.

Nitrofurantoin, a commonly prescribed urinary bacteriostatic antibiotic, is a member of this hormone-disrupting family. It is of real concern that we as urologists have given women long-term antibiotic therapy with this agent not knowing its potential affect on our hormones. You see, until recently, there were no tests which could determine if a chemical affected our hormone receptor sites. As a result, many approved drugs have never been evaluated for this potential side effect.

Chronic antibiotic therapy has been shown to alter gut absorption, slowing excretion of hormones fed to livestock. These elevated hormone levels are passed along to humans in the form of the meat we ingest. Due to the antibiotic influence, some of the estrogens recycle through animal body systems, and then our own, potentially causing early onset of menarch, or the beginnings of a girl's menstruation cycle. Remember too that this family of compounds can deplete the female body of estrogen by accelerating its breakdown, potentially causing premature or early onset of menopause.

Dioxon, an estrogen disrupter, and other hormonal pesticides, have been linked with endometriosis. This might explain the epidemic of this problem in countries formerly dependent upon its usage. Fungicides, used to treat the vaginal infections often caused by chronic antibiotic therapy, interfere with hormone production by inhibiting the synthesis of fatty compounds call sterols. Humans form steroid hormones from another member of that family—cholesterol. Without sterols, cell membranes become unstable, or "leaky" allowing toxic chemicals to invade the cell. Literally hundreds of agents could be implicated in the prevalence of interstitial cystitis around the world. One would expect the incidence to vary from country to country, as it does, since different environmental factors are at play.

The work I do never seems to stop. There is an ever evolving understanding of cell membranes and how to stabilize them. No single method will make everyone well. We are engaged in solving a great mystery. Each patient must observe her symptoms and environment to see what triggers or ameliorates each attack. That way, we can keep filling in missing pieces of the interstitial cystitis puzzle.

THREE

Interstitial Cystitis: Clues for Getting a Correct Diagnosis and Treatment Plan

IF you were to come to me for a diagnosis of interstitial cystitis, we would look for numerous indications. In my opinion, the symptoms known as urethritis can be an early sign of the disease. To have interstitial cystitis, you do not have to have a shrunken, ulcerated bladder. I maintain that if lost bladder capacity were the only hallmark of interstitial cystitis, 77 percent of my patients with the disease would never be diagnosed as having it. If I depended on just one factor in making a diagnosis, I would miss many patients. For example, Marilyn went to a leading urologist for help with her symptoms of constant bladder burn. He refused to treat her, however, because she did not have urinary pain. He said flatly that she did not have interstitial cystitis.

The first step to diagnosis, of course, is to take your medical history.

- What diseases have you had?
- What problems, if any, run in your family?
- When did your symptoms begin?
- Have you noticed what agents make you feel better or worse?
- Do you have digestive problems?
- Are you a chronic dieter?

Next we would take a urine sample and run some tests. We would want to make sure you do not have an infection. We would note your urine pH. If it is alkaline, I would like to know if you take calcium supplements that are buffered with bicarbonate. If you do not, a highly alkaline urine could be a sign of interstitial cystitis.

We would draw blood and measure your white blood cell count. A low count would indicate that your immune system has been activated. We would test for Epstein-Barr virus activity and thyroid function.

Once all this information is collected, I usually can tell within 98 percent certainty whether or not you will have interstitial cystitis. But to determine which type, I must look directly into your bladder and obtain tissue for the various tests we've described.

This has to be done in the hospital operating room. For people with healthy bladders, a cystoscopic procedure can be done in the office. But for those with interstitial cystitis, cystoscopy is unthinkable without general anesthesia. The pain of distending the bladder could not be tolerated by a conscious patient.

The cystoscope is a lighted tubular instrument that I insert into your bladder. I would first look for visual signs of angiogenesis, those corkscrewlike capillaries. After filling the bladder to full capacity with water, I would drain it and measure the volume. This tells me your true capacity, and from it we can calculate your normal voiding range. Generally healthy people void at about half of their anatomic capacity.

I would look to see if the last bit of water draining from your bladder contains any blood. More important, when I look back in, are there bleeding sites, hemorrhages, striations (streaks), or even ulcerations on your tissue?

The next step is to photograph your bladder. I do this for every patient. It gives us a record of what your bladder looked like when you were first diagnosed.

I would then snip out some tissue for immunofluorescence and the staining technique described in Chapter Two. This will help us determine which variety of interstitial cystitis you have and help tailor therapy.

At this point, I would also start you on a basic treatment I have devised to help your bladder tissue heal in the face of a hostile environment—that is, your urine.

Regenerating Bladder Cells

In thinking about leaky cell membranes (see Figure 2-1, Leaky Urothelial Cell, p. 67), I began by looking for ways to stabilize cells. How might one stop the membrane from interacting with urine?

It has been demonstrated that cells duplicate, divide, and grow when the intracellular pH (that is, the pH within the cell) increases to above 7.2. Classic studies of sea urchin eggs show this dramatically. When the eggs are placed in a medium with a high pH, they duplicate and begin regeneration all by themselves, without fertilization.

My approach to interstitial cystitis was inspired by this natural phenomenon. I reasoned that the bladder cells of interstitial cystitis patients had been burned by acid. Therefore the intracellular pH was no longer in the correct range. If I could raise the pH above 7.2, the damaged cells could at least have a fighting chance to regenerate. They might begin to repair themselves naturally because pH-dependent enzymes and other metabolic intermediates in the cell could then begin functioning. This is akin to throwing on the switch to the generator inside a bladder cell. But how to turn on the cells, how to raise their pH when the tissue is still exposed to the very environment that is destroying it?

Since 1978, a by-product of the paper industry has been approved for the treatment of interstitial cystitis. The drug is called *dimethyl sulfoxide,* or DMSO. Although it was not a cure for the disease, it was found to offer symptomatic relief for many patients. As time wore on, however, the beneficial effects of DMSO would lessen. Often the drug simply seemed to stop working.

I began to investigate other properties of DMSO. Researchers had found that DMSO can penetrate normal barriers, even skin, and quickly get into tissue. And if DMSO were combined with other drugs, the DMSO would piggyback those drugs directly into tissue. As such, DMSO was a natural transport mechanism for carrying drugs into the body. One group of researchers, for example, found that a steroid drug mixed with DMSO could be transported into tissue at $\frac{1}{1000}$ the dosage required systemically.

Moreover, DMSO itself only exerted transient effects on tissues it penetrated. In all of the diseases for which it was tried there were no long-lasting effects. But if you consider it to be a carrier, not a treatment in itself, DMSO could be very handy.

My goal was to stop inflammation and raise intracellular pH in damaged bladder cells. The first criterion could be met with steroids, anti-inflammatory drugs used widely to help stabilize membranes of the body. But DMSO and steroids alone will not do the trick. Steroids require an alkaline pH to remain active. When placed in the bladder, acid in urine can easily inactivate a steroid, resulting in no prolonged effect on bladder tissue. Therefore a buffer was required. The obvious answer lay in a box of Arm & Hammer baking soda.

Bicarbonate of soda, as noted, is alkaline and helps stabilize the tissue of burn patients. Also, sea urchins require bicarbonate to raise pH so they can multiply and divide. By incorporating sodium bicarbonate into the mixture, I could hope to buffer the steroid and induce cellular regeneration.

Thus the Gillespie cocktail was born. Placing this trio of drugs—DMSO, steroid, and sodium bicarbonate—into the bladders of interstitial cystitis patients had dramatic results. In one subset of patients, those who were only missing the protective GAG layer, the bladder tissue stabilized within a few weeks.

This treatment has also proved effective for patients with what is called *radiation cystitis.* Molly, for example, was cured of cancer of the cervix through intense radiation therapy. The treatment stopped one disease and started another—namely, interstitial cystitis. Molly's bladder lining was severely damaged by the radiation. She experienced pain, burning, cramping, urinary frequency, and other hallmarks of interstitial cystitis. She saw many doctors before I made the diagnosis of radiation cystitis because Molly simply neglected to tell her doctors that she had been treated for cervical cancer with radiation. I found out from the questionnaire she filled out and treated her, successfully, with the Gillespie cocktail.

How Can We Arrest Abnormal Capillary Growth?

There were patients, however, whose bladder tissue was more severely damaged. Although helped by this cocktail, they did not remain stabilized. These were women who showed massive capillary growth, or angiogenesis, in the bladder. They tested positive for one particular antibody within these very same capillaries.

The capillaries of the interstitium serve as a filtration mechanism for the contents of urine and extracellular fluid; they drain away impurities. In one subset of interstitial cystitis patients, this filtering mechanism is out of balance. They experienced continuous capillary proliferation.

Although I received two U.S. patents, one European patent, and one Australian patent for the bladder treatment I developed, as well as for a new oral medication that had already shown preliminary success in stopping capillary growth, major pharmaceutical firms could not justify spending the estimated $54 million necessary to bring a new drug to market for the relatively small number of individuals affected by interstitial cystitis. Pamela Sue Martin, however, was grateful for the opportunity she had in 1984.

"Ever since my treatments I have been fine," Pamela said recently. "Only when I am under severe stress do I feel little twinges, but nothing like it used to be. But now I understand what is going in my body. I stayed on a low-acid diet and I reduced my stress. I have a wonderful son and I keep myself healthy."

Noninvasive Treatment for Spine Problems

Less than 10 percent of patients whose problems originate in the spine require spinal surgery. The majority of spine problems can be helped through changes in body dynamics. Be aware of your environment and the many ways in which you can place abnormal stress on your lower back. If you sit at a computer, be sure the height of your chair and back support are appropriate. There is a back rest called The Better Back (see Appendix A) that can be placed in any chair to help support the normal alignment of the spine, whether you are sitting at home, in a restaurant, or in the car. Get up and stretch every hour if you can.

Women who ride horseback take a beating on their lower backs. For every movement up from the saddle, there is an equal and opposite movement down into the saddle. The impact is forced right up the spine, where it is absorbed by your "shocks," the disks, at the two lower lumbar levels. If you have intermittent pelvic pain, I'm not suggesting you should give up riding if it's your one pleasure in life (though I certainly hope you have more!). Simply understand the reason for your pelvic pain and take action by faithfully performing back exercises to keep nature's shock absorbers in shape.

There are various resistance exercise programs, such as Pilates or Nautilus, that when done properly can strengthen your back and stomach muscles so that you are not "toasting" that marshmallow of an injured disk when you move. Deep muscle massage is another potenially beneficial technique, but I would recommend that you only use a licensed massage therapist for proper treatment.

If you have a feeling of pressure in your pelvis, you might ask your doctor to prescribe nifedipine (Procardia), a heart medication. It was discovered that the fibers which keep the disk contained in its space can "leak" a neurotransmitter, called calcitonin gene-related peptide (CGRP), when irritated. This can cause pressure feelings in the bladder. By taking just 10 milligrams of Procardia at night, you can block this response. Again, sensory nerves are responsive to small amounts of medication, so don't overwhelm them by taking too much!

The patient with the unstable back may have difficulty starting to urinate. I have successfully used the drug Klonopin at night in its lowest dosage for this problem. This medication was originally used to control nonspecific seizures, especially in children. It decreases the ability of the sympathetic nerves (remember they run down the front of the spine) to respond to stretch signals and allows the bladder neck to open easier. Some doctors are afraid to use this medication because they believe you can become addicted. Although in higher doses this is possible, I have never

---

EBV Titers

There are four aspects of EBV titers:

- The IgG titer tells us whether or not you have ever been exposed to the virus. If positive, you probably had mono at one time and recovered. You are supposedly immune to it.
- The IgM titer indicates recent infection. You most probably had this infection within the past six weeks.
- The early capsid antigen titer tells us you have active disease at the moment. The virus is busy duplicating in your body.
- Finally, the Epstein-Barr nuclear antigen (ebna) titer tells us your disease is at least several months old.

If you were to test one thousand people at random, 90 percent would show IgG and ebna titers. But, as we have recently discovered, many interstitial cystitis patients show chronic active titers. That is, they have titers showing previous exposure (IgG and ebna) plus early capsid antigen titers. The virus has become reactivated.

---

found a spine patient to need more than the minimal dose. Again, overwhelming nerves with higher doses prevents them from responding altogether!

How the Environment Can Aggravate
Your Immune System

When Teddy Epstein discovered the Epstein-Barr virus in the 1950s, he said he felt it would be the Rosetta Stone of cancer. I believe it may be part of the code breaker of inflammatory disease as well. EBV is the most common cause of infectious mononucleosis. It makes you tired and weak, and your lymph nodes swell. After two months, your immune system inactivates the virus. You develop antibodies that prevent infection.

Or so it is with most people. Some people have chronic, constant infections. The diagnosis can be made by looking at what are called blood titers, which are measures of infection in the blood.

How the virus gets reactivated is a current area of medical research. We know this virus can live in damaged epithelium, the special protective cells that line cavities and organs such as the lungs and bladder. What fascinates me is that interstitial cystitis patients have a large epithelial organ, the bladder, which is damaged.

What does the virus do to interstitial cystitis patients? Let's assume the virus is in your bladder tissue. It rests there quietly, without mishap, until something comes along to activate it. Such activators may be substances, such as phorbol esters and other chemicals, from the environment. The substance stimulates the virus to go from a quiescent to an active, destructive phase. In the quiescent phase the virus "sits back." In the destructive phase, it ruptures cells and destroys them.

One patient got sick within fifteen minutes after arriving at work every day. She then discovered that her office shared an air-conditioning duct with two neighboring cabinetry shops. The chemicals they used on furniture wafted into her office and activated her virus. Blood tests revealed high early capsid antigen titers. When she went home at night she soon felt better.

But the toll on her was emotionally devastating. She grew more and more depressed, more and more tired. Like so many interstitial cystitis patients, she thought her life was out of control. She even thought of suicide.

Therapies That Hurt More Than Help

Because patients are so often desperate, urologists have tried some fairly drastic therapies to treat interstitial cystitis, therapies that in my opinion tend to do more harm than good. For example, although I am trained and certified to use lasers in the treatment of bladder disease and elsewhere in the body, I have found this technique to have no lasting benefit in treating interstitial cystitis. A laser is basically a fancy instrument used to cauterize tissue. Ulcerated portions of the bladder are simply burned away. But this process actually creates more damage to bladder tissue and increases capillary growth. Lasers are not a satisfactory way to deal with interstitial cystitis.

Another therapy is called *bladder augmentation*. Basically, the top of the bladder is lopped off surgically. Only the bladder neck, trigone, and ureters are left. Then a piece of bowel is excised and refashioned to form a new top half of the bladder. The goal is to restore bladder capacity in patients whose bladders are shrunken and scarred from years of unarrested interstitial cystitis.

Bladder augmentations work for a small percentage of patients, namely those who do not have disease in the base of their natural bladders. But for most patients, this is not the case. They get the new bladder, only to find that their old symptoms of burning, urinary frequency, and pain have not been alleviated. They then wind up with two different membrane surfaces in their bladders. It becomes very difficult to apply cell stabilization techniques to this hybrid tissue. The outlook for many "augmented" patients is not good.

The last resort for some women is total cystectomy, or removal of the bladder itself. The ureters are joined and made to drain passively through a hole on the stomach, either into an external bag or into an internal pouch that must be catheterized.

When a woman with interstitial cystitis comes to me for treatment, I make her a promise: I will never, under any circumstances, remove her bladder. (It may well be, however, that her disease is so far progressed or her bladder has been so damaged that I cannot stop the disease process and cannot save her bladder. In these rare instances, urinary diversions, leaving the bladder, may be the only answer.) The reason I make this promise to patients is that I am determined to find a way to stabilize every bladder that crosses my doorstep. A patient needs to know this, so we can work together to solve his or her particular piece of the mystery of what causes interstitial cystitis.

My orientation to this disease is to discover the origin of a patient's pain and to treat the cause, not the symptoms. It is a daunting diagnostic process.

What the Mind Can Do to Help Heal the Body

Whatever the cause of your interstitial cystitis, you are faced with the daily task of coping with this devastating disease. It is not easy. The depression in patients I have seen is usually dominated by a tremendous sense of loss and feelings of grief. Losses aren't something to be taken lightly. If you have a medical problem that interferes with your desire to excel, you can be placed in a state of emotional turmoil. You must learn to accept wisely that *today* you are limited, but think about what you can do, rather than what you can't. Be gentle with yourself. Learn to love yourself and do what you can today and leave tomorrow alone until it is today.

A few of my patients, in fact, are clinical psychologists. But even though they are experts in helping people resolve problems, they were unable to apply their training to help themselves.

Martha, for example, refused to look me in the face on her first three visits. How she dealt with her own patients at this time still mystifies me. As a practicing psychologist, she had convinced herself that her pain was psychosomatic. She underwent sex therapy to try to cope with the pain of intercourse. She worked every minute of the day to dissociate her body from her mind.

After several treatments, however, she changed. She looked me in the face. She smiled. And she admitted that the pain had driven her to avoid facing the world around her, including her patients, her family, and her physician.

I have watched many patients undergo such changes, transforming from destitute, emotional cripples into functioning adult women.

My goal is to give back to each patient the control over her life. I ask her to be responsible for her own health. It requires a lot of work on her part. In talking to patients about coping with interstitial cystitis, I am reminded of a story my mother told me when I was a schoolgirl:

Once there were two frogs that had fallen into a pail of cream. The sides were slippery and steep so that despite all their efforts, they could not escape the pail. One frog decided it was hopeless. She gave up, sank to the bottom, and drowned. The second frog refused to give up. She kept churning away with all her strength. Suddenly, she let out a satisfied croak because there she was, sitting on a pat of butter churned up through her own efforts.

If you believe, as some interstitial cystitis patients do, that there is no hope for a cure, you will sink to the bottom and psychologically drown in your own sorrow. But if you take each day and decide that you're not going to let the disease conquer you, you will find a way to get on top of your own pat of butter.

Anger won't help. Some interstitial cystitis patients are furious with the medical profession for not having solved the puzzle of this disease. I believe anger is a self-defeating emotion. You cannot change your disease by ranting at people who treated you, in good faith, years ago. Medical knowledge changes over time. So I encourage you to put your anger behind you and concentrate on today.

Will There Ever Be a Cure?

I had a patient with interstitial cystitis who came into the office recently and the first thing she said was, "Is there a cure for this? What is the cure?" I had to sit her down and give her my "Semantics of Cure" lecture.

"What does the word *cure* really mean?" I asked her.

She said, "Well, it means your problem is gone forever."

"Does it mean there is no evidence that the problem ever existed?" I wondered.

"Oh," she said. "When you put it that way, there is no cure for anything."

"Exactly right. There is no cure that eradicates all evidence that a disease was ever there. The cure for appendicitis is an appendectomy, but you still have the scar. For every medical problem, the best a physician can do is to help you gain control over it."

I do not like the word *cure*. My goal is to have you, the patient, control the disease process rather than having the disease process control you. Your goal is to resume a normal life. To do so, you must take responsibility for your health. But if you consider yourself "cured," you might well go out and undo all the things that made your bladder stable. You might think, "I'm completely well. I can eat what I like, take diet pills, carry fifty pounds of dog food into the house because I'm cured!" And, of course, by exposing your bladder to harmful environmental factors you could start the disease process all over again.

The patient who came into my office asking for a cure failed to understand that the power to heal was in herself. Thus, she set herself up as the victim.

How to Stop Being a "Victim"

Throughout this book, I have tried not to use the word *victim*. I do not buy into the idea that women with interstitial cystitis have been victimized by the medical profession or by life in general. The women who come to me with the need to be treated as victims are the ones I cannot help; I will never be able to help them until they learn to break the trap of self-victimization and take responsibility for their own health.

On the other hand, I can understand why they feel this way. People with chronic pain, especially when it lasts over six months, sometimes tap into very primal needs. But the victim mentality is self-defeating. The victim has capitulated to the disease. She may even begin to rely on her role as victim for a sense of self-worth.

I will never forget one afternoon when two patients with severe, intractable pain from back injuries were both lying on a couch in my office. The man, who gasped audibly with each bladder spasm, was trying to reach his shoelace, which had become undone, but collapsed back in pain with each attempt. Three other patients in the room ignored his plight. Suddenly, without saying a word, the woman in equal pain got down on her hands and knees and tied his shoes. She had begun to heal herself through a simple act of kindness to another human being.

I urge you to examine your feelings about interstitial cystitis, should you have this disease. Victimization encourages anger, self-pity and lack of responsibility, all of which will get you nowhere. When you view yourself as a victim, you are doing nothing to help yourself.

And there are, as you have seen in this and the previous chapter, many things you can do to begin to help yourself. While there is no "cure" for interstitial cystitis, there are dozens of ways you can help yourself, medically and psychologically.

Support groups can be of benefit, but you need to be careful about "toxic people." These are the individuals who become negative about another's success or discourage others when they have begun to take positive steps toward learning about themselves. That is why I recommend that support groups be monitored by a licensed therapist. A lot of harm can be done in groups as well as good. If you feel depressed instead of encouraged by your support group, seek private counseling to get yourself back on track.

It is important that you believe in the power of yourself as a healer. As a doctor, I can only guide you along the path. But I have seen on many occasions the power of faith and conviction in understanding what is true regardless of what others say. I often tell patients to internalize, or bring a recommended therapy into their subconscious. If they feel anxious about following that choice, I encourage them to reject it and consider another, perhaps less ideal way of treating their problem. In this way, there can be no victims, only empowered healers.

VIRGINIA

Virginia has run several group therapy sessions of interstitial cystitis patients in the Los Angeles area. As a marriage and family psychotherapist with the disease, she understands interstitial cystitis in a way that most urologists do not. I think you should read her story:

"I had a lot of pain the first year. But unfortunately for me, I had a mother who was a hypochondriac. She loved every illness. And I was so determined that I would not also become a hypochondriac that I assumed the pain was all in my mind: I must be crazy; they could not find anything wrong with me.

"So I started a search. I would figure out why my psyche was harming my soma. I would be the clever psychologist and cure myself. Whenever I came to the end of a day, completely exhausted, I would say, 'Yes, it's true, I'm not dealing well with life.'

"The search continued through years of therapy until I finally began to realize, 'Wait a minute. I am not a crazy human being. I hurt. There is pain.'

"So I started a new search. I went to physician after physician. My husband was absolutely convinced that I was a hypochondriac like my mother. Our relationship began to develop a lot of problems.

"Even though I was a therapist and I felt psychologically okay, I began to have suicidal thoughts. I began to think I could only go through so many more bad weeks, then if I cannot find relief, I want to die. For me, the important thing is not the length of life we live; it is the quality of life. And I want quality. I want to dance. I want to play and have fun.

"One day my husband saw Dr. Gillespie on television and he called me. 'C'mere. This is what you have. Listen to what she's saying.'

"I listened hard and the next day went to my urologist and explained to him what I had heard. And he said, 'Oh, that's a horrible disease. You don't want it.'

"Now, he's a lovely man. He said, 'Okay, I'll put some DMSO into you. If it helps that will be fine. We'll go from there.' He put in some DMSO and it really helped. But when it came time to go back, I decided to try Dr. Gillespie herself.

"After we went through the full diagnosis and she told me what it was, I cried. I started sobbing because of the years and years I had thought I was nuts, headed for the loony bin, knowing no one could find anything. I think I cried for a week.

"But next there was a feeling of absolute relief that someone had heard my agony. Someone had heard my pain. I was not nuts. And there was hope.

"Then the fear started. The anguish, not out of sadness, but out of the knowledge I have something really unknown. My first response was, 'Well, the understanding of this disease is in its infancy stage. We don't know what we're going to do. I'll probably be a guinea pig.

"But then I did what psychologists do. I reframed the issue. I thought, 'Isn't this wonderful! My disease was found out when research is just beginning so I can be in on the adventure. I'm going to get well!'

"But then I locked into a new psychological trap. In getting my first treatments of the Gillespie cocktail, I locked on to the phrase 'six weeks.' Instead of hearing Dr. Gillespie say, 'The first course is six weeks,' I heard instead, 'It will be cured in six weeks.' I wanted it to be over in six weeks. And of course, it was not over so quickly. But it was much better.

"The next lesson I learned was how to deal with setbacks. This happened to me when I experienced a potassium loss and had to stop treatments until my potassium levels could be restored to normal.

"I felt real terror. 'Oh, my God, I may never get back into control.' All the questions about how to deal with this disease came back. And then I had another setback, an infection. Every time I had a setback, I tried to fight the feelings I was having. I tried to say, 'I'm not depressed! I'm going to lick this.'

"Then I tried a new tactic. I had read literature suggesting that people who handle disease with a sense of anger or a sense of positive well-being do better than others. Accordingly, I decided to deal with my depression. I was furious. I was wallowing in depression. And I called it a snit day. I am allowed to have snits. For twenty-four hours that I'm depressed, I allow myself to feel sad. I don't try to tell people I'm okay when I'm not. If my husband doesn't like it that day, I suggest he go into another room. Because if I'm going to be in a snit, I'm going to be in a snit. When I finally realized that depression is only anger directed at yourself, it only took twenty-four hours to return to normal.

"And I began to understand that even in my snits, I was better off than in the earlier days of my disease. I had whole nights when I could sleep. I had days without pain. Was that not glorious?"

Interstitial cystitis patients like Virginia have done remarkably well. They are also willing to extend a hand to others, to help them cope with the stress of this disease. But in so doing, many have noticed an odd psychological problem. When women who are not doing well talk to women who are doing well with this disease, communication can break down. It is as if some patients do not want to hear that others are doing well. They feel anger, jealousy, and fear. Why is she better and not me?

On the other hand, my patients say some women they talk to (who were not diagnosed, treated, and educated at my clinic) seem not to be willing to take responsibility for their own health. "A woman called me from Boston," said Judy, "wanting to know how I was doing. I told her about all the things I have done and she didn't want to listen. She wanted to complain."

On the other hand, some interstitial cystitis patients who are stabilized want to forget this whole miserable episode of life. They refuse to talk to women who are not doing well because it reminds them of their former agony.

I believe we should all support one another. Those who do well should help those in pain. The women in pain should not resent those who do well.

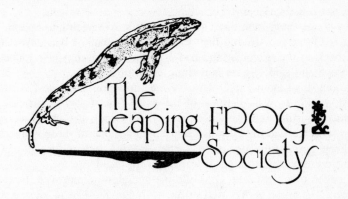

The Leaping Frog Society

There is always hope and there are people who have been freed from the ravages of interstitial cystitis. In fact, my patients who remain free of symptoms for six months or longer have formed the Leaping Frog Society. At this writing, many of them have become pregnant and delivered healthy babies. Several others have sent in their wedding announcements. They all churned up their pat of butter and got out of that slippery pail. As their stories reveal, it was not an easy journey.

PAULA

"About six years ago I started to have burning in my bladder. I thought it was an infection and trotted off to the urologist. He said it was typical for women my age to have a little pain in the bladder caused by stress. He then gave me thirteen silver nitrate treatments. Even though these hurt a great deal, he kept giving them to me. And I got worse.

"For the next two or three years, I felt so much pressure and burning that I lived on pain pills. Many days I could not get out of bed. I saw three more urologists. The fourth one told me my pain was all in my head. He said I was basically crazy and would have to accept that.

"Finally, as I was too sick to get out of bed for months, my gynecologist said I needed a hysterectomy. He thought I might have endometriosis. But before surgery, he sent me to a famous urologist for a workup. This, the fifth urologist, performed cystoscopy under anesthesia. Later, he told me, "The good news is that you do not have cancer, you have a normal bladder." My gynecologist had mentioned the term interstitial cystitis and

I asked the urologist about it. He said it was such a rare disease that I could not possibly have it.

"So at age thirty-nine I had a hysterectomy. Everything came out. I felt better for three months and then the pain came back. I was devastated. I went back to the urologist and had a second cystoscopy. He looked me in the eye and said, 'There is nothing I can do for you.'

"About this time my internist gave me antidepressants and I went back to bed, unable to walk because of the pain. Then I saw an article about interstitial cystitis and Dr. Gillespie's clinic. I took the article to my internist with tears in my eyes. He said, 'You are one of those women who will keep going from doctor to doctor, looking for an answer you will never find.' He, too, thought it was all in my head.

"I began treatment with Dr. Gillespie and slowly improved. It was not an overnight miracle. We tried different things and had to keep working on it. I'd say it took eighteen months for my symptoms to be brought under control.

"And I can say today that I am pain free. I am beginning to eat some of the foods that I could not eat before. It's such an unbelievable feeling that I think I should knock on wood so as not to break my good fortune. But I know, deep inside, it was not luck that made me better. It was hard work."

ESTHER

"I developed a burning in my bladder in August 1981. It did not feel like the cystitis I had had before so I went to a urologist. He dilated my urethra, which did not help at all. It made me worse.

"The second urologist told me my symptoms could be connected with incipient multiple sclerosis. He gave me antibiotics and Valium. Neither helped.

"The third urologist insinuated I had sexual problems with my husband and that this was the cause of my bladder pain. I have been happily married for twenty-five years and couldn't believe he was saying such a thing. He sent me to a biofeedback therapist and began treatments with DMSO and silver nitrate. None of it helped.

"I flew to other cities and saw top specialists in my search for help. One, a leader among all urologists, told me that it sounded like interstitial cystitis but that without the symptom of frequency (I only had burning) I could not possibly have interstitial cystitis.

"I have always loved to entertain. But for over two years I could not do anything. I resigned from all my volunteer work and spent my days lying down with a heating pad. I had a hysterectomy. And the bladder pain continued. I must say I resented it. It completely interfered with normal life. I could not trust myself to feel well and was afraid to plan anything. If I had a dinner party, I might have to leave in the middle of it and go lie down. And the way the doctors treated me was humiliating.

"When I first went to Dr. Gillespie, I was contrite. I had always been told I was creating this illness. I told her I felt helpless, humiliated, and that maybe I was losing my mind. And she said, 'The problem is not in your head. You're sitting on it.' I couldn't believe her at first. I had been to the so-called top specialists in the country. And she then proceeded to prove it to me.

"I am definitely improved. I can entertain and go on family ski trips. I'm not yet cured in the sense that there is never any discomfort. But the quality of my life has returned. The feeling is wonderful."

AMELIA

"I had interstitial cystitis for twelve years. Over much of that time I was treated nearby at an excellent diagnostic clinic—excellent, that is, for most diseases except interstitial cystitis. In all the time I went there, they never explained my disease to me. They always said the same thing: 'You are doing well. Keep up the good work.' They suggested hydraulic stretching of my bladder to make it bigger.

"Meanwhile, I had reached a point of desperation. I asked my doctors if there was something more we could do. All the medications I had taken were not making my bladder well. I took opium suppositories for pain near the rectum. It was so bad that I could not sit or stand any pressure in that area.

"Also, the disease was so erratic. There were days when it got better and days when it was excruciating. I asked what about diet? Is it something I am doing? Is it something I'm eating or drinking? They would always assure me it had nothing to do with food. It was then that my doctors described different kinds of surgery. The alternative was to remove my bladder or augment it with bowel. The very thought of surgery put me into a terrible depression.

"About this time, a friend saw Pamela Sue Martin on television talking about her bladder problem. I called the station and they gave me Dr. Gillespie's name and address. I called and talked to her nurse, who explained the basic treatments to me and the attention I would have to pay to diet and vitamins.

"Since I live in New England and Dr. Gillespie was so far away, my husband suggested I simply get some DMSO treatments from a local physician. But I was fascinated by the diet connection. I wanted to go to

Letters

A LETTER FROM MARY ANN

It's been one year this month since I finished the treatments for interstitial cystitis and I can't tell you how wonderful it's been to have a pain-free bladder. I didn't write any sooner because I wanted to make sure that tomorrow wouldn't be different. This is the first pain-free year I've had in at least ten or fifteen years.

A LETTER FROM MOLLY

I have felt better in the last five months since coming to your clinic July 10 than I have in about seventeen years. Now I believe in miracles. I tell my friends and family I am like a song, "I Have a New Body, Praise the Lord, I Have a New Life." As I told you, a famous urologist in Texas had told me I had to have my bladder removed. A neighbor's son talked to four urologists for me and they said that it was all I could do for an advanced case like mine. Now, after your treatments, I have gone from about ⅓ cup capacity to ¾ cup capacity.

A LETTER FROM CEILA

I think we each must have within us the power of curing. It takes strong faith. The doctors are there to help us.

A LETTER FROM ALMA

This was the best Christmas I had in a long time. I actually enjoyed the rush of shopping!

California and get the whole story for myself. In October 1984 I made my first visit to her clinic.

"As I was waking up from the anesthesia after my first treatment with the Gillespie cocktail I remember feeling horribly groggy. I asked, 'Is my bladder worth saving?' She said, 'You bet it is!' and I felt incredible relief. The talk of surgery had frightened me. She assured me that I could keep my bladder, and she helped set things up with another urologist near me who would continue treatments under her guidance. My hometown urologist said the treatments made a lot of sense. He was happy to do them.

"In the meantime I started to watch my diet. I saw there was a definite relationship between pain and foods. I love fresh tomatoes in season. It was nothing for me to eat three or four a day out of the garden. I used to drink iced tea with lots of lemon.

"Now I have not had anything acidic for over a year. Although I still have the disease, I feel wonderful. Now I know I'm healing.

"I did have one setback, however. I developed terrible pain and assumed my interstitial cystitis had come back forever. It turned out I had a bacterial infection. Once it cleared up, I was back to a more normal condition. I know I am making progress now."

DENISE

"On a scale of one to ten, with ten feeling the best you ever have in your life, I'd say I'm a seven or eight. This is fantastic. I went back to exercising and taking aerobics four times a week. The constant yeast infections I've always had are now gone. And some really good news is that I now have normal sex without fear of being hurt."

DEBBIE

"So often when someone provides assistance, even though it's appreciated, it goes unthanked. But I had to thank Dr. Gillespie for the insights she gave me into my bladder problems. When I originally came to Dr. Gillespie, I think I hadn't had a day in a year without some level of pain, usually moderate or severe, and infection after infection. Today, I still have bladder problems from time to time but now it's minor occasional pain and only infections two or three times a year (not perfect, but to me that's a world of difference). I've read every article that comes along on bladder infections, but Dr. Gillespie gave me the most insight. She explained why some things I did from time to time caused problems or made matters worse—like when I was in severe pain and drank a gallon of cranberry juice a day and then thought I was *really* going to die from the pain. She was the only doctor who had the answers on why this was a mistake and didn't help with my bladder problems."

DARLEEN

"For the past nine years Dr. Gillespie has been my lifeline and has kept me going many times when I would have simply given up. I'll never easily forget two years ago when I was down to 80 pounds and Dr. Gillespie was visibly rattled by my situation. She sat me down and explained I was at death's door, and I would die if things did not improve and do so quickly. She saved my life that day and I thank her from the depths of my being.''

ELEANOR

''The results from my surgery are quite overwhelming. There are days when I do not suffer any discomfort, and times when I do, the discomfort has only been slight. For years the pain had been ever present and severe. I never thought there could be anything to help my condition, but now there is a smile on my face that hasn't been there for years. Lupus is easier to deal with. I thank Dr. Gillespie from the bottom of my heart. Her compassion and dedication have given me back my sense of well-being.''

KATHY

''It has been two years since Dr. Gillespie performed my surgery, and I want to thank her for making me feel like a normal, healthy woman again.

''Before I went to her, I had suffered for so long with bladder problems that I was skeptical of most treatments, yet desperate to be healthy again. After reading her book and hearing her speak, I was drawn to her positive approach and her desire to find the reason for various bladder problems, including interstitial cystitis, from which I suffered. All of my other doctors (of which there were many) did not seem to be making any progress toward helping me, and the approach they took was 'You'll have to live with this for the rest of your life.' This negative, resigned attitude left me with much frustration.

''Because of her positive, helpful attitude, I felt comfortable placing myself in her care, even though I was still apprehensive about surgery. After my surgery, I prayed that I would be better, at the same time wondering how long my improved condition would last.

''I am happy to say that I continue to feel healthy, strong, and practically pain free. I was once told I would have to lessen the quality of my life by living with a debilitating disease. I now lead a full life and feel a sense of renewal. I exercise regularly to strengthen my back and know my limitations where my diet is concerned.''

WOODY

''This was one of the most difficult times of my life, and Dr. Gillespie really put me at ease. I never felt that the situation was out of control, but rather that together we were solving a puzzle, with a successful outcome not in doubt.

Years ago I was hired to record a piano performance by a very religious Jewish man. He had a prayer for everything, even thanking God after each trip to the bathroom. At the time I thought he was crazy. Now I'm not so sure. . . ."

CAROLE

"Dr. Gillespie gave me respect and knowledge, which no other physician had given me. Her treatment taught me how to take full responsibility for myself, which has served me well over the last ten years."

DIERDRE

"Dr. Gillespie has been a teacher to me. She has taught me the art of rationally and clearly defining what is wrong, instead of throwing temper tantrums—which is how I was when I first met her. When I first came to her I was a mess. My bladder was causing me so much pain that I felt like jumping out of my skin. It was truly unbearable. I had been to a half-dozen urologists and a few gynecologists, but no one had any answers. The pain seemed to run my life, making me feel angry and more upset each day. The pain continued for several years. I began to think there really wasn't an answer out there. However, being determined to find one, I stumbled upon her.

"The urologists before her had no solutions to my problem, except for total removal of my bladder, which seemed completely insane. When I went to Dr. Gillespie, she gave me hope. The wonderful part was, the hope turned into a reality and my bladder became at least 99 percent better, if not more!"

KAY

"Compared to my symptoms prior to surgery, I have improved dramatically. I do not experience the abdominal or pelvic heaviness or urinary frequency. I realize that my situation is related to lower back instability.

"I am grateful to Dr. Gillespie for her skills and expertise to deal with my complicated case. 'The RN with four ureters' was treated with compassion and personal concern."

FOUR

How to Talk So Your Doctor Will Listen

I like to go to the waiting room to greet each patient and escort her personally into my office. In this way, I let the patient know that she is coming to someone who wants to help her in solving her urological problem as a partner.

If you were my patient and this was your first visit, I would put you to work before we talked. When you came in, my nurse would hand you an eight-page questionnaire. It is geared to give me basic information, helping me orient and organize my thinking about you as a patient. And it forces you to organize your thoughts and orient yourself as a partner in our consultation.

Although the questionnaire is simple, if you are like some of my patients, it may take you an hour to fill it out. Before you come to the office, you should organize your thoughts and make a detailed list of your symptoms. Be prepared.

Believe in Lists

You probably don't go to the grocery store without a shopping list. Why shouldn't the same be true for a visit to a doctor?

It seems that many physicians have been taught to beware of patients carrying lists because list makers have a reputation for being phobic. It is not known where this stereotype originated but recently, a family practitioner from Alabama, Dr. John F. Burnum, debunked it in the prestigious *New England Journal of Medicine*. The *Journal* rarely runs nonscientific articles, but Dr. Burnum's article was anecdotal, based on his own observations that list-writing patients were quite sane. The editors believed the subject extremely important and thus ran the article as a way of alerting physicians to this point of view.

"Traditional medical wisdom holds that patients who relate their complaints to their physicians from lists are, ipso facto, emotionally ill," Dr. Burnum wrote. "DeGowin and DeGowin in their venerable textbook on diagnosis say that note writing is 'almost a sure sign of psychoneurosis. The patient with organic disease does not require references to written notes to give the essence of his story.' But," said Dr. Burnum, "note writing is a normal, honorable practice that can be used to advantage in patient care."

Dr. Burnum decided to observe seventy-two list-writing patients. "I found no association of emotional disorders with list writing in men," he reported. "Women list writers are more apt to have nervous troubles, but the majority were emotionally normal. Almost all of these emotionally normal list writers had serious physical disorders. Patients with organic disease, therefore, do refer to written notes to give the essence of their story—and not because they are peculiar or crazy."

Note writers simply want to get things straight, he said. Even though they may be anxious and distraught, they are nevertheless seeking clarity, order, information, and control, and to avoid wasting the doctor's time.

Most lists seen by Dr. Burnum consisted of the patient's symptoms and logical questions they wanted to ask. Most contained five or six items, but an emotionally stable executive had written a twenty-point list.

"Lists comprise the same thousand-and-one subjects discussed by all patients: skin blemishes, gas, chest pain, my sister has cancer, do I? shots for foreign travel, why does my blood pressure fluctuate? family or job troubles, diet, vitamins, medications and exercise," Dr. Burnum said.

"Notes may be of great help in the orderly transfer of information to the physician. Medical care turns on communication. Whatever helps patients express themselves and helps physicians understand patients is acceptable."

I agree wholeheartedly with Dr. Burnum. Many list-writing patients do have complicated disorders. It takes time to diagnose such cases, and it requires considerable skill on the part of the physician to interview such patients.

In fact, many physicians do not know how to coax patients into revealing important information—especially small things that the patient may think are inconsequential but which turn out to reveal aspects of a disease process. In medicine, as in other walks of life, there are few skilled interviewers.

* * *

I have my own little black binder in which I keep daily lists, projected lists, lists of unfinished work, and lists of concepts and ideas. When a patient bearing a list comes to see me, I take it as a sign of how complicated her disease process has become and how well prepared the patient is.

One extraordinary patient put together a virtual book on her disease, complete with index tabs. It included her medical history, copies of her lab tests, her independent observations, things other doctors had done, her husband's views, lists of questions, and treatments tried.

When she took this compendium to one well-known urologist, he refused to look at it. When she brought it to me, I asked for my own copy so I could underline parts, refer to it, and use it in arriving at a diagnosis. It indeed held the key to her problem, which was treated, and she is now pain-free and doing very well.

You don't have to go to this extent in making lists but coming prepared to every office visit makes economic and medical sense.

How Women Can Get the Best Help: The FEMALE Formula

Here's what you need to get organized when preparing for a visit to the doctor. Remember the "FEMALE" formula. Each letter stands for an important aspect of preparing to establish a successful partnership with your physician:

- Facts
- Evolution
- Medications
- Associated problems
- Laboratory records
- Emotion

Facts

Before you go to the store to spend your money, you sit down and assess what you really need. Before going to a physician, you should assess what you really want the doctor to do for you. What do you need from this physician and how are you going to get it? Do you need an investigator to unravel a mystery, or does the problem seem pretty clear?

You should be organized when you go. As you would take an inventory of what's in your cupboard before shopping, you should take an inventory of what you've observed. Identify the facts by thinking about these questions:

- Tell me, does it hurt before, after, or while you urinate?
- Does it hurt at night or is it associated with lifting, coughing, running, sneezing, or jogging?
- Is there a burning sensation associated with voiding?
- Is there a pressure or cramp?
- Where is the pain located, what causes it, what relieves it?
- Does it get better or worse when you eat certain foods?
- What is the color of your urine?
- Is there debris in your urine?
- Have you seen blood in the urine or is the blood only on the tissue paper when you wipe?
- Do you get pain down your leg? Do you have lower back problems? Do you have pains that go into your hip, your leg, up your spine?
- Do you leak urine when you run or jump in place, cough, or sneeze or does it leak all the time?
- Do you get fevers with any of the symptoms you're describing? Have you recorded those temperatures?
- Do you have a watery green discharge from the vagina as a symptom or is there a thick, cottage cheeselike material?
- Has your sexual partner had any problems?
- Do you get infections whether or not you have intercourse?
- Do you void with a good stream? Does it stop and start?
- Does it burn on the outside of the urethra or in the vagina when you void?
- Does it feel like your insides are falling out?

I know that women are extremely accurate observers of fact. They are very aware, in great detail, of what hurts them. But many of the facts might not get through to the doctor unless they have thought them out and written them down ahead of time.

Evolution

Once you have put down the facts, it is important to note the chronological evolution of your symptoms. This will help us find out how your problems may have come about. I begin interviewing each patient with, "You were perfectly fine until . . . ?" I want her to focus on when her body started to change.

I get many surprising answers. One woman immediately realized, with the help of her husband, that her problem began four years earlier than she had thought. She had thought her problem started after she took medication prescribed by a doctor the year before. Her husband recalled that while they were out camping four years earlier, she had needed to void frequently and was tired for several weeks. Her problem, we eventually found, was related to those earlier symptoms.

As discussed in Chapter Two, many fairly common diseases, including strep throat and mononucleosis, may leave you immunologically vulnerable for future problems. You probably now appreciate the importance of going through your medical history. Any disease, no matter how commonplace, may be a precursor to your present bladder problems.

You should also record all the surgery you have had. Which tissues were removed? Many times I see patients who complain of pain in their lower abdominal right quadrant. It could be a number of things, including an ovarian cyst or appendicitis. Some of these patients have had an ovary removed but don't remember if it was the right one or the left one. They may remember what hospital they were in but not the name of their doctor.

It is simple to obtain the records of any past operations by calling the hospital records office. Your doctors, too, will release your medical records if you sign a consent form requesting it. Keep copies for your own records.

In studying the evolution of your disease, take note of how medicines, especially antibiotics, affected your symptoms. When treated with antibiotics, did your symptoms abate after one or two days or not until a week or ten days later? Were your symptoms better or worse? Did you become allergic to any of the medications?

The idea of evolution forces you to organize your medical history sequentially, not randomly. Follow the process through as you've experienced it. It may help to use birthdates, anniversaries, jobs held, or schools attended as points of reference to recall facts and developments.

Each person's medical evolution is unique. No one can figure it out for you, and only you can organize it properly. As we discuss what's happened, I may be able to ask some questions that will remind you of events that you thought were unrelated and that you left out. But we have to work together to get the whole story.

Medications

It's frustrating to have a patient tell me that a doctor gave her a medication, but she doesn't know the name of it. Perhaps all she knows is that it was a little white pill and that it made her sick to her stomach.

Vagueness about medication is ill-advised. Always keep a record of the drugs you take. Either keep the empty prescription bottle or jot down the name of the drug in a little notebook kept in the medicine cabinet. Otherwise, you might get confused.

For example, one woman knew that a purple pill she once took had made her sick. She thought it was Pyridium, a drug sometimes used to treat urinary tract infections, when in fact it was a sulfa drug. When she was later prescribed a sulfa drug for a bladder infection—because she said she was allergic to Pyridium—she got sick!

If you don't know the name of a medicine you've taken, call the doctor who prescribed it for you and ask the nurse to check your medical records. Always keep an up-to-date list of any allergies you have. If a medication gives you unwanted side effects, let all your physicians know about it. Keep everyone who treats you aware of any changes in your body's reactions to drugs and medicines.

We need to know the names of all the medications you take for any health problem. Medicines are excreted in urine and hence may affect bladder tissue, causing urinary tract problems. For example, some antidepressants can keep the bladder muscle from working properly. Medications that relax the intestinal muscles for people with colitis may also cause the bladder muscle to relax and not empty completely.

Keep a record of the exact dosage of all your medications. I know of a woman who didn't realize she was taking an estrogen supplement. As part of the therapy for a bladder problem, a different physician prescribed estrogen therapy. For several weeks, the woman took a double dose of estrogen. She was unharmed but the mistake could have been avoided had she been aware of what was in her pills.

What medicines had no effect? I may be ruminating in the back of my mind about one drug over another to try on you. But if you can tell me that a certain drug previously had no effect, it can save us both time and save you prolonged discomfort.

Combinations of medicines can have untoward effects. Every time a patient tells me she is taking medications that I am not familiar with, I look up the drugs in a reference book and read about all possible drug interactions. Drug interactions do cause urinary tract problems.

For example, Mary Jo regularly took decongestants for her allergies. Later she developed a bladder problem and needed bethanechol chloride to help her void efficiently. The bethanechol chloride stimulated her bladder muscle. But the decongestant tended to close her bladder neck, affecting tissue there much the same way it affected tissue in her bronchial tree. The interaction of bethanechol chloride and decongestant made voiding difficult for Mary Jo. She developed hesitancy and was unable to get her urine stream started while on both medications.

If you take many different medications, I recommend that you go to the library and check out books on prescription drugs and drug interactions. You might want to buy one for home reference. Ask your physicians about drug interactions. It's better to be safe than sorry.

Also, keep a record of the side effects of drugs. Some side effects can be beneficial. I prescribe an anti-seasickness drug (transderm scopolamine) because, as a side effect, it inhibits bladder contractions and spasms in interstitial cystitis patients. Side effects in general are the price you pay to restore your body's health. They include headache, dizziness, nausea, and tiredness. Some side effects can be avoided by switching medications.

Have you tried home remedies for your urinary problems? It's important to let your physician know everything you're taking, including vitamin pills. Many times I see patients with highly alkaline urine and discover they consume large quantities of calcium carbonate, a calcium supplement for postmenopausal women. All home remedies, including cranberry juice and herbal teas, could potentially contribute to your symptoms. If you have a urothelial membrane leak, acidifying your urine may increase your pain and discomfort. Over-the-counter drugs that you take for colds, allergies, or other common ailments could also be implicated. Take time to make your lists and don't leave anything out.

Associated Problems

Family diseases and other medical problems interrelate in ways that patients never suspect.

Whenever a new patient comes to my office for an evaluation of cystitis, I always ask if she has lower back problems. I'm often greeted with a look of utter surprise, as if I were a Houdini who X-rayed her spine with my eyes. Most women never correlate lower back problems with bladder dysfunction. And, although the correlation between the nerves in the lower back and nerves in the bladder is well-known in urology, many physicians fail to make the association, especially in younger women. But relatively minor back stress, along with other factors, is frequently enough to cause cystitis.

You should know your family's medical history. Are there cases of heart disease, cholesterol problems, diabetes, kidney disease, or anatomic problems with the urinary tract? While interstitial cystitis is an environmental disease, caused by external factors rather than inborn biologic factors, a genetic factor may be involved. I have treated a mother and daughter with interstitial cystitis as well as a daughter and father with the disease.

Many inheritable diseases can interact with the urinary tract. Diabetes is a classic example. Because a diabetic often loses sensory perception, her bladder may lose the ability to sense when it is full. The bladder enlarges and eventually loses the ability to contract and empty properly. Leftover urine promotes the onset of infections.

A diabetic whose disease is not controlled also experiences insatiable thirst. As she drinks more, her bladder walls stretch and the muscle tone deteriorates. I have a patient who develops severe voiding problems every time her insulin fails to manage her diabetes. The rest of the time, her bladder functions normally.

Gout, which involves a buildup of uric acid in the body, is hereditary. It can lead to a class of kidney stones that are difficult to detect by a single radiographic X ray. This condition requires an intravenous pyelogram (IVP), which is described in Appendix E.

What is your family's cancer history? There is increasing evidence that some families may be prone to a particular type of cancer, which may be the result of genetic deficiencies in tissue growth and protective layering.

What are your other medical conditions? Do you have colitis, arthritis, or neurologic problems? Asthmatics often take medications that can affect the bladder and prevent efficient voiding.

When you were treated for an earlier disease, did your doctor prove the diagnosis or only surmise the problem? For example, some patients diagnosed as having pelvic inflammatory disease (PID) have no positive cultures. These patients may have interstitial cystitis. Patients said to have endometriosis likewise may never have had a laparoscopic examination to confirm the gynecologic suspicion of this problem. Many women are told they have a gynecologic problem when in fact it is urologic. And vice versa. The point is that *diagnostic proof should not be ignored.*

I have a patient who was told for two years that she had a chronic uterine infection. But cultures of her urine and cultures of her vagina proved she had no infection at all. Rather, she had interstitial cystitis and went untreated because of poor diagnostic work. If your physician says he has the impression you are suffering from X, Y, or Z, ask, "How do we go about proving that is the problem? What do you recommend to prove a diagnosis?" Laparoscopy proves endometriosis. A positive urine culture proves cystitis. And so on. Be sure your physician treats you for a *real* condition and not for a *probable* cause of your symptoms.

Lab Work

How many times have you been X-rayed? What did those X rays show? Unless you have records of your laboratory tests, you may forget important findings. People tend to misinterpret or misrelate facts told them about such tests. For example, one person told me her white count was low. In fact, when we got the test records, it was normal. A different blood measure had been low.

Lab tests are useful for determining when a disease process may have begun. Again, test records are available from hospitals, clinics, or the doctors who ordered them. If, for any reason, a physician refuses to release your medical records you can get the records from other sources. It is your legal right to have copies of all your medical records. Personally bring them to the new doctor's office. Don't mail them ahead of time for they might get lost.

Some tests need to be done only once. Avoiding unnecessary repetition of tests saves you time, money, and discomfort. For example, many cystitis patients undergo an IVP, an X-ray study that shows the kidney anatomy and bladder placement (see Appendix E). Once this test result is normal, it rarely needs repeating; people certainly don't need several IVPs as one might need an annual chest X ray. Moreover, people who are allergic to shellfish should not have an IVP done, since they are likely to be allergic to the iodine used in the procedure. Frequent exposure to radiation in reproductive females should be avoided unless absolutely warranted.

Other tests, such as uroflows and urine cultures, might need to be repeated often, as they reflect current functional status. It depends on the individual's problems. But not knowing what's been done to you in the past makes it hard for the physician to understand the present and difficult to assess the future.

Emotion

Emotion has been the undoing of women through the ages. It is what makes some women with valid debilitating urologic disease end up in psychiatric hospitals being treated for what is considered an imaginary disease.

The plain fact is that most physicians do not deal well with emotional females.

I have less of a problem getting my women patients to focus on facts because emotion is something that I live with every day. But to many of my male colleagues, an emotional woman is a complete enigma. She is "hysterical" and her complaints make no sense. This has been particularly true of stubborn and, until recently, seemingly causeless and mysterious problems of the female urinary tract.

In my experience, men tend to speak from fact, women tend to speak from emotion. When you tell me that the pain in your bladder is ruining your marriage and destroying your life, you are not giving me factual detail about the pain in your bladder; you are telling me the effects of the problem, not helping me get to the root of it.

THE SAME STORY TOLD TWO WAYS

To show you what I mean, here is the way two women related their symptoms of urinary incontinence during an office visit:

Patient A: "Dr. Gillespie, my problem first seemed to begin after I had my second child. I noticed I was having problems controlling the urine but it was not so bad. I only needed to wear a small protective pad when we went out in the evenings. When I was at home, I could usually put my hands between my legs or quickly cross my legs if I was going to sneeze or cough. But lately things have been getting worse. Now that I'm back working again, I find I can't manage the problem the same way. I don't have to get up at night, but one time I did have some pain and burning. I had to get up three or four times. I went to my gynecologist and got a urine culture. It was positive and I was treated with Ceclor [cefaclor] for three days. The burning problem went away but I'm still left with the leakage. I'd like to know what can be done."

Patient B: "Dr. Gillespie, I just don't know what I'm going to do in a situation like this anymore. I can't go to my friends' houses anymore. All my friends are sort of staying away from me. I think it's because I ruined my best friend's dining room chair when we were playing cards. When I laughed at a story, before I knew what happened there was a wet spot on the chair. I could feel it on the back of my dress. Well, I really didn't know what to do. I never got asked back. I'm having to wear four or five pads during the daytime and I'm so isolated. I don't know what to do about it anymore."

Patient A gave me accurate, helpful facts without emotion. She knew when she leaked, how much, and what could arrest it. The impact on her life is clear, but the emotion does not cloud or distort the facts. As a physician, I would easily know in what direction to proceed to help this patient.

Patient B has not given me helpful facts. I've heard everything except the kinds of observations that would help in making a diagnosis. Not only did she waste some of our time, but she failed to give me any accurate evidence of her problem other than the fact that she leaks urine when she laughs and she has to wear pads. Evidently she wanted help because her incontinence was ruining her social life.

It may be very hard to separate emotion from observed fact, particularly if you've been to numerous doctors, all of whom failed to find a reason for your symptoms. But don't feel as if no one will ever listen to you.

Many sufferers of chronic cystitis have this outlook on their visits to new physicians. But you need to take each visit with an open mind. If you don't get satisfaction at one place, go to another. An astonishing number of people today are well informed about medicine. Doctors are finding that if they don't give straight answers, the smart medical consumer will take his or her business elsewhere. You don't need to stay with a physician who promotes ignorance, won't explain side effects, or keeps you overmedicated as a way to keep you quiet.

Be aware, however, that chronic pain affects emotional stability. You "trigger" more easily than you would if you were pain free. Pain makes you more sensitive and unable to tolerate suggestions or inferences that may be relatively benign. Try not to respond to a physician's questions in a way that infers your problem is psychiatric or emotional.

I sympathize with your agony and pain, but we must concentrate on the facts of your situation if I am going to help you. Women with interstitial cystitis, for example, live day to day with a kind of unrelenting torture. When they try to relate their symptoms to physicians, understandably they typically focus on their mental anguish. Many physicians then diagnose these women as having a psychosomatic disorder. Thus many women do not get the kind of rational medical treatment more readily given to male patients.

But, as I've stated, women tend to be extremely accurate observers of fact and can use that skill to advantage in their health care. When preparing for your next visit to a doctor, remember the acronym FEMALE. If you relate facts before emotion, your observations will help to establish a valid interaction with the physician.

How to Tell If Your Doctor Is Paying Attention

I have often heard from patients that "they just don't think their doctor is *listening* to them." How can you tell if your doctor is paying attention to your problem?

First, I strongly recommend that *all* visits begin in the doctor's office and not in an examining room. The reason is simple: In the exam room, you are usually naked and placed in a situation where you feel vulnerable and on less than equal standing. Second, in the office the doctor has to sit to talk; standing isn't an option. A doctor standing in the doorway of an examining room while the patient asks questions is somewhat akin to the idea of "eating at a trough" instead of sitting down with your family for a meal. The impression the patient has is that time is short. How often have you been placed in a room with a drape sheet and had to hail your doctor "like a taxi" in order to get your questions answered? As a medical student I was instructed to keep my hand on the doorknob so as to ensure that patients would be "quick" about asking their questions. With the changes in today's health-care systems, we may see more of this deplorable habit.

When the doctor/patient relationship fails, it is generally owing to a lack of communication between the two. So here are eight warning signs that you need a more caring, interested physician:

You Need to Consider Finding Another Doctor If:

1. Your doctor seldom makes eye contact with you.
2. When you offer information that might influence or change the diagnosis your doctor has made, he or she rejects it and seems to rely solely on his or her expertise.
3. The last time you were emotional your doctor maintained a polite, unemotional distance.
4. When your doctor explains something to you, you get a lecture instead of a chance to discuss things you don't understand.
5. You question your doctor's proposed diagnosis and he or she becomes defensive, or worst of all, reminds you which one of you is the doctor.
6. After a visit, you find that you didn't mention all your symptoms because you felt rushed.
7. Your use of a list or other organized method of reporting your observations is not given due consideration, especially if your questions or observations are unusual.
8. Your feelings toward your doctor are slightly angry or fearful.

Keep looking until you find a connection with a doctor, a partnership that can become a healing relationship. You will not only discover a friend, but a better, healthier you.

FIVE

Anatomy Is *Not* Destiny

A model of the female urinary tract sat on my office desk. It took up space, got in my way, and I knocked it over from time to time. But for one very important reason it never left my desk in the sixteen years that I practiced urology: Most women do not know what their urogenital system looks like. If a picture is worth a thousand words, a model is worth a novel.

To overcome cystitis, you must have a mental picture of how you are built. And so, as part of getting you started on the road to understanding, I am going to discuss your anatomy in the same way as I would sitting with a patient in my office.

Believe it or not, knowledge of the female lower urinary tract is still evolving. Many earlier assumptions about the way women are constructed have been overturned in recent years. Please remember that urology, like other medical specialties, is a fast-moving discipline in which exciting discoveries and new treatments arrive on the scene virtually every month. Our knowledge is not static and even information about basic human anatomy can change.

Your urinary tract is exquisitely adapted for bearing children. Its primary function—the elimination of the body's liquid wastes—is usually carried out effectively and efficiently.

If you encounter problems with your bladder or urinary tract, you may unwittingly be altering nature's design. You may do things or introduce agents that interfere with normal function.

Why Women and Men Must Be Treated Differently

Because men's and women's urinary tracts share the same primary function, the transportation of urine, they are often analyzed according to common assumptions and principles. Naturally all urologists recognize that men and women are anatomically different, but in the final analysis of what can go wrong with the urinary tract, the similarities between men and women often have been held to be more important than the differences.

But the differences are significant (see illustration page 140). The male urinary tract serves a major sexual function while the female tract serves but a secondary sexual function.

Consider the male urethra. As a rule, it measures ten inches from the bladder to the tip of the penis. Its job is to carry urine but also to transport semen during sexual activity. Concepts of physics tell us that the best way to transport a liquid is to move it through a round, smooth channel that holds its shape. The male urethra is ideally designed for this purpose.

The female urethra measures about two inches from the bladder to its opening just below the clitoris. Its primary job is to transport urine. Its sexual role, moving out of the way during childbirth, is secondary. Thus the female urethra is a corrugated tube with a large surface area that can stretch and flatten out when it needs to.

"The Rape of the Female Urethra"

The female urethra has a different, evolutionary function from the male urethra and needs to be studied, examined, and treated differently. When it is not, the consequences can be painful.

For example, the male urethra has a well-defined external sphincter located in front of the prostate gland. The sphincter is a muscle whose job is to close and open like the on-off valve of a garden hose. When open, fluid passes and when closed, fluid cannot pass. The muscle is under somewhat voluntary control.

Unfortunately for men, their urethras are easily infected by certain bacteria, such as gonorrhea. When this happens, scar tissue—called a stricture—forms. The stricture prevents a man from urinating freely. The solution is to dilate or rupture the scar tissue by inserting gradually larger metal rods into the urethra. As you can imagine, this procedure can be very painful.

For decades, some urologists have viewed and treated the female urethra as essentially a shortened version of the male urethra. In this view, challenged only recently, women would also be subject to bacterial infections

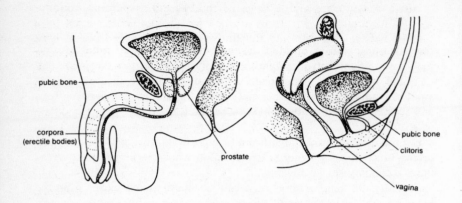

pubic bone

corpora
(erectile bodies)

prostate

pubic bone

clitoris

vagina

Figure 5-1, Male and Female Anatomy

that create strictures in their urethras. Although women do not get gonorrheal urethritis that causes scarring, they do suffer other bacterial invasions. Thus a common treatment is to stretch open the female urethra to free it of so-called strictures.

Unfortunately, what urologists have been breaking open in women is not a stricture. It is the female external sphincter, which many physicians believed women did not have. As a result, normal tissue is needlessly traumatized and often scarred. The practice is what many urologists now term "the rape of the female urethra."

How Could It Happen?

How could we have not known? One reason is that if you compare the male and female urethras, centimeter per centimeter, it appears that the external sphincter *is* missing. The urethra is not long enough to contain the external sphincter at the same site (see illustration page 142).

But women do have an external sphincter in the urethra. It is a muscle within the wall of the urethra itself, but many urologists believed it to be a birth defect marked by a 'lack of growth as a woman matured, which supposedly resulted in poor flow and infections in adulthood. Unfortunately, urologists only saw women with infections and never had healthy women in their offices for comparison. All women have this muscle; it is not a birth defect.

Female children found to have bladder infections were frequently diagnosed as having birth defects. Their sphincters were then ruptured by dilation.

Adult women were said to have the child urethral syndrome. Unfortunately, the urethra is frequently blamed for the problems caused by a bladder muscle that does not function properly, often because of back problems that need to be investigated (see Chapter One). If your doctor insists you need a urethral dilation, I advise you to ask for further evaluation, including a uroflow. If the doctor still insists, you might want to get a second opinion.

It should be noted that in a very few children there is a type of abnormal tissue called a *Lyon's ring.* It may cause infection and reflux. When the ring is dilated, the infection stops. But this is a rare condition and can be picked up with an X ray. As such, it rarely persists into adulthood.

Women also have some voluntary control over this external sphincter. When you tighten this muscle, you can feel it pull up through the vagina. You can consciously keep the sphincter closed, even when your bladder is uncomfortably full, until you are ready to urinate.

About the only thing that can go wrong anatomically with the female urethra is rare. In developing countries, where some women deliver babies that are too large for their birth canals, the urethra can be ruptured. This rarely occurs in developed nations and should not cause you concern.

More Comparisons and More Differences

Again, comparing men and women, both sexes have glands in the urethra that put out wetting agents to reduce surface tension and let urine pass smoothly over the tissue. These identical glands—called *Skene's glands* in women and *Cowper's glands* in men—are located in pairs at the opening of the female urethra. *Littre's glands,* which also lubricate, are found within the urethra itself. Men alone have the *prostate gland. Prostate* means ''guardian.'' Located below the bladder, it is the gateway through which sperm enter the urethra. It also produces fluid for semen.

Another belief stemming from the comparison of men and women is that the female urethra can be in the wrong place, that it may be too high or too low. There is a birth defect called *hypospadias* that is much more common in men than women. In men, the urethra may not reach the tip of the penis. In this case, it must be surgically extended to restore normal appearance and the flow of urine. In female hypospadias patients, the urethra does not grow long enough and it opens into the vagina. This, too, can be surgically corrected.

Unfortunately, some urologists have taken this concept of a misplaced urethra and extended it to healthy women. The idea is that recurrent infections are promoted or exacerbated by a uretheral opening that is too high or too low. The urethra, they say, is dragged into the vagina with

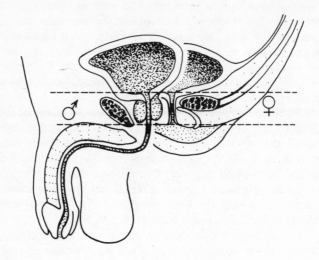

Figure 5-2, Comparing the External Sphincter in Men and Women

intercourse and this increases bacterial infection. It is ''too low'' and needs to be raised surgically up out of the vagina. This doesn't make sense. If you can see your urethra on the outside, it's in just the right place.

In all women, the urethra is in the same place—just below the clitoris and above the vagina. Since these openings share common tissue, it is unlikely for them to be in the wrong place. Nevertheless, physicians have surgically cut and repositioned urethras in the hope of stopping infections.

The Bladder Neck

Moving up the urinary tract, features become identical, functionally and anatomically, in men and women. First is the *bladder neck*, located at the bottom or opening of the bladder. *Neck* in this sense means small opening, like the part of a balloon that is tied off. The bladder neck is also called an *internal sphincter*. It, too, is composed of tiny muscles that open and contract like the pupil of an eye.

Your bladder neck serves as the first lock for keeping urine in your bladder. It is not under voluntary control—that is, you cannot consciously cause it to open or close. When a woman's bladder neck is injured, urine can leak out after a cough or sneeze if the external sphincter is not strong enough. However, if she increases her pelvic floor tone by contracting her buttock muscles, she can tightly close the external sphincter to prevent urine from leaking all the way out.

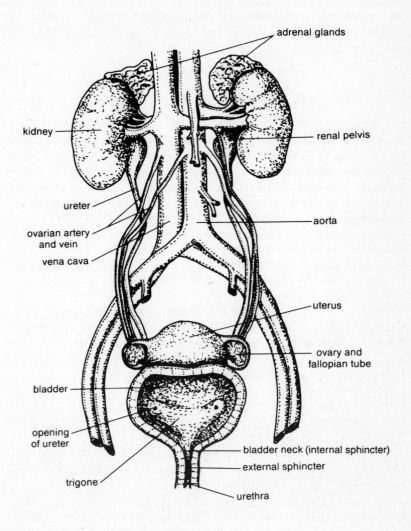

Figure 5-3, The Complete Female Urinary System

These sphincters—and indeed the entire urinary tract—are laced with networks of nerves that control their action. Nerves leading from your brain are connected to your urinary tract along networks that arrive, via the lower back, at your bladder. One set controls the external sphincter, another the internal sphincter, and others lead to the bladder itself.

These nerves are important to your urologic health, and we will come back to them later.

The Bladder and How It Works

Your bladder, which can be viewed simply as a bag for holding urine, also contains a main sensory area, rich with nerves, that signals you when it is time to urinate. Called the *trigone* of the bladder, because of its roughly triangular shape, its tissues derive from a group of parent cells in the developing embryo different from the tissues in the rest of the bladder. The trigone is special. It is the "signal to void" area of the bladder and its message must be heeded.

The *bladder* itself is like a balloon. Somewhat Y-shaped when empty and spherical when full, it holds a maximum of between 12 and 16 ounces of urine. In general, comfortable voiding volumes are half this. For reasons as yet unknown, female bladders tend to have larger capacities than male bladders.

The outer part of the bladder is covered with a membrane lining found throughout the abdominal cavity. The bottom is supported by the floor of the bony pelvis. In front, the space between the pubic bones and bladder is filled with loose, fatty tissue. And at the top of the bladder, a strong fibrous cord connects the bladder with the navel.

In order to empty, your bladder must force out fluid, so it is endowed with strong muscular tissue, called the *detrusor,* within its walls. The detrusor must generate enough pressure to cause complete emptying. When it is activated, urine is forced out of the bladder.

Nerves to this muscle also arrive from the lower back. You could compare them to battery cables in your car. These nerves conduct an electrical current to the bladder and stimulate a contraction.

The inside of the bladder, as well as the urethra, is covered with a lining of what are called *urothelial cells.* This lining is protected by a mucous layer that prevents the tissue from being burned by the acid contents of urine. The *GAG layer,* as discussed in Chapter Two, acts as a wetting agent that keeps the lining smooth so that it will be an effective fouling barrier against the acid elements in urine.

The Ureters: Elegant Channels to the Bladder

Urine comes into your bladder through two strawlike structures called *ureters*. About twelve to fourteen inches long, these tubular structures go straight up to your kidneys. Your ureters enter the bladder near its bottom on either side of the trigonal sensory region.

Ureters are simply urine transport channels, but they move liquid in an elegant fashion. It is important that urine cannot move back up into your kidneys, even when you stand on your head. The backward flow of urine can cause damage to kidney tissue by overdistension and by transporting bacteria from the lower urinary tract. This can result in pyelonephritis.

To ensure that fluid moves in only one direction, your ureters make use of special clamplike muscles that contract in waves. Tiny amounts of urine are propelled ever downward by the undulating muscles. A stream of urine spurts into your bladder every ten to thirty seconds. At the entrance to your bladder, again there are strong muscles that prevent urine from going in the wrong direction. At the point where they enter the bladder, the ureters become somewhat thinner, enabling them to collapse and close off as bladder pressures rise.

The Kidneys: Your Purification Machines

Your ureters enter each *kidney* (see illustration page 146) in twin structures that resemble the cup of a lily. This area is, in fact, called the *calyx,* which is Greek for the cup of a flower. The calyx is a boundary region between your kidney and ureter. You can think of it simply as a funnel. There is a junction between the bottom of the funnel (the opening to the ureter) and the region above (the top of the funnel) for collecting liquid.

Urine rolls through a catchment area composed of lots of little cuplike structures. There the urine is finally captured and drained away.

One of your body's vital organs, the kidney, delivers all urine to the catchment area. Luckily, we are each born with two kidneys. If one is damaged, we can survive with the other.

Your kidneys serve as the body's purification machine. Your body works much like a factory. You take in "raw materials" (food and drink) and from them extract energy and materials to build the products your body needs. This process creates wastes. Solid wastes are excreted through the colon while liquid wastes are carried through the bloodstream until they can be removed.

Your kidneys filter such wastes from blood. They are incredibly efficient filtration devices that extract toxins, acids, and other undesirable products small enough to be carried away in the blood.

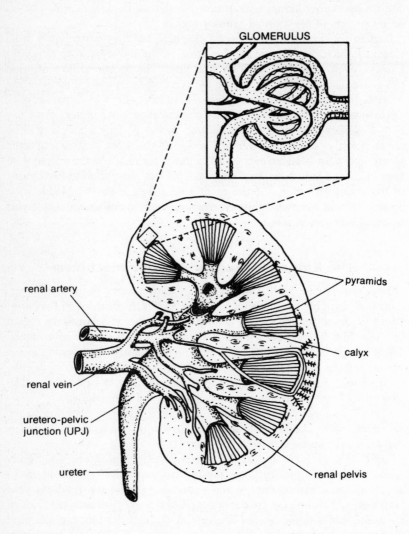

GLOMERULUS

pyramids

calyx

renal artery

renal vein

uretero-pelvic
junction (UPJ)

ureter

renal pelvis

Figure 5-4, A Normal Kidney and Its Small Filtering Units

Kidneys also maintain a constant volume of blood circulating through your body, regulate fluid balance, control pressure relationships between blood and tissue, and maintain the body's electrolyte system—the relative amounts of sodium, potassium, and water required by every cell in your body.

Every twenty-four hours, the kidneys filter more than 45 gallons of blood plasma. Most of the materials carried in the plasma can be reused. The kidney's small filters, called *glomeruli,* take out such materials and then return them, in perfect balance, to the circulatory system. About 1 percent of the 45 gallons that are filtered daily—1.6 quarts—is removed as waste, or urine.

Your urine should be somewhere between pale and darkened yellow, and clear enough so you could read a newspaper through it.

How Much Water Should I Drink?

The volume of urine produced in a day, of course, depends on your environment. In hot, dry climates, a certain amount of your body's liquids is eliminated as perspiration. The wastes are then concentrated in a smaller amount of water. The idea that you should drink eight or more glasses of water a day makes little sense in view of this regulatory mechanism. You should drink as much as feels comfortable, given your level of activity, the climate, and your diet. Use common sense. On an average, we need 32 ounces of fluid a day.

Each kidney is shaped like a bean and measures 4½ inches long, 2 inches wide, and 1 to 2 inches thick. They are located on either side of your spine in the middle of your back and above your waist, under the shoulder blades (see Figure 5-5). If you feel pain in your lower back, it is not a kidney infection. The top of each kidney is in fact attached by strong fibers to the diaphragm, and both kidneys rise and fall somewhat as you breathe. Blood is delivered to the kidney by *renal arteries.* (*Renal* just means "pertaining to the kidney.")

Each kidney has, at a minimum, 1 million glomeruli, or tiny filtration units. They are the result of one of nature's finest designs.

A Run Through the System

Now let's run through the system from the top down. Suppose you drink a glass of water. It is absorbed into the bloodstream, where it performs numerous jobs before reaching the kidney as a constituent of plasma. Some of the water is extracted as urine and drips, as dew cas-

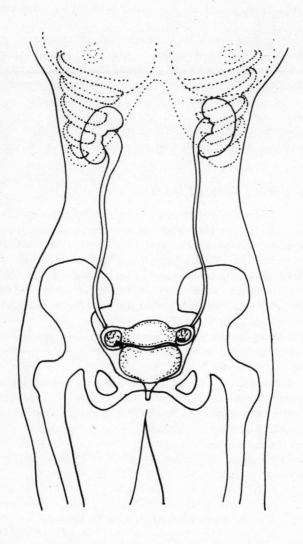

Figure 5-5, The Normal Position of Kidneys

cades among leaves, down a lubricated pathway to the top of the funnel, or renal pelvis.

When this area collects about a quarter of an ounce of urine, the ureteropelvic junction opens and the urine is propelled down the ureter, in wavelike contractions, to your bladder. A second valve opens and the thimbleful of urine is pushed into the bladder near the trigone area.

Slowly, in this way, your bladder fills from bottom up.

When it is about half full, the trigone begins to stretch under the weight of the accumulating urine. The urine also sends signals to special nerves in the bladder lining. These events signal your brain that you need to consider allowing time to get to an appropriate place to void.

A very complicated, integrated series of functions follows. When you are ready to go, the bladder muscle begins to generate an increase in pressure. As a result, the bladder neck opens and the external sphincter shuts down any activity. You relax your pelvic floor and the bladder muscle contracts. As this happens, the trigone contracts so that your ureters are shut tight, and no urine can flow the wrong way despite the head of pressure.

Voiding is an act of changing pressure gradients. Continence, or staying dry, is the result of the pressure in the urethra being greater than the pressure in the bladder.

The urethra generates its own pressure, which can be measured with instruments. Let's say, on average, it measures "4" on a pressure scale.

The bladder fills passively. As it fills, it does not generate any pressure of its own. Once the bladder is full, however, it does begin to exert pressure that typically, on the same scale, may measure 30. Voiding or urinating occurs when bladder pressure is greater than pressure in the urethra.

As you urinate, pressure in the bladder steadily falls: It goes from 30 to 29, 28, 27, and so on, down to 10, 9, 8, and on down to 5, 4, 3.... When it falls below the urethra's pressure—to below 4 on our pressure scale—the urethra's pressure dominates once more. The sphincters close. You stop voiding and, slowly, passively, your bladder begins to fill up again.

You may have noticed that if you hold urine for a very long time, against pressures that can really hurt, you may have trouble, when you finally do go, emptying your bladder completely or voiding with a good, forceful stream. Small amounts of urine may continue to dribble out for a while. This is because you have distended your bladder and it cannot generate its normal head of pressure. If you blow up a balloon a second time, making it bigger than it was, the balloon loses elasticity. Your bladder operates under similar principles.

Kidney Malformations and Diseases

Some congenital kidney problems are serious and some are not. I find it fascinating whenever a patient comes in and says, "I have been followed for years by my other doctor for my traveling kidneys." I try not to laugh and ask, "Oh? Where did they book a ticket?" Or, "How far have your kidneys traveled this year?"

The look on the patient's face is quite interesting as I then explain that "traveling kidneys" are normal. The top of each kidney is attached by strong fibers to the diaphragm, so that the kidneys rise and fall during breathing. Some rise and fall, or "travel," more than others. It used to be that surgeons would operate to reposition a traveling kidney. That operation is no longer in vogue because now we know that the position of the kidney has no bearing on its function. If you're told you have a traveling kidney, don't worry. It won't leave you.

An unusual birth defect is the *horseshoe kidney*. During fetal development, both kidneys fail to rise up to their proper place under the rib cage. They lie, like a horseshoe, in the pelvic cavity. Fortunately, the condition rarely bothers its owner; despite the odd placement, the kidneys work fine.

Another birth defect is the *solitary kidney*. One kidney fails to develop and the other, or solitary one, acts as a kind of super kidney. The main drawback of this arrangement is that the owner does not have the protection of two kidneys in case the one is damaged.

An inherited disorder called *polycystic kidneys* can slowly destroy both kidneys. For reasons unknown, numerous small cysts develop in the kidneys and hold urine, as in little sacs. The kidney tissue is ultimately destroyed.

Yet another kidney disease, *fibromuscular hyperplasia,* is more prevalent in women than in men. In this disorder, the main artery going to the kidney takes on the appearance of a string of beads. Blood flow is impeded. As kidney function is impaired, the patient tends to develop high blood pressure. The condition can be corrected by placing a balloon catheter through the artery, thus opening it up and restoring normal blood flow.

Diabetes is probably the best-known kidney disease. With this condition, in which insulin is not taken up properly in the body, excess glucose is circulated in the bloodstream. As the kidneys clear and filter blood, the extra glucose is dumped into urine. In this process, tiny capillaries in the kidneys may eventually become scarred and damaged. Ultimately, the kidneys may lose their ability to clear toxins and other substances from the bloodstream properly.

Another well-known problem is kidney stone disease. Stones may develop in women who repeatedly dehydrate themselves by jogging and other exercise. Dehydration promotes the formation of tiny crystals in the kidney that later pass through the ureters. Other people may develop stones as a result of abnormalities of the parathyroid. Birth control pills, which decrease the availability of B_6 in the body, may lead to kidney stone formation. Finally, as will be discussed in Chapter Eight, it is not uncommon for stones to pass in some women six weeks or so after childbirth.

Urologists, by the way, have long violated the Hippocratic oath when it comes to dealing with stones. Hippocrates said, "Never cut for stones." Yet, up until very recently, stone surgery has been a mainstay of urologic practice. A machine called a lithotriptor, developed in Europe and now available in major hospitals in the United States, promises to change forever the ways stones are managed. The lithotriptor uses high-energy shock waves generated outside the body to disintegrate stones inside the body while the patient sits in a tub of warm water. Within a few hours, the resulting stone particles—about the consistency of coarse sand—begin to pass naturally from the urinary tract. I believe there can be no better way to understand the pain and torture of passing kidney stones than to have one yourself. I would recommend that if you, or someone you know, has suffered from kidney stones to read *The Kidney Stones Handbook* by Gail Golomb, who understands first-hand how to help you take charge of this condition. See Appendix A for more information.

Toward a New Understanding of Women's Bodies

You might think that everything there is to know about human anatomy has already been discovered. But that is not the case. As researchers refine their tools and develop greater understanding of how the body functions, they are discovering new nerve networks and systems.

Urology in particular has been somewhat handicapped by its male-dominated view of the urinary tract, but things are changing for the better. Many urologists, both men and women, are coming to understand how function and design differ between the sexes. The better you understand nature's design, the better you are able to care for your body and know when something has gone awry.

SIX

You Don't Have to Live with Incontinence

MILLIONS of adult Americans—no one is certain how many—suffer some degree of urinary incontinence. That is, they do not have complete control over their bladders. To their never-ending embarrassment, they leak urine.

Incontinence is a common problem, yet, until the pharmaceutical industry saw it as a potentially large market to be exploited, you never heard much about it. Talk shows didn't deal with the topic. Women's magazines and newspaper health columnists rarely wrote about it.

To my constant amazement, incontinence remains one of the most taboo subjects in American culture. People are willing to talk about their hemorrhoids, constipation, and sexual dysfunction but they do not, in public or private, talk about their incontinence.

Perhaps we, as a society, are fixated on continence—the ability to stay dry—because of our early toilet-training experiences. Children are taught that continence is a virtue. It symbolizes our first encounter with self-control. Continence is so deeply intertwined with our unconscious memories of parental approval and disapproval, perhaps we will never be comfortable with the subject.

The statistics are staggering. Incontinence, or the leakage of urine, occurs in people of all ages, but is particularly common in older people. At least one in ten persons age sixty-five or older suffers from incontinence. This condition affects women in far greater numbers than it does men—fully 85 percent are women. On average, women with this condition first experience leakage at age forty-seven, yet three in ten develop incontinence before the age of thirty-five. As baby boomers turn fifty this year, it is estimated that 8 million community-living women will struggle with this problem, and 11 million fifteen years from now.

A study sponsored by two different pharmaceutical companies showed 23 percent of women with this problem put off seeking medical attention because of embarrassment, waiting an average of four to ten years. One in six never discussed urine leakage with anyone, and more than a third of those who did waited a year or more after the condition developed to discuss it! Sadly, close to half of all women with incontinence had to change their lifestyle.

It is not an insignificant problem. For the elderly, incontinence is a major medical, psychological, and social problem. It has been estimated that nursing homes spend up to $1.5 billion a year coping with incontinence. About 40 percent of all the sanitary pads sold in this country are used for incontinence. It may surprise you to know that the average woman uses nearly three pads a day. That's more than one thousand pads a year!

As a urologist, however, I can make the claim that incontinence is treatable. There are numerous ways to deal with the problem so that whatever the cause, incontinent adults can become fully functioning adults. The more we talk about incontinence, realizing it is not something to be hidden, the more people will discover the treatment that is best for them.

Types of Incontinence

Judy's Story: Urinary Stress Incontinence

Judy is a fifty-six-year-old medical librarian with four grown children. "Life is supposed to get easier after your children leave," she told me one day last year, "but for me it got worse." Judy leaked urine whenever she laughed, coughed, or sneezed. Her condition, called *urinary stress incontinence,* caused her to leak urine whenever a "stress," such as a sudden sneeze, took her by surprise. With warning Judy could tighten up the muscles on her pelvic floor and sometimes prevent the leak. But most of the time, she could not.

"The problem first began about twenty years ago," she said. "I thought it was just because of childbirth. Unfortunately, women were just led to believe that this is just one of the things that happen to us. I was told not much could be done."

The problem affected Judy's life. "It was minor when it started, but as time went on, it became very difficult. I couldn't do exercises. I was constantly aware of where the restroom was, but it didn't make any difference. It was very difficult.

"Imagine what it's like walking into the dry cleaner's hoping his wife is on duty because you have to explain that you have urine all over your pants or all over your skirt. You have to tell them it's urine. They use certain stain removers and certain cleaning processes for that.

"This went on year after year and I tried doctor after doctor. But often I was patted on the head and told, 'Well, this is what happens to women when they undergo labor.' "

Urinary stress incontinence is the most common type of incontinence for a very simple reason. More often than not, it is a consequence of childbirth. Forty-seven percent of women with incontinence associated the onset of urine leakage with a major life event, such as childbirth. Given the number of American women who have given birth, it is understandably a widespread problem.

Stress incontinence, like many disorders, follows a continuum. It can be mild or severe or anything in between. It usually develops slowly in women ten years or so after they have finished having children.

As a baby moves down the vaginal canal during birth, its head lodges underneath the bladder neck. It rests there temporarily before final expulsion through the vagina. If the baby stays in this position for very long—perhaps because its head is big for the mother—stress is imposed on the ligaments that support the bladder neck.

By and large, this stress has no immediate consequences. A few women experience more severe compression to nerves in the vaginal canal and are unable to void twenty-four hours after delivery. Permanent damage is rare, however, and most women quickly resume normal urinary function.

But years later, once gravity begins to affect muscular tone, the bladder neck may slowly start to descend into the vaginal canal. As it does so, it pulls along a small portion of the bladder and forms a protrusion called a *cystocele*. A cystocele holds urine. When you void, your bladder does not empty totally because there is always a little bit of urine resting in the cystocele. You have a fallen or dropped bladder.

HOW TO TELL

You can tell if you have a cystocele if you put your fingers in your vagina and then purposely cough or strain. If something comes down and touches your fingers near the opening of your vagina, you have a cystocele.

Another way to tell is by noticing how you void. If you wait a moment and another little squirt of urine always comes out, you probably have a cystocele. That little squirt is the cystocele emptying.

Cystocele means "bladder hernia." It is simply a saclike protrusion of bladder tissue that isn't located higher up, where it belongs. When a cystocele holds urine, the weight of the urine tends to tug on the bladder neck. Under this strain, the bladder neck is unable to generate its normal closing pressure.

When you laugh unexpectedly, sneeze, or run in place, a shock wave is sent through the bladder neck. A normal bladder stays closed under such everyday stress. But a bladder neck weakened by childbirth and pulled upon by a cystocele just opens up. You leak.

When a person with stress incontinence has forewarning, say, that a sneeze is coming, she can sometimes prevent urine from leaking by clamping down consciously on her pelvic floor muscles. But when there is no warning, which is most of the time, she leaks.

Many women with this problem practice what are called Kegel exercises to strengthen the muscles in the pelvic floor. These isometric exercises are simple to do. Feel your buttock muscles tighten and relax as you pull up and inward with your vagina. I recommend that women do them every day while they brush their teeth. That rolls two habits into one. With improved muscle tone, a woman who sneezes can exert enough external pressure on her urethra to prevent urine from leaking out.

But many women aren't sure if they are contracting the right muscles, so I have developed a foolproof way to perform this exercise correctly, called *Vaginetics*. Look at Figure 6-1. First lay on the floor with your legs bent. Now raise your pelvis so that your hands act as a counterbalance. This tightens your stomach and back muscles at the same time. The uterus will fall back into the pelvis, and you will find that as you pull up and inward with your vagina, the *only* muscles you can contract are the pelvic floor muscles.

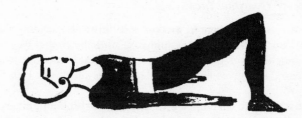

Figure 6-1, Illustration of correct position for Vaginetics

I find this exercise so intense I can only do five ''reps'' at a time. It certainly beats trying to ''squeeze'' in one hundred repetitions in any other position!

I'm convinced that women who have very rapid baby deliveries and who have very flexible perineums do not generally develop stress incontinence. But those with less flexible perineums, who tend to need episiotomies to help deliver their babies, are candidates for this type of incontinence. Much also depends on how long a fetus's head rests against the bladder neck before the transition stage of labor begins. Of course the number of children borne is also a factor. Many women develop stress incontinence after a third or fourth baby is delivered.

Women with stress incontinence leak different amounts. In my mind, it doesn't matter how much you leak—I don't care whether you wear four maxipads or one minipad each day—at issue is the loss of bladder control. Some urologists will tell you that unless you soak eight pads a day, your problem is not serious enough to fix. I do not concur, because incontinence is treatable, and no one should have to put up with it unnecessarily.

Pity Great-Grandma, for this was not true for past generations and it is still not true for women in many developing countries. When a woman gives birth without medical assistance to a baby that is too large for her body, she may develop tears in her urethra that are called *fistulas*. Forceps deliveries can also traumatize urethral and rectal tissues. Women with fistulas leak urine continuously. The leak may be small or large. Some women must wear adult diapers to accommodate the problem.

There are, however, several surgical techniques available to close and repair fistulas. The tears are carefully layered and stitched in such a way that urine cannot find its way past the sutures.

In past generations, women had to live with fistulas. They devised many techniques for catching urine or for masking its odor. Their techniques became as secretive as the cause of their problem.

Kate's Story: Overflow Incontinence

Kate is a forty-one-year-old account executive at a leading advertising agency in New York. She has a mild case of diabetes that was diagnosed after her daughter was born seven years ago. Kate carefully watches her diet, exercises, and gives herself regular insulin injections. Her diabetes is under control.

But last year, Kate developed a vexing bladder problem. She sometimes found that when she got up from her chair, she had leaked. Other times, she had not. When she bent over to pull on her panty hose or tie her sneakers, she sometimes leaked. Other times bending over, she did not. Then there were times that she leaked while lying in bed, flat on her back. There was no warning. No sensation of "I have to go now." No pattern to predict when the leaking would occur.

Then, in one month, she developed two bacterial bladder infections, one right after the other. She went to her doctor and got a physical exam. Her insulin levels were correct and her blood sugar was in normal range. But to her great dismay, the surprise leaking continued. What could be causing it?

Kate suffers from what is called *overflow incontinence*. The name refers to the fact that her bladder muscle is not functioning properly. While it can happen to anyone, it often plagues diabetics or those with severe lower back problems.

Diabetics encounter two problems with their urinary tracts. One is that they lose sensory perception to many nerves, including the nerves that send signals to the bladder muscle. The bladder gets only weak signals that it is time to contract. The second problem is one of overdistension. Diabetics are constantly thirsty when their system is out of balance and they drink copius amounts of water. This causes the bladder muscle to distend and lose tone. Some diabetics' bladders hold twice the normal amount of urine—as much as 1,000 milliliters—because of this stretching.

Imagine Kate's bladder as a bucket that is filled to the top. Because she has lost sensory mechanisms, she can void only with a pressure that empties a quarter of her bladder each time she goes. Her bladder never empties completely and it does not take long for her bladder to overfill. Since she has lost the feeling to know when to void, Kate begins to leak. As her bladder never empties completely, she is susceptible to cystitis. If her blood sugar were not controlled, the resulting high sugar content of her urine would be especially conducive to bacterial growth.

Unlike Elizabeth, who only leaks when she sneezes, coughs, or is otherwise stressed, Kate leaks without any warning. She has a functional problem, not an anatomic problem. Her bladder neck is intact and all the angles of her urinary tract are correct. Thus surgery is the wrong way to correct Kate's problem.

Kate's problem is a weakened bladder and weakened "battery cables" (nerves to her bladder). The first step in treatment is to restore neural transmission through oral doses of synthetic acetylcholine called bethanechol chloride. This drug is a carbon copy of the body's natural chemical transmitter, acetylcholine. Flooding her "battery" (the bladder) with "battery acid" (the drug) strengthened the weak transmission of the charge from her nerves, and her bladder began to empty more efficiently.

In addition to keeping her diabetes under control, Kate put herself on a voiding schedule. At home she wore a small kitchen timer around her neck that rang every two hours. At work she was able to remind herself within other scheduling routines. With time, she regained some of her original bladder tone.

* * *

Overflow incontinence also affects people who do not have diabetes. A woman came to my office last year saying she had to wear nine or ten pads on the days she leaked most. Some days were better than others. Most of the time when she leaked, she did not have any warning. She also leaked when she coughed or sneezed.

I asked her about her back. She said she had some small discomfort. An X ray showed there was compression of her fourth and fifth lumbar vertebrae. Another X ray study, a voiding cystourethrogram, showed that her bladder neck had lost support. As with many incontinent people, there were multiple aspects to her problem.

I gave her bethanechol chloride to help correct the bladder muscle problem. By augmenting neural transmission to the detrusor, her overflow incontinence was brought under control.

To correct the bladder neck problem, we tried another medication called *ephedrine,* a decongestant that causes the bladder neck to close down.

This patient responded very well to "chemical surgery." She did not undergo corrective anatomic surgery because her problem could be controlled by medications alone. If we had corrected only her neural problems, she would have remained with stress incontinence. If we had surgically repaired her bladder neck, she would have been susceptible to repeated bladder infections because she would still have been unable to empty her bladder.

It is very important that your physician differentiate all the causes of cystitis and incontinence because several problems can occur simultaneously and therefore multiple treatments may be required. The urinary tract is composed of multiple units, and one or more parts can go awry.

Melissa's Story: Urge Incontinence

Melissa has a different kind of problem called *urge incontinence.* The first time she experienced it, she was at the movies. Halfway through an engrossing film, she realized she had to void. She made her way to the bathroom, only to find a line. The urge to go became greater and greater. Before she could get to a stall, the urine poured out of her and thoroughly wet her clothing.

People with urge incontinence experience strong bladder contractions at unexpected times. The bladder empties of its own accord. If you have a severe bladder infection, for example, you may experience tremendous urgency and spontaneous voiding, as the bladder tries to expel the infected urine. More commonly, the problem tends to be caused by damage to nerves in the upper back, above the fourth and fifth lumbar. Back injuries,

Voiding/X rays

This is a photograph of an X ray of the bladder and bladder neck of a patient with urinary stress incontinence. See the little beaking at the bottom. That's her open bladder neck. When she coughs or sneezes, I can observe the contrast media in the urine going through the bladder neck.

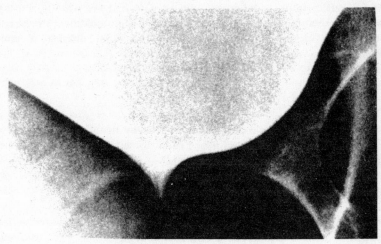

Figure 6-2, Stress Incontinence

strokes, and diseases such as multiple sclerosis can lead to such neural damage.

As a result, there is a lack of inhibitory fibers that release an enzyme that stops the activity of acetylcholine. Inhibitory signals are blocked and only activating signals get through to the bladder, telling it to contract. Then the urge to urinate is uncontrollable.

This type of incontinence is treated with medications that block acetylcholine transmissions. Probanthine (propantheline bromide) or oxybutynin chloride work by relaxing the bladder muscle in an attempt to keep it from responding to the excess signals to void. If a spine problem is involved, such as narrowing of the spinal column by arthritis, the drug Klonopin may be more helpful.

These are secondary management approaches that treat the symptoms rather than the cause of such incontinence. The cause, in many of these cases, may be a stroke or other brain damage that cannot be corrected. Many times injured backs and damaged disks cannot be repaired. Thus medications are often the best route to controlling such incontinence.

In Melissa's case, she was found to have "writer's neck" caused by vertebral instability that was putting pressure on her spinal column. Surgery relieved this compression and her voiding returned to normal.

Choosing the Right Treatment for Incontinence

If you suffer from incontinence, you need to find out what is causing the problem before you have any treatment. When incontinence has anatomic causes, surgery may be the answer. When it is caused by a functional problem, medication, prosthetics or even exercise may be the answer.

Surgical Procedures

There are many surgical procedures to prevent incontinence caused by anatomic problems. Like incontinence itself, these operations run a gamut from uncomplicated to very complicated.

COLLAGEN ANYONE?

For patients with mild stress incontinence, there is a simple technique that can be done in the doctor's office. It is about twenty years old and was first developed in Europe. When the procedure was first developed, they used a paste of teflon, the same material that lines nonstick cookware. It was injected directly into tissue to give it added volume. This technique has been used to thicken the vocal cords of people with paralyzed larynxes. Urologists used it to thicken the bladder neck in the same way.

However, a compound called collagen is now the preferred material for injection. The collagen treatment is not for everybody. It tends to work on women who have small cystoceles and mild stress incontinence, called Type 1. This is the woman who leaks with exercise but uses a mini panty liner or at most one sanitary pad in the course of the day. Women with large cystoceles cannot be helped this way because enough collagen cannot be packed into the tissue without the added weight of urine pulling open the bladder neck.

Before injecting the collagen, I anesthetize the urethra with a cotton-tipped swab soaked in a liquid anesthetic. I then place a longer swab with anesthetic up to the bladder neck. All the pain sensation nerves in the urethra, up to the bladder, are then paralyzed. If your doctor knows how to anesthetize the urethra (and unfortunately many do not!), you will feel no discomfort.

Although some patients would prefer to have "heavy drugs" or a general anesthetic, I find that local anesthesia produces more satisfactory results. When I was taught how to do this procedure in Europe fifteen years ago, it was always done under general anesthesia. But upon returning to the States and thinking it over, I decided to alter the procedure. When the patient is awake, she can cooperate. By coughing or sneezing, she can help me determine how much collagen is needed to close off her bladder neck and whether or not we have achieved total continence. I have given injections in this manner to more than twenty women and all are doing extremely well or better, I think, than if they had not been awake to help.

During the procedure, I pass a cystoscope through the urethra to view the bladder neck. Using a long special needle, I then inject collagen into the musculature of the bladder neck. The amount varies, depending on each woman's anatomy. The goal is to bring bladder neck tissue together in order to duplicate the normal anatomy of continence.

Once the collagen is injected, the patient never feels it.

Results using collagen instead of Teflon need to be evaluated over the long term. I personally believe that women with Type I incontinence would best be treated by vaginal exercises instead of office surgery. This is not a popular opinion, as everyone wants a "quick fix." But by selecting a candidate properly, excellent results can be obtained.

Judy, for example, was an excellent candidate for the surgical procedure. She was so happy after her surgery, in fact, that she appeared with me on the *Hour Magazine* television show to tell women all over the country about her experience. How did it change her life?

"It's been a year now and it's just remarkable," Judy told her interviewer. "To have gone from a constant awareness of the possibility of a problem—heavy sanitary pads, be sure to wear cotton clothing if you're going to be gone a long time, always the fear of odor, and so on—is just remarkable. Now I've thrown away all those heavy old things. No problem! Exercise is fine.

"There's no pain, no difficulty. When it's over, it's sort of like getting up from the table and throwing away your crutches. But I tossed away something else."

Now that aerobic exercise is popular, many women are finding that they leak when they run in place or do jumping jacks. Some trot off to the bathroom in the middle of the exercise routine while others wear pads. (Running and jumping do not *cause* incontinence. However, such exercise can unmask an anatomic problem that is already there.) The collagen treatment is well suited to such women, who tend to have a mild form of stress incontinence. But again be aware that there is the potential for an allergic reaction to collagen, so try Vaginetics first, or some of the other noninvasive techniques I will discuss at the end of this chapter.

A FACE-LIFT FOR THE BLADDER

When the bladder neck is wide open and the cystocele is what we would term moderate, the success rate for collagen surgery decreases markedly. If this is your problem, there are other approaches we can take. You may be a candidate for what amounts to a face-lift of the bladder.

The goal of this surgery, known as an *anterior repair,* is to tighten the vaginal tissue underneath the bladder. The surgeon, usually a gynecologist, cuts some vaginal tissue and pushes the cystocele back up. He or she then gathers the vaginal tissue, tucking in some of its wrinkles, and sews it up tightly. This gives more support to the bladder's base so that the bladder neck is often brought back into alignment.

The procedure is designed to correct cystoceles, not to correct major problems of the bladder neck. Patients with large cystoceles but minor bladder neck problems find great success with this surgical approach.

An advantage of this operation is that it leaves no readily visible scars because everything is done through the vagina. However, anterior repairs—like face-lifts—may need to be redone after several years.

Keep in mind that your problem may change with time. A cystocele may be controlled while a bladder neck problem worsens. Remember that each part of the urinary tract has many subunits that can fail. Different problems occur at different times.

HOW RECONSTRUCTION TECHNIQUES CAN BRING DRAMATIC IMPROVEMENT

For many people, bladder control is lost because supportive tissue that normally helps close down the bladder neck is out of alignment. With the system askew, there is no pressure available to help close the bladder neck.

The ultimate cause of this problem is gravity. As women age, there is loss of muscle tone in the bladder neck. Because of neurologic damage from pregnancy and childbirth, the bladder neck falls. The aqueduct opens. There is no resistance in the pipeline to keep the water back inside the dam. Urine flows like water through a pipe whose faucet is stuck open.

Women with this problem tend to have severe incontinence, requiring more than one or two pads a day to maintain dryness. It is for this kind of incontinence that urologists do reconstructive surgical procedures. The idea behind each technique is to create compression and resupport the bladder neck area. By altering pressure gradients, continence can be restored. Continence, if you recall from Chapter Five, occurs when pressure in the urethra is greater than pressure in the bladder.

An early technique, called the *Marshall-Marchetti-Krantz procedure,* was developed by three surgeons to correct incontinence in a man. It was found to work so well in women that it is used exclusively for stress incontinence (which men rarely have).

Unlike the anterior repair, this surgery requires an abdominal incision. The surgeon then sutures the tissue supporting the bladder neck and urethra to the pubic bone for support. This pulls the bladder neck forward, angling it much like a Chinese finger trap. When you cough or sneeze, the pressure flowing from your abdomen is directed into the pubic bone, not down the urethra. With this added support, you stay dry.

However, this procedure requires that you have a well-functioning bladder muscle. If the bladder neck is obstructed but the bladder muscle is not strong enough to empty the bladder, you could trade your incontinence for cystitis. Before undergoing this operation, *it is important to have a uroflow and cystometrogram done to document how well you void.* Patients have to realize that once continence is restored, they may have to fine tune or adjust the system back into balance, much as they do with the color on a television set.

This operation is a major form of surgery that must take place in a hospital. The stay is a week. The incision is usually made from below the belly button down to the pubic bone. It leaves a longitudinal scar.

As with any surgery, be sure that you choose a physician who is experienced with the procedures and knows when they are indicated and how to select patients for each approach. If you find someone who has performed this operation several times, your operation is likely to have fewer complications.

Another type of operation, with several variations, is done through the vagina. It is called a *Stamey urethropexy* or a *Pereyra procedure.* Unlike the Marshall-Marchetti-Krantz procedure, an incision is made in the vagina. Tissue on both sides of the bladder neck (called the *endopelvic fascia*) is then grasped and sutures are placed through it. Next, a tiny cut is made just above the pubic bone, alone the pubic hair line, and a special instrument is passed through the hole to pick up the sutured material down below the vagina. Like a crochet needle, the instrument pulls the sutures up to the abdominal wall. The sutures are cross-tied for support. You now have a suspension bridge mechanism for supporting the bladder neck.

During surgery, a tube is put through a hole in the lower abdomen in order to drain urine. In this way, a catheter between your legs is eliminated while swelling caused by the operation subsides. By turning the spigot knob on and off, voiding can be practiced and it is easy to tell how much urine is left behind. Once normal voiding resumes, the tube is removed.

This procedure requires only a one-day stay in the hospital and is very successful. I performed this surgery on one of my sisters, which shows what confidence my family has in me. Within a week she was back at work and she never lost a drop!

New Minimally Invasive Techniques

The changes in laparoscopic equipment I described in Chapter Two have had a significant impact on the surgical treatment of incontinence. Christopher Chapple, a urologist in England, developed the concept of using retropubic (behind the pubic bone) CO_2 to dissect the area around the urethra without having to enter the abdomen. After learning this technique, I found it to have several advantages over the vaginal needle procedures just mentioned.

The patient undergoes a general anesthetic and a tiny needle is inserted just behind the pubic bone. The gas is infused into the area, which separates the small blood vessels and nerves from the surrounding fat. This results in far less blood loss and minimal trauma to your tissue. The laparoscope, which has a magnifying system, is inserted and the sutures are placed under direct vision into the periurethral tissue, unlike the vaginal needle procedures, which are done blind. The patient can go home the same day and the catheter is removed from the urethra the next day.

Fibrin glue is also being considered for this surgery. Much like Super Glue for the body, fibrin can be injected through the laparoscope and the vaginal tissue is "sealed" around the urethra, much like you would glue two pieces of fabric together. Although still under investigation, I suspect that fibrin glue sutures will become commonplace in the near future. This glue is already used widely in Europe and Japan in order to control blood loss and seal leaks in the lung tissue. This procedure is not new. I used this same glue during my residency over fifteen years ago to remove multiple stones from the kidney. It is another example of my thinking on medical advances: Nothing is truly new!

Prostheses to Support the Bladder Neck

As you will recall, one of the most common causes for recurrent urinary tract infections in the sexually active female is the use of an overly large diaphragm. But could this knowledge be of benefit in treating incontinence?

Michelle's Story

Michelle had multiple sclerosis, or MS, a debilitating and destructive disease of the nervous system. Although she had courageously adjusted to the many handicaps of this disease, she just couldn't accept that she would be unable to attend the theater or play cards with friends because she couldn't recognize when her bladder was full. She came to me looking for an answer.

We discussed how agile she was with her hands and that we needed a device she could manipulate in and out of her vagina as needed. She began to laugh when I recommended that she try using the largest size diaphragm made to obstruct her bladder neck. "I thought I'd never have to use one of those things again!" However, it worked and she has been enjoying shopping and her new life, now that she has control back.

There are new prostheses currently under investigation that work on the same principle as the diaphragm. One such prosthesis is "fingers" made of silicone placed on either side of the urethra that exert pressure to close the bladder neck. As incontinence is a $10-billion-a-year health-care burden, more research dollars will be spent in the development of better temporary devices.

Nonsurgical Procedures: Medicine Only, Please

Many cases of incontinence are not caused by anatomic problems. If your problem is caused by functional or neurologic problems, you should never have surgery without first undergoing a complete urodynamic evaluation.

If lower back injury, diabetes, or any other disease is preventing chemical neurotransmitters from reaching your bladder, you may respond to medicines to correct the deficiency. I prefer to assess what can first be done functionally for a patient. I'm constantly surprised at how effective the right combination of medications and exercise can be in restoring continence.

Patients with overflow incontinence, caused by bladder muscle underactivity, may require 100 milligrams of bethanechol chloride a day. That's four 25-milligram pills a day. Someone with urge incontinence may require an antispasmodic medication such as Pro-Banthine at 15 milligrams four times a day.

The two most commonly prescribed drugs for incontinence are bethanechol chloride and Pro-Banthine. One stimulates smooth muscle to contract while the other inhibits it. As you might expect, these medications have opposite side effects.

Bethanechol chloride may cause blood pressure to increase a bit whereas Pro-Banthine may drop blood pressure. Bethanechol chloride may cause some people to sweat and it increases the heart rate. Pro-Banthine dries the mouth and slightly decreases the heart rate.

As with all medications, whether they are blockers or augmenters, you need to modify dosage as therapy progresses. I do this by monitoring the patient's condition with repeat uroflows. If I find that your bladder is generating too much of a contraction, causing you to void too often, the dose of a stimulating drug is too high. In contrast, the dose of an anti-spasmodic medication may be too high if you are having difficulty in voiding. We then adjust the dose accordingly, which allows you to void more normally.

There is another medication that was developed to treat bed-wetting in children, called desmopressin acetate (DDAVP). This nasal spray works by changing the signals in the hypothalamus that tell your kidneys how much water to clear, especially at night. I have used this spray in adults with nighttime urinary control problems. If you have this type of incontinence, ask your doctor for a trial prescription.

If you are postmenopausal, or in the perimenopausal phase, which can last for ten years, loss of estrogen could be responsible for your incontinence or urgency. Ask your doctor to check your estradiol level at mid-cycle, that is, halfway between the first day of your period and when you estimate your next period should begin. If your estradiol is less than 200, you are showing signs of changes in ovulation. A small application of vegetable-derived estrogen cream, such as Ogen, can be applied from Day Five through Day Twelve of your cycle. This will help raise your estrogen levels back to normal and your incontinence may resolve. For a more detailed discussion about hormones, please read the next chapter.

Some postmenopausal women are helped by combining estrogen therapy with a weak antidepressant, called imipramine (Tofranil). By taking only 10 milligrams of Tofranil at night along with one-quarter applicator of Ogen, 70 percent of women using this therapy reported improvement in their symptoms.

As you can see, there is no "one therapy treats all" approach that will work in dealing with incontinence. The medical treatment of incontinence requires understanding the needs of the person, not just treating the problem. My goal in treating incontinence and cystitis is to correct the root of the problem. If there is any way we can correct the primary cause, such as through exercises to strengthen back muscles, you will not need to use medications forever. By stabilizing the lower back and relieving pressure on the nerves to the bladder, many women can throw their medications away.

Learning to Adapt

Doris is seventy-two years old, and although she has had many experiences, last year was the most embarrassing time of her life. She has been incontinent for several years now, as the result of a lower back problem and the legacy of childbirth. And like many people her age, Doris is not a good candidate for surgery. She has had to learn to live with incontinence.

But last year took the cake. During her golden wedding anniversary, with all her friends around, she leaked. Every time she got up to dance, the urine spot on the back of her dress grew bigger and bigger. Everyone noticed, but she didn't discover the spot until later and she thought she would die of embarrassment.

When Doris came to me, she was in tears. Some days she was using only two pads, but on other days she needed six. She really didn't care how many pads she had to use. She just didn't want to leak all over her clothes, she wanted to diminish the odor, and she was tired of having her skin burned by urine.

A combination of techniques helps people like Doris. One was devised by another patient who solved part of the problem by designing a half-slip out of plastic that neatly covers the back of her dress or skirt. When she's out to dinner or playing cards with friends, she can laugh and have a good time without worrying that she'll wet the chair. Anyone can fashion such a half-slip, and I guarantee that it works!

To prevent the odors that build up when urine is concentrated, I recommended to Doris that she drink a lot of water. Although she continued to leak, and she had to use more pads, there was less ammonium in her diluted urine, so the odor did not cause further embarrassment.

Many incontinent people are always wet, and their skin becomes leathery from exposure to urine. Such tissue is easily cracked, causing it to bleed. When acid urine comes into contact with such wounds, the pain is indeed terrible. To protect her skin from being burned by urine, Doris began using a cream containing vitamins A and D. Like creams used to protect babies from diaper rash, it provides a molecularly balanced barrier against urine and works to heal ammonia burns.

Doris stopped by to see me several months after we first met. She showed me photographs of her two grandchildren and said that her life was much improved. Using these methods, she was now comfortable in social situations.

People are starting to demand that something be done about incontinence. Self-help organizations have evolved over the past ten years, forcing industry to pay attention to this devastating problem (for a list of these

Ten Warning Signs of Bladder Problems

- Leakage of urine that prevents desired activities.
- Leakage of urine that causes embarrassment.
- Leakage of urine that began or continued after an operative procedure (hysterectomy, cesarean section, lower intestinal or rectal surgery).
- Inability to urinate (retention of urine) following an operative procedure.
- Urinating more frequently than usual without a proven bladder infection.
- Needing to rush to the bathroom and/or losing urine if you do not arrive in time.
- Pain related to filling of the bladder and/or pain in relation to urination (in the absence of a bladder infection).
- Frequent bladder infections.
- Progressive weakness of the urinary stream with or without a feeling of incomplete bladder emptying.
- Abnormal urination or changes in urination related to a nervous system abnormality (stroke, spinal cord injury, multiple sclerosis, etc.).

Remember: Incontinence is not a disease. It is a symptom of an underlying condition.

organizations, see Appendix A). More women get information on new treatments for urine leakage from the news media than from their doctors! That situation is just another example of the problem with communication in medicine. But before progress can be made, both patients and doctors need to understand their obligations in the matter better. If you are ashamed to discuss the problem, no one will be able to help you. If a physician doesn't take your complaints seriously, or worse, doesn't want to listen when you want to discuss the topic, change doctors.

In many instances incontinence cannot be ''cured'' in the sense that the problem disappears forever. But incontinence can be well managed so that people may lead normal lives. This is certainly better than the alternative of being frightened and lonely, unable to be with friends.

As a urologist, I will do my best to bring the subject of incontinence into the arena of public debate and consciousness. It is a problem that has been overlooked and ignored far too long.

SEVEN

How Menopause and Aging Affect Your Urologic Health

IN the Cameroon highlands of West Africa, there lives a sixty-two-year-old grandmother named Mami Estah, whose attitude toward life is most instructive. Until she was fifty, Mami Estah's primary role in life was that of wife and mother. She raised eight children, cooked, tended her farm, and sold extra crops in the market. Her life was dominated by duties and routines.

But when Mami Estah entered menopause, everything changed. She was liberated. She left her husband, bought two cases of beer, and opened a bar. She rented out a back room. As the bar became successful, Mami Estah entered local politics. She became the eyes and ears for friends in the capital and grew so powerful that the prime minister paid her many visits. As was the custom for women of her status, Mami Estah took "wives" to grow her food, cook, and clean for her. The wives took male lovers but the children were "fathered" by Mami Estah. Eventually she ran for office and became powerful in her political party.

In Mami Estah's culture, premenopausal women have very defined roles and little opportunity to move outside prescribed tasks. But once a woman enters menopause, the restrictions are lifted. She is free to operate in society much as a man. With her childbearing years behind her, she can do whatever she pleases.

Somehow, in our supposedly more advanced culture, American women tend to fear that life is finished after the children are gone. The empty nest syndrome strikes. Menopause is not a time of celebration and liberation. It is not perceived as a life passage that brings opportunity and challenge. Instead, many American women become fearful and mournful upon entering menopause. Many fail to plan for this period of their lives and fail to take up new challenges. Mami Estah would certainly pity them.

What is it about menopause that frightens so many of us? The word itself comes from Greek and means "ending of the monthly." Around the age of forty-five or fifty, regular menstrual cycles become increasingly irregular and then stop. Before menopause, we ovulate and are capable of having children. After menopause, we stop ovulating and can no longer have children.

The most significant medical consequence of menopause is loss of estrogen, which can drop by 75 percent. As I have noted, estrogen is related to maturity of the secretions that protect the urinary tract. When, in menopause, estrogen levels decline, the bladder lining and vaginal tissues become more prone to bacterial adherence. The vagina is less elastic. During intercourse, tissue may be abraded. The vagina may contract, actually shrink in size.

While this may sound frightening, you do not need to worry. Our sex lives do not come to an abrupt end at menopause. There are currently more than 30 million postmenopausal women in the United States. Each woman can expect to live about a third of her life, and a full and vibrant third, after menopause.

Nevertheless, modern medicine still has much to learn about the natural biologic transition of menopause. Scientifically speaking, it is a phenomenon full of mysteries. Neither the male nor the female reproductive tract is fully understood. Research about both sexes is active.

The study of the male urogenital tract falls to urologists. That is, we study and treat a man for problems of his reproductive system as well as his urinary tract. But, as far as the medical profession is concerned, women require two kinds of specialists. Gynecologists study and treat problems of the female reproductive system. Many of them also practice obstetrics, which involves the special needs of pregnancy and childbirth. Urologists, however, treat the woman's urinary tract only; her reproductive system is someone else's business. There is no textbook for urologists on menopause, let alone a chapter on the subject in any urology book. The only material I could find was a chapter in a gynecologist's textbook on obstetrics!

Because pregnancy and childbirth are complex, it is easy to understand why specialties arose to handle those processes. But, in contrast to the treatment of the genitourinary system in males, there *is* an overlap between specialties in handling the female urogenital system; urologic and gynecologic problems are not mutually exclusive.

Menopause is primarily a gynecologic event. Yet you would be surprised how many women come to urologists with problems that can be traced to their menopause. Menopause most definitely has urologic implications. On the other hand, many women go to a gynecologist for basic urologic problems, such as incontinence. The point is that your reproductive tract and urinary tract can affect one another. This seems especially true in menopause.

What Happens When Estrogen Levels Drop

Your vagina has a layer of protective coating, the layer that keeps bacteria from adhering to its surface. The coating is dependent on hormones. When you lose estrogen, the coating decreases. You can develop vaginitis (inflammation of the vagina), yeast infections, or vaginal bacterial infections. You may feel itching or experience urinary frequency.

Such symptoms are sometimes treated with antibiotics. *But this may only worsen the problem.* The vagina possesses a delicate balance of what you might think of as "friendly bacteria." One, called lactobacillus, is known to help prevent harmful bacteria from adhering to tissue. Antibiotics can wipe out the defensive lactobacilli along with any "unfriendly bacteria" that may have caused your infection. In any case, after taking an antibiotic, you need to restore lactobacillus balance as soon as possible.

There are several ways to do this. One is the old home remedy of douching with yogurt. It works because yogurt contains lactobacillus, the same bacteria you need in your vagina. If you find this too messy, you can douche with a special acidophilus-lactobacillus preparation that is sold in health-food stores. It does not help, however, to take lactobacillus orally, in products such as acidophilus or raw milk. The human gut digests or destroys these helpful bacteria (which are good for you), but none make it to your vagina through this route. You must add the lactobacilli externally to help your vagina. It works only temporarily and does not restore the lactobacillus to the tissue permanently.

In general, douching is not a good practice. Some women are told to douche to prevent the vaginal odor that sometimes accompanies menopause. But regular douching can dry vaginal tissue, giving bacteria a better surface on which to adhere. Constant douching can even lead to cystitis when vaginal bacteria make their way into the bladder.

Nowadays most gynecologists recommend estrogen replacement therapy to healthy women entering menopause. Since menopause is a gradual process, changes of vaginal tissue can also be gradual. Thus you may start out replacement therapy with an estrogen cream applied directly to the vagina. Later, when estrogen levels have fallen more, you may need oral doses of estrogen. Two hormones, estrogen and progesterone, are often given together.

Estrogen or Estrogen and Progesterone?

Many women are confused about the pros and cons of estrogen therapy versus estrogen/progesterone therapy. And no wonder. Studies show there are dramatic trade-offs. It is a confusing picture.

For example, a highly respected long-term study found that women who took estrogen may have a lower incidence of heart disease than women who took no hormones. Estrogen appears to raise what is termed your body's good cholesterol, which is a factor in preventing heart disease; the implication is that estrogen replacement is good for your heart. Another study showed that estrogen helped prevent osteoporosis, which means it is good for your bones. Indeed, the relationship between osteoporosis and estrogen deficiency has been known for almost half a century.

But other studies have shown that estrogen replacement therapy increases your risk of developing cancer of the uterine lining, called the *endometrium;* the implication is that estrogen replacement is bad for your uterus. Indeed, if you have ever had cancer of the breast or uterus, your physician will most likely not prescribe hormone replacement therapy, but even that practice is changing, as you will read below.

But for healthy women it is a different story. To counteract the risk of endometrial cancer, about ten years ago many physicians began prescribing progestins along with estrogen. The logic? Since estrogen causes tissue maturation, it builds up the endometrial lining. Progestins have the opposite effect, causing loss of maturation and breaking down the lining. In other words, progestins breaks down what estrogen builds up. On the double hormone therapy, you resume menstruation and have regular periods.

The medical profession is divided on the question of hormone replacement therapy. Although evidence strongly suggests that estrogen users are at increased risk for endometrial or breast cancer, the magnitude of that risk is quite low if certain precautions are taken. Endometrial cancer is a rare disease. Estrogen users have the same risk of getting it as do nonestrogen users who are obese. Furthermore, endometrial cancer is a slow-growing cancer with minimal invasion into the uterus. It is usually diagnosed early and survival rates for women with the disease are high. In fact, overall, estrogen-associated cancers do not appear to cause a decrease in life expectancy.

The question remains: Will the double hormone therapy be good for both your heart and your uterus? The answer is not yet clear. People have not been taking the estrogen/progestin combination long enough for researchers to find the answer. Despite the lack of answers, it is popular today to take progestins with estrogen to decrease the risk of endometrial cancer.

I consider the double therapy comparable in terms of risk to taking oral contraceptives. Progestins may, in fact, negate the beneficial effects of estrogen and result in a higher health risk (for heart disease, osteoporosis, and strokes) than taking no hormonal therapy at all. It is known that progestins can actually raise triglycerides, increasing your risk of heart disease. Furthermore, progestins may increase your resistance to insulin and cause you to crave carbohydrates, which can lead to excess body fat. Progestins also modify the turnover of the biogenic amines, tryptophan, tyrosine, tyramine, and phenylalanine, altering sympathetic nerve responses. In patients with interstitial cystitis, amine turnover is already a problem responsible for many episodes of sudden bladder pain.

The same is not true of progesterone, a natural hormone. Progesterone is produced in large quantities in the eggs you ovulate when you are still menstruating. However, it is also produced by the adrenal glands. Progesterone causes smooth muscle to relax, increases body temperature, and decreases blood pressure. It is also important in the production of *myelin,* the fatty insulation surrounding nerves.

Hormone Therapy and Urinary Problems

If, like Meryls, you have chronic bladder disease, there is no question that progestins can be harmful. Meryls is a patient of mine who was treated for interstitial cystitis and remained symptom-free for one year. "I was doing great when *bam!* I ran right into menopause!" Her gynecologist ordered her "the usual"—oral estrogen followed by ten days of progestin therapy. Her life quickly changed for the worse. Whenever she took the progestin, Meryls developed cramps, bleeding, and migraine headaches. Her bladder hurt and her urinary pH shot up.

She came to me for help with her bladder. It was clear that the estrogen was increasing cellular maturation in her bladder and helping form the protective layer on the bladder surface, because she had no symptoms when she was taking estrogen *only.* But a commonly prescribed progestin, Provera, was making her bladder tissue more "leaky" by increasing the amount of harmful byproducts in her urine produced by abnormal metabolism of the biogenic amines (more on this in Chapter Eleven). Meryls's bladder was abnormal and it could not tolerate the double hormonal therapy.

Unfortunately, Meryls's doctor refused to give her estrogen. She said

Meryls had to be cycled monthly on the progestin regardless of her bladder problem, explaining, "If I give you estrogen only you'll get breast cancer, and you don't want *that!*" The doctor also refused to acknowledge that the migraine headaches were associated with progestins (although such a link has been made in several studies).

Fear of Cancer

Unfortunately, many doctors try to intimidate women by using the threat of cancer to get them to follow their proposed course of treatment. However, the fear of cancer has been greatly exaggerated in our culture. According to a study done by Karen Steinberg, a molecular biologist at the Centers for Disease Control and Prevention, women who took estrogen alone for fifteen years had a 30 percent increase in the risk of breast cancer. This risk was tripled for women who had a family history of the disease. But let's put this into perspective. Instead of the average woman's 10 percent chance of developing breast cancer sometime in her life, the risk of a woman on estrogen for fifteen years might bump up to 13 percent. *And any woman who took the drug for less than five years had no increased risk at all!* Malcolm Pike, an epidemiologist at the University of Southern California argues that for each additional breast cancer death caused by hormones, eight deaths from heart disease could be prevented!

The argument goes even further for women who are breast cancer survivors. In an editorial in the *International Urogynecology Journal* in 1995, Dr. P. J. DiSaia, from the University of California at Irvine, demonstrated that estrogen therapy given to seventy-seven breast cancer survivors failed to "fuel the fire" of recurrent disease. He reiterated my feelings that a "sea of emotion" exists when dealing with cancer. "Every urogynecologist understands the benefits of local and systemic therapy to women who suffer from urinary incontinence. Women deserve a comprehensive explanation of the positive effects of hormone replacement therapy. Because freedom from recurrent breast cancer can never be guaranteed, some women will develop recurrences coincident with any new hormone exposure; patients must understand this possibility. Patient and physician education will be necessary to change these patterns. The patient must understand that everything we do in medical practice involves a risk/benefit analysis. However, she must be properly informed so that she can make her own decisions regarding this important therapeutic tool."

Meryls conferred with an endocrinologist (an expert on hormones) and was given different options. She could take estrogen only, which was good for her vagina and bladder, and if she should develop abnormal bleeding, an endometrial biopsy could easily be performed in the office. She would undergo mammography every two years to be certain there were no changes that could indicate a developing tumor. Another option was to use the progestin for only five days three times a year. In this way, the potentially thickened lining of the uterus would be shed, and her risk of endometrial cancer would be reduced to normal. A third option was to try natural estrogen and progesterone therapy in addition to diet, nutritional supplements, and exercise.

Meryls chose the second option and found a new gynecologist who would follow her closely. She tallied all the risks and actively took responsibility for her health.

In general, women with chronic bladder problems or interstitial cystitis should think twice before taking progestins. Consult with your gynecologist and ask for help in working around all your health problems when choosing any hormone replacement therapy.

In general, any therapeutic decision you make should be agreed upon by you and your doctor. You assess the risks and then work with your physician to minimize them through a health management program. Your preferences count. You may have to shop around to find a doctor who will join you as a partner in your health care, as opposed to the type of physician who says, "Do as I tell you and don't ask why." But the search is worthwhile, and the doctors-as-partners are out there if you look.

Urethral Dilations in Menopause Can Be Harmful

During menopause, many women develop bladder infections for the first time. When they go to the urologist they are told they have a stricture that must be dilated. In this procedure, the urologist inserts gradually larger rods into the urethra and stretches, or dilates, it open. The idea is that you have an obstruction in your urethra that has to be broken open. When urine flows freely, the theory goes, your bladder infections will stop.

As discussed in other chapters, urethral dilations are rarely called for. The procedure is generally useless and painful, and in menopausal women, it can create incontinence.

There is, however, a historical basis for why urologists would believe a postmenopausal woman needs urethral dilations. With the loss of estrogen, a small ring of fibrotic tissue can form in the opening of the urethra. A generation ago, when estrogen replacement therapy was not widely available, some older women would develop this band. It probably was not a prevalent cause of bladder infections.

Nowadays I rarely find this fibrotic ring in older women. Estrogen replacement therapy is prevalent and we just don't see it. But the practice of dilating postmenopausal women has endured. A patient recently said that a urologist told her, "My God, woman! You have the urethra of a three-year-old child!" The patient said she certainly was puzzled by this. How come her urethra had found the Fountain of Youth while the rest of her still looked over sixty-five? In my experience, older women are much less likely to buy this story than are younger women. After all, wouldn't you be skeptical upon learning that you've lived fifty years with a child's urethra and never noticed it before?

If you develop bladder infections at this point in life, assess the situation carefully. Your urethra is probably not guilty. More likely at your age are other problems such as osteoporosis or lumbar strain and lower back problems that prevent your bladder from emptying efficiently. As discussed in Chapter One, back trouble is a prime source of bladder trouble.

If you are dilated, you could temporarily find yourself leaking afterward. As we get older, our bladder necks open up a bit, but the external sphincter comes to the rescue and keeps urine from leaking out. A urethral dilation can paralyze the external sphincter and leave you incontinent for a few days. The leakage goes away but your bladder infections could easily continue.

ANNA MARIA

When Anna Maria went in for her annual gynecologic checkup, she got a terrible fright. Microscopic amounts of blood were found in her urine. At age forty-nine, she was experiencing hot flashes and had planned to discuss that problem with her doctor. Instead, she heard a whole discourse on what it can mean when blood is found in urine. The worst case was cancer.

In not the best of spirits, Anna Maria came to me for a urologic examination. While it is true that blood in the urine is one warning sign of cancer, other things can cause this symptom.

I asked her if she ever noticed blood in her underpants.

"Why, yes," she answered. "When I wipe myself, I sometimes see small amounts of blood on the tissue. It hurts to wipe. Sometimes I just dab the outside."

"Do you feel a little burning sensation after you urinate?"

Surprised, she said, "Yes, it does burn. It feels better if I apply a little pressure to the spot that hurts."

"Have you ever seen any blood in your urine?"

Anna Maria was firm. "Absolutely never. And my gynecologist told me the lab test showed very few blood cells. But she said I should have you check me out anyway."

"Do you smoke?"

No, she had never smoked. Nor had she ever worked around known carcinogens that have been associated with bladder cancer.

On the examining table, I took a close look at Anna Maria's urethra. The cause of her problem was immediately evident.

Like the vagina, the urethra has its own protective layer. When children get what is called bubble bath syndrome, the chemicals in the product inactivate this bacteria-resistant layer. Loss of estrogen can also result in degeneration or loss of this layer, leading to what is called a *caruncle.*

A caruncle is a little growth of tissue stemming from an inflammation at the opening of the urethra. Like a little red tongue, it is an outgrowth of irritated tissue.

I had Anna Maria sit up and look at her urethra with the help of a mirror. Although her caruncle was small, she could see it sticking up like a little flame. It was the source of the minute amount of blood in her urine and the light staining in her underwear. It was the source of the burning sensation she felt when she urinated. "The burning is on the outside," she said, "but I never thought to look for anything with a mirror."

A caruncle is a hallmark of estrogen deficiency in women. But what nature takes away, medicine can sometimes give back. Anna Maria put a dab of estrogen cream on her finger and rubbed it into the caruncle. This was like giving her urethra an artificial protective layer. After several weeks of treatment, the caruncle shrank. Sensitive urethral tissue no longer interacted with the environment. Potential causes of inflammation, such as bacteria from the vagina, would not take hold at the opening of the urethra.

Sometimes caruncles grow too large to be treated with estrogen cream. In that case, the tissue around it can be anesthetized locally in the doctor's office. The caruncle is then snipped off.

Blood in urine is a relative finding. In my opinion, if there are twenty to forty red blood cells in a urine sample looked at under the microscope, full diagnostic tests would be wise. But if there are only two to three red blood cells seen in a typical assay, something less serious may be the cause. The loss of estrogen can, for example, thin the walls of the urethra itself. During and after menopause, the urethra is more fragile and subject to having tiny capillaries burst. These are temporary but may lead to a finding of blood in the urine.

One urinalysis should probably not be the criterion for alarm, especially if the patient has never seen blood in her urine. But if the finding is repeatable and in larger concentrations, the possibilities of more serious diseases should be evaluated.

BETTY

Betty came to see me with a common complaint of early menopause. She felt the need to urinate frequently. Where before she could drink lots of fluid and wait hours before voiding—''I've always been a real camel,'' she said—she now found herself wanting to run to the toilet every half hour. She could repress this urge if she just told herself it was a false signal. But if she gave in, only a little urine came out. It began, she said, ''to drive me crazy.''

On standard tests, Betty's bladder looked great. Her bladder pressure and flow rates were normal. She could indeed move dirt across the sidewalk. Her back was not troubling her and there were no caruncles. She looked normal.

But her problem could be traced back to that loss of estrogen that accompanies menopause. There are estrogen receptors in the trigone, the triangular area in the base of the bladder. The trigone (fully described in Chapter Five) arises from different embryologic tissue than the rest of the bladder and strongly responds to estrogen. The tissue has what are called *receptor sites,* which are like keyholes to molecules of hormone. When an estrogen molecule encounters a receptor, it locks on. The estrogen then helps maintain a protective GAG layer on the trigone.

As your bladder fills, the trigone is shielded from urine by this protective layer. But when the bladder is half full, tiny molecules in urine stimulate sensory nerves in the trigone that it is time to void.

But when you lose estrogen, the GAG layer thins and it takes only a small amount of urine to defeat the barrier. The result is urinary frequency, as Betty was experiencing.

''You know,'' she said, ''I wet my bed when I was a kid and I had to go to the bathroom all the time. I felt like this back then.'' Betty had reverted to what I call the teeny-weeny bladder club.

Many women with urinary frequency have insufficient protective lining in their trigones. This can be caused by different factors but the result is almost always frequency.

The solution to Betty's problem was straightforward. When she went on oral estrogen replacement therapy, her symptoms disappeared. The estrogen induced her protective GAG layer to thicken and restore normal bladder function. As Meryls did, she decided to avoid progestins because they upset what estrogen builds back up in the bladder.

Many women past menopause also have a problem with their thyroid hormone. I believe this is an issue that is not carefully evaluated by many gynecologists. Thyroid hormone is important for cellular maturation and may be linked, in a complicated interaction, with estrogen and other sex hormones. It exerts very real effects on bladder tissue. I find many patients' symptoms of urinary frequency disappear when they take medication to put their thyroids back into normal range.

DENA

Loss of estrogen can lead to bladder infections along circuitous pathways. One of my favorite examples of this is Dena. She was a tornado of a woman who bore and raised thirteen children. Dena never sat still. She talked fast. And, as you might expect, she voided fast.

By her own account, Dena sat on the toilet as little as possible. After urinating, she'd dash to her feet and be off to do something more important.

But then Dena developed what some physicians call menopausal cystitis. She had never had a problem with her urinary tract in her life. Then, boom! menopause changed all that.

Actually, Dena had symptoms of bladder trouble all her life. But she could usually stave off infections by forcing herself to drink quarts of liquids and urinating often. She only used antibiotics when desperate. Moreover, Dena voided with a hard, fast stream thanks to her powerful abdominal muscles. She had used these muscles all her life to help her urinate. And like most women who bear several (in this case thirteen!) children, Dena had a cystocele, a protrusion or hernia of her bladder wall that held a small amount of urine. Like most cystoceles, Dena's never gave her any trouble, thanks to her strong bladder neck, and she never knew it was there.

Then three things combined to do in Dena's urinary health. First was loss of estrogen, which caused her vagina to lose its tone or elasticity. Then, more than a weak bladder, she really had a weak vagina.

Second, as she grew older, the supporting ligaments that held Dena's bladder in position began to lose tone. Both her bladder and her cystocele gradually fell. The cystocele began to sag into her vagina. Her bladder changed shape as its angle of suspension altered.

Third, Dena's bladder never worked right in the first place. She had compression in her lower spine that affected the flow of neurotransmitters to her bladder. But Dena had never had a problem because of her sensational abdominal muscles. These, in effect, made up for her poor bladder function. But when the bladder fell, the abdominal muscles could only push in one direction. They could no longer force her bladder to empty.

Now she was set up for infections. Because she never sat on the toilet long enough to let her cystocele drain, residual urine was left in her bladder. Her bladder did not work properly. Dena got recurrent urinary tract infections.

She responded to bethanechol chloride, a drug that enabled her bladder to contract fully. And she learned to sit on the toilet for an extra thirty seconds or so. If you have a cystocele, you will notice there is a little spurt of urine that comes out after you finish voiding. As the bladder empties, it pulls the cystocele up last, and flattens it. The urine in the cystocele is the last urine out. By squeezing your pelvic floor, you can pull up the bladder muscles and hasten the cystocele to empty.

DOROTHY

As we have seen, loss of estrogen affects the vagina, urethra, and bladder. It also affects bone, which is actually an organ of the body.

Dorothy was in her early seventies when she came to see me. She was spry with a jolly outlook on life. But she did have a problem. For seven years, Dorothy had been combating recurrent urinary tract infections. They came with unsettling regularity. She said she felt as if she were the backbone of the antibiotic industry.

Dorothy's gynecologist held to the school of thought that cystitis is "no big deal," Dorothy explained. "He told me not to worry about it. He said the infections are caused by my thin bladder. Is there such a thing?"

She was worried that bacteria from her bowel could pass through this alleged thin wall and cause her a lot of grief. I assured her that thin bladders are not a cause of cystitis. Her uroflow was abnormal and led clearly to a diagnosis: Her infections could be traced to a lower back problem. "I've always had twinges of discomfort in my back," Dorothy said. "But I ignore it. I'm not a complainer."

Many women suffer silently as Dorothy did. But menopause is a time to speak out about back discomfort. Younger women can experience temporary injury to vertebrae and nerves traveling the spine. Older women can develop osteoporosis, a permanent anatomic change. Between 15 and 20 million American women have this problem, which tends to accelerate around the time of menopause. It is three times more common in women than in men.

Osteoporosis means "porous bone" and is not a single disease but likely the end result of many disorders. If you think of normal bone to be like Swiss cheese, a bone with osteoporosis has bigger and bigger holes. Such bones grow fragile and eventually collapse. The disks may also degenerate and dry out, compressing nerves in the spine. Osteoporosis is brought on by a chronic gross deficiency of calcium. Because many older people are sedentary, they cut back on total food intake. Unfortunately, they also cut back on vitamins and minerals.

Calcium is an element that is stored in bone. Our bodies use it for a host of basic cellular functions. Whenever the body needs more calcium, it is withdrawn from bone tissue. If for any reason you do not get enough calcium or calcium absorption is impaired or the borrowing goes on too long, the bones lose out. The body keeps withdrawing calcium, which it must have to live, and the bones degenerate.

Everyone begins to lose bone by the age of thirty-five—some say as early as fourteen—but it is gradual. Then at menopause and for about eight years after menopause, bone loss can be very rapid. Some women lose up to 10 percent a year of the bone in the spine. Then the loss resumes its gradual pace.

Osteoporosis is associated with increased fractures of the hip, back, and other bones. White women who undergo premature menopause with hysterectomies and thin women seem to be at highest risk for such fractures. A woman entering menopause has about a 15 percent chance of sustaining a hip fracture in her remaining lifetime. About 40 percent of postmenopausal women who fracture a hip do not return home from the hospital, either dying or remaining in long-term care facilities.

As the holes in bone keep getting bigger, the spaces between the vertebrae collapse. The vertebrae are pressed against each other. Such changes in the spine affect urinary voiding. Thus menopausal women with urinary problems need to have the health of their backs evaluated.

What happens to the bladder when the vertebrae collapse depends on whether the problem is in the upper back or the lower back. When it happens in the upper back (a condition known as ''dowager's hump'') (see Figure 7-1), nerves that travel to the bladder are squeezed. The bladder does not get the message to inhibit voiding and the bladder contracts on its own. The primary symptoms are urinary frequency and urgency. As noted earlier, frequency can be brought on through changes in estrogen receptors to the trigone. But osteoporosis of the upper back is another cause.

The lower back presents a different story. When vertebral disks lower down are compressed, the bladder can be completely knocked out of action. Nerves are squeezed and the bladder does not get the message to contract. Urine stays overlong in the bladder and, like a stagnant pool, invites organisms to thrive. The primary symptom is chronic urinary tract infection. Overflow incontinence can also develop.

With osteoporosis these changes are permanent. No amount of exercise or yoga classes will rectify the problem and estrogen therapy will not replace bone mass. However, there is a new nasal spray, calcitonin-salmon

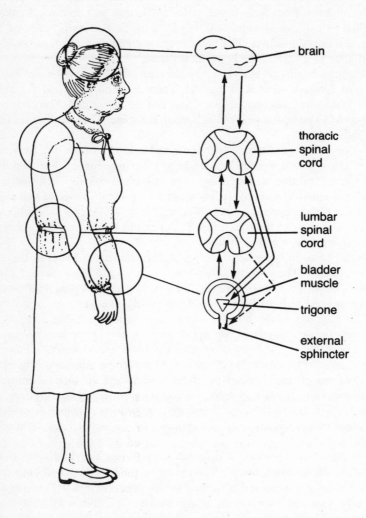

Figure 7-1, Areas of the Body That Can Cause Urinary Problems

---

Foods Containing Natural Estrogens

A number of different foods are sources of natural plant estrogens. The following is a list of the food sources highest in estrogen. These foods are also high in vitamins, minerals, fiber, and essential fatty acids, and they are low in saturated fat.

alfalfa	fennel	red beans*
anise seed	flaxseeds	red clover
apples*	garlic	rhubarb*
baker's yeast*	green beans	rice
barley	green squash	rye*
beets	hops*	sage
cabbage	licorice	sesame seeds
carrots	oats	soybean sprouts
cherries*	olive oil	soybeans
chick-peas	olives	split peas
clover	papaya*	squash
corn	parsley	sunflower seeds
corn oil	peas	wheat
cowpeas (black-eyed peas)	plums*	yams
	potatoes	
cucumbers	pumpkin	

Foods with an (*) should be avoided by women with interstitial cystitis.

(Miacalcin) which can halt further progression of bone loss and even increase bone mass in some instances. This therapy is especially indicated for women who chose not to take estrogen or cannot tolerate it. Dorothy began this therapy and was also greatly helped by bethanechol chloride, which helped her bladder contract, and the infections cleared up. She also took calcium supplements and learned to eat foods high in calcium, such as leafy dark green vegetables, yogurt, and cheese. For a list of foods containing natural estrogen, please see above.

Degenerative arthritis and cracked vertebrae (spondylolisthesis) can also lead to recurrent urinary tract infections. Another woman in her seventies, Hattie, told me proudly that she could hold urine longer than any of her friends. But she developed cystitis precisely because her bladder was not emptying completely. Her uroflow showed abdominal straining and her cystometrogram showed poor voiding pressures. Her problem was traced to degenerative arthritis of the lower spine, a common site of arthritis.

RUTH

The bladder is one of the most sensitive indicators of neurologic health. In postmenopausal women, it can forewarn of strokes and other damage to the brain and nervous system.

Ruth was the first person who demonstrated this to me. She was in her seventies and healthy, when all of a sudden she became incontinent. She would feel a cramping sensation and urinate uncontrollably. Oddly, whenever she put her hand in cold water, she urinated. This was very inconvenient for washing dishes and doing other household chores.

Ruth's internist, however, could find nothing wrong. Her blood pressure was a little high but not worrisome. The urologic workup in my office, however, showed that her bladder was experiencing uninhibited contractions. It was "firing" all on its own. She urinated when she put her hand in cold water because she was stimulating a well-known but not at all understood feedback mechanism in her nervous system. Nothing was wrong with her back and it was hard to know how to help her. Two months later she had a major stroke.

Ruth was proof that the bladder is one of the most sensitive indicators of neurologic problems. Before her stroke, numerous brain cells had begun to be cut off from oxygen and ceased to function. Some of these nerve cells were involved with her bladder function. As the cells slowly died, her bladder was gradually affected. Finally, the stroke became acute and Ruth went into urinary retention. That is, her bladder ceased working entirely.

Fortunately, Ruth recovered. She went through a physical therapy program and regained control over her bladder.

Since Ruth came to me I have seen several patients, both male and female, with similar symptoms. They are older and previously healthy with bladders that overreact for no discernible reason. Within a few months, they have strokes. I am now convinced that this pattern of urologic findings can predict strokes in some individuals.

In such cases, patients might want to take a baby aspirin every day. This helps prevent blood platelets from clumping together and may ward off a stroke. If you believe you may be at risk, you should discuss with your physician current thoughts on stroke management and prevention.

ELLA

Ella was another patient who really stumped me for a time. She was fifty-two, had just gone through menopause, and was not taking estrogen replacement therapy. Although she had had uterine cancer and undergone a hysterectomy, she looked fabulous. "Except for these bladder infections," she said, "I feel better than I ever have."

Ella had no history of bladder infections before menopause. Her uroflow and cystometrogram were normal. Her bladder generated adequate pressures. She had no problems with her back and her urethra looked fine.

Why did she get infections? The only clue was that the infections were related to intercourse. They happened after she and her husband made love.

Ella reaffirmed for me the value of being a woman physician. I have found that women are comfortable confiding in other women. After much discussion, Ella said she was worried about not having enough lubricant in her vagina. "I know women my age dry out and I don't want that to happen. I read in a woman's magazine that one way to avoid infection is to be well lubricatred," she said. Ella then described the lubricant she put on her husband's penis before lovemaking. Ella was following that uncommendable concept, "If a little is good, a lot is better." She frosted his penis with the goo.

The jelly was indirectly responsible for her infections. During intercourse, bacteria adhered to the lubricant that then would be deposited in her urethra. As it stuck to her tissues, bacteria had a chance to collect, grow, and travel to her bladder.

To eliminate infections, Ella learned to use the lubricant appropriately. She put a dab at the vagina's posterior forchette (see Figure 1-7, p. 34) where it would do the most good. This curve at the bottom of the vagina is where most trauma occurs. Here the vagina is vulnerable to tears if the angle of penetration is too high. But if the forchette is lubricated, the vagina is protected.

A word here, too, about sexual positions during menopause. At this time, your urethra is more vulnerable than ever to improper technique. The urethra lacks protective layers and can be traumatized by high angles of penetration. It is not as resilient as it was when you were younger.

Fortunately, there are many positions other than the missionary approach (male on top) that will not hurt your urethra. When the man enters from the side, the angle of penetration is ideally aligned to the vaginal opening. You can sit on top of him or have him enter from behind as you rest on your hands and knees. Anything that keeps the angle of penetration from stressing your vagina and urethra is fine.

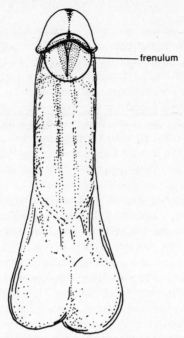

Figure 7-2, The Main Sensory Area of the Penis

It may help you to know how a man is stimulated, so that you can experiment with his anatomy and yours. The main sensory area on his penis is the *frenulum,* a little skin bridge between the head of the penis and the shaft below (see illustration above). It is this part of his penis that needs to be stimulated for him to achieve orgasm. The shaft of his penis is not his erogenous zone. The frenulum can be stimulated without a lot of up and down pumping action. Moreover, the penis does not have to be fully inserted and thrusted for him to feel pleasure. If you hold his penis just partway in your vagina with your pelvic floor muscles, even a slight rocking motion will feel good to you both.

FLORENCE

While loss of estrogen is a major factor in the urinary troubles encountered in menopause, it is not the only problem. The incidence of incontinence rises with age. It is fair to say that women after menopause are leakier than women before menopause. Of course menopause does not *cause* incontinence. But the factors that lead to incontinence are more prevalent the older we get. (See Chapter Six for a detailed discussion of urinary incontinence.)

Around menopause, the overlap of gynecologic and urologic problems seems to increase. My advice is to choose your specialists carefully. Just as you would not want a urologist to deliver your baby or insert an IUD, you may not want a gynecologist to treat your urinary problem with gynecologic procedures.

Florence's story illustrates this point well. She is a fifty-five-year-old grandmother who took up jogging shortly before her fiftieth birthday. "I finally succumbed," she said. "My husband is a runner and now I'm as addicted as he is. I may be slow but I'm steady. I probably do ten to fifteen miles a week and I love it."

Florence is not alone. My first office looked out on a road in west Los Angeles that is still famous for its jogging path. Hundreds of runners went by all day long. Many, I noticed, were women Florence's age.

Two years ago Florence noticed that she was leaking urine while running. The problem had been there to a minor degree before, but now it had become worse. She had what is termed mild urinary stress incontinence, a strictly physiologic problem involving loss of support to the bladder neck.

Without thinking much was wrong, Florence went to her gynecologist. She knew women her age tended to leak. She wanted to know if it could be stopped. She certainly did not intend to give up running.

The gynecologist examined her and said, "So you leak urine?"

"Yes," said Florence. "But only when running."

"Well," the doctor said, "the reason is that you have a fibroid [a benign growth] on your uterus. The uterus is pressing down on your bladder, creating the problem. Your bladder can't fill properly against the mass."

"How big is it?" asked Florence.

"Well, it's about the size of a tennis ball."

Florence thought back to the times she was pregnant. A fetus gets a lot bigger than a tennis ball and doesn't cause this problem. She did not have any cramps or bleeding from the fibroid. Why should it cause trouble?

"This fibroid is taking up space," the gynecologist said. "Your bladder is too weak to push against it. You're no spring chicken. It's this constant pressure from the fibroid that's making you leak urine when you run."

Florence did not like hearing this. Then the doctor said, "The best solution is a hysterectomy. You're past the age when you're going to have kids. I guarantee with your uterus out, you won't leak. It's the best course if you plan to keep running. Otherwise, you'll get more leaky." The doctor then added, with a wink, "After I take out your uterus, I'll tighten up your vagina. Your husband will like that."

Florence was now very worried. Her uterus, despite the fibroid, was healthy. It did not bother her. Did she really need a hysterectomy? Did she need to be tightened up?

It is highly unusual today that I see a woman in her sixties who still owns all her parts. There has been a predilection in recent years for removing uteruses on the following grounds: Why keep it if you're not going to have any more children? What's the difference? (Of course, the corollary to this operation in men is highly frowned upon. They do not undertake such drastic steps when they decide to have no more children.)

Having your uterus removed *does* make a difference. For some women, it creates major medical problems. The uterus and bladder are closely aligned; they share supporting ligaments. The uterus is meant to "press" on the bladder and, as the British urologist Richard Turner-Warwick says, when the uterus is taken away, the bladder misses it. Any time the uterus enlarges, it does so without altering bladder function. This is an important point to remember.

Just as the urethra is often incorrectly blamed for bladder problems, so the uterus is often blamed for a bladder problem.

There is a widely held myth concerning postmenopausal women and fibroids of the uterus. Uterine fibroids, as Florence's doctor said, enlarge the uterus and thereby press on the bladder. He believes that this causes symptoms of frequency because the bladder is unable to fill properly, or that it causes the bladder to leak. This theory is not correct. The biggest "fibroid" of all is a 9-pound fetus. Such enlargement of the uterus is perfectly normal and does not alter bladder capacity. As will be discussed in Chapter Eight, you may urinate more frequently when pregnant because you are "voiding for two," but the size of your bladder does not change. It does not make sense that a fibroid would have a different impact on the bladder than pregnancy does. Both enlarge the uterus. And like pregnancy, fibroids have no bearing on bladder function. Hysterectomies have never made a bladder function better.

Why does this belief—that the uterus is to blame for a leaky bladder— persist in gynecology? There is a probable answer. In the extreme condition of uterine prolapse, the uterus falls and pulls the bladder down with it. The bladder neck is opened and women leak urine. The most effective treatment for this condition is to remove the uterus. But I believe that many gynecologists have applied this principle to uteruses and bladders that are in proper position. The extreme case has been generalized for all cases.

At the same time, many gynecologists were taught that urinary frequency during pregnancy is a function of the uterus pressing on the bladder. As will be discussed in Chapter Eight, this is really not the case until the very latter stage of pregnancy; women urinate frequently in pregnancy for other reasons.

Gynecologists view the bladder from the perspective of the uterus and tend to overlook the urologic explanations for incontinence. It is only as more gynecologists become interested in the bladder (which seems to be happening) that these "gynocentric," to coin a word, explanations will become less common.

Florence's problem was with her bladder neck. If you recall, we stay dry when the pressure in the urethra is greater than the pressure in the bladder. When support ligaments to the bladder neck lose tone, the bladder neck starts to pull open. Then only the external sphincter in the urethra keeps us dry, and a sudden stress such as coughing, laughing, sneezing, or the pounding motion of jogging can be enough to let urine past the sphincter. Then we leak.

Fortunately, Florence came to me for a second opinion. She had never had surgery in her life and was not anxious to undergo the scalpel. I explained to her that fibroids could be removed through the laparoscope, and she didn't need to lose her uterus if this was the cause for her problem. She had only a mild "fallen uterus," which could be treated by resuspension rather than removal. The treatment also helps restore support to the bladder. After the procedure, Florence kept running, and in fact sometimes waved as she passed by my office.

ALICE

When Alice was forty-seven, she began to have trouble urinating. Her gynecologist said her uterus was enlarged and it had best come out. "He did find tumors and I am convinced it was a necessary operation," she said. But six weeks after surgery, she developed intense bladder pain. It was a relentless, burning pressure that left Alice devastated.

The ancient Greeks thought there was a connection between a woman's emotions and her genitals. The Greek word for uterus is *hystera,* and thus we call the surgical removal of the organ a *hysterectomy.* Hysterectomies are the most frequently performed major operations in the United States. In 1984 alone, 700,000 hysterectomies were performed in the United States. Despite widespread awareness that many of these operations are unnecessary, that number has decreased by only 100,000 since!

Some physicians routinely take out the ovaries at the same time they remove the uterus. The attitude is that once you've had children, the uterus and the ovaries become useless, bleeding, symptom-producing, and potentially cancer-bearing organs. But there is now clear evidence that the ovaries are important throughout your life, even in old age. They should not be removed unless they are diseased. If they are taken out, you will experience what amounts to man-made menopause.

There is confusion over the terms used for this operation. Most people think of a ''total hysterectomy'' as removal of the uterus, fallopian tubes, and ovaries. In medical terminology the removal of both fallopian tubes and ovaries along with the uterus is a ''total hysterectomy and bilateral salpingo-oophorectomy.'' When the uterus and cervix are removed it is properly called a ''total hysterectomy.'' In a ''subtotal hysterectomy,'' the cervix is left in.

The uterus can be taken out in two ways, through the vagina or through an incision in the abdomen. The vaginal procedure is indicated when the uterus is small enough and pelvic ligaments large enough to allow easy access through the vagina. Laparoscopically aided vaginal hysterectomy is another technique that helps to prevent injury to the ureters through direct visual dissection.

If you refer to Figure 5-3, The Complete Female Urinary System, page 143, you will notice that the ureters (the tubes that carry urine from the kidneys) cross the ovaries on their way down to the bladder. One well-known complication of a hysterectomy is accidental cutting of the ureters. This is usually recognized immediately and repaired, but if it is not, fever and pain occur on the injured side right after surgery. If still not recognized, within one or two days the symptoms of a kidney infection can arise.

Another complication is not so well-known. It involves the network of nerves discussed in Chapter Two that carries chemicals first identified in the brain—the neurotransmitters serotonin, norepinephrine, and acetylcholine. These nerves run from the brain, to the heart, to the gut, to the bladder, and to the clitoris. Target tissue along the pathway contains receptor sites, the exact locations where the neurotransmitters bind. The pathway of nerves is highly coordinated by the brain and controls the body's fight-or-flight response. Signals are sent to stimulate or prevent transmission of these substances.

As I discussed in Chapter Two, my research in developing the LUVE procedure revealed the location of these nerves as they travel to the bladder. As pointed out, on one side, nerves go to the trigone. Another set goes to the erogenous G spot in the vagina. The nerves then continue to the urethra and on out to the clitoris. Injury to the upper pathway, or superior ureterovesical plexus, may result in difficulties with sexual function, while damage to the lower or inferior ureteral plexus can affect blood flow into the trigone and the G-spot of the vagina.

Many women complain they lose vaginal sensitivity after a hysterectomy. Some have problems achieving orgasm. I believe that overzealous dissection of the ureters during a hysterectomy may be to blame for this result. Patient's observations have real, physiologic answers. They are not imagining these problems.

Interestingly, these nerves have been found and fully traced in men. When the nerves are cut accidentally during a prostate operation, men become impotent. Thus urologists have learned how to avoid damaging the nerves of men. But urologists have had little interest in proving the existence of these nerves in women and learning how to prevent damage to them because they do not perform hysterectomies.

Of course, not every woman who has her ovaries and uterus removed will suffer damage to these nerves. Many are lucky. But, as my office charts attest, the problem is far from rare.

MARILYN

Within days after her hysterectomy, Marilyn experienced intense burning in the lower part of her bladder. We knew it was too soon for loss of estrogen to create this symptom. And she experienced no frequency and had no infections; the problem was burn.

She had developed one variation of the disease that we call interstitial cystitis. There were other contributing factors to Marilyn's problem but the main precipitating event was her hysterectomy. The nerves conducting the fight-or-flight neurotransmitters to her bladder had been injured, most likely by being put on too much tension. This would alter the balance of those transmitters in her bladder, as I discussed in Chapter Two on pp. 99–100. Certainly one of them, serotonin, has been implicated with burn to tissue.

Within a few months, Marilyn began to notice that certain foods made the burning more intense. Wine, cheese, and chocolate were at the top of the list. These foods contain substances that are converted into serotonin by the body.

Working on the assumption that a nerve feedback mechanism might be out of sync, I prescribed a medication that blocks the action of serotonin. Marilyn went on a diet low in serotonin-promoting foods. Her burning improved markedly. (See Chapter Eleven for more good news about how diet can help.)

In the meantime, gynecologists are pioneering new methods that should make hysterectomies less prevalent. Using a technique called hysteroscopy, doctors can now look inside the uterus to see if internal fibroids or polyps are present, eliminating unnecessary dilation and curettage (D+C). For example, uterine bleeding can be treated with lasers that cauterize or seal the bleeding sites; the uterus does not necessarily have to come out. Thus physicians are learning how to heal from within the organ.

Women today are much more assertive about their health care. This is particularly true in menopause, as women take responsibility for their health. It is never too late to do so. With information about how your body changes, you can enter menopause with a very positive mind-set. Like Mami Estah, you can plan new beginnings, do the things you never dared or had time for, and create a satisfying lifestyle.

Many of today's fifty-plus women are excellent role models for younger women. They choose to live full lives that their daughters are proud of and will choose to emulate when they grow up. If you look around, you will see this gift that flourishing older women are giving to younger women everywhere.

Although the road to becoming your own health advocate is difficult at times, you will discover a new source of power within yourself, that is the power to heal.

EIGHT

Avoiding Cystitis During Pregnancy

When Miriam was six months pregnant, her obstetrician found bacteria in her urine. She had just gone in for her regular checkup and her urinalysis tested positive for *E. coli*. Her physician telephoned her immediately. The instant that bacteria such as *E. coli,* enterococcus, or proteus are seen in a pregnant woman's urine, an alarm is sounded. It is well-known that infected urine is associated with premature labor, and sometimes the fetus does not survive. Therefore, this condition is not to be taken lightly.

It was Miriam's first pregnancy and by every routine measure she was doing extremely well. She looked and felt fine. She had gained the right amount of weight. She continued her work as a city attorney, and other than needing more sleep, her life had not changed much because of her pregnancy.

But now her doctor told her there was true cause for concern. He called her in for another examination but could find nothing wrong. A second urinalysis also tested positive for bacterial infection. Thinking an expert in urinary tract function could shed light on the matter, he referred Miriam to a urologist.

When Miriam came to my office, she was upset. She didn't really want to see another physician but she did want her baby to be healthy. Her "problem," she said, was that she felt fine. She didn't feel as if she were ill.

After I asked some questions, Miriam finally blurted out, "But I feel perfectly well! You'd think that if I had an infection I'd feel some symptoms. What is it about pregnancy? Does being pregnant somehow take away the symptoms of cystitis?''

Miriam was concerned and I couldn't blame her. Every woman referred to me for asymptomatic cystitis during pregnancy is greatly distressed. It is a confounding problem. You don't want to take a chance of promoting premature labor. But if there are no symptoms, what could be the matter?

I told Miriam to give me another urine sample, cautioning her to make sure she caught the urine in midstream. Then I took a urine sample from her bladder using a catheter. The next day, there was good news: The urine in her bladder was sterile, but the urine she had caught for culturing was contaminated. Therefore, it was only something in the way she had voided that was causing the contamination.

The Shelf Syndrome

Unlike most urologists, I have been pregnant and have delivered a baby. This experience has afforded me a different perspective on questions of urologic health during pregnancy.

When I was about six months pregnant, I began to notice that I had damp underwear most of the time. I was immediately concerned. Was I becoming incontinent? You're not supposed to leak urine when you're pregnant. I wasn't feeling any unusual urges to urinate. In fact, like Miriam, I felt great.

Then one day, as I was sitting on the toilet mulling over the damp underwear problem, the answer struck me. There I was, sitting back on the seat, with my hands folded on my abdomen. I called this my "shelf," that little bridge between your chest wall and the uterus. This shelf allows you to do all sorts of unique things such as balancing books on it or hiding needed surgical instruments from the scrub nurse in the operating room. And it stays with you to the end of your pregnancy.

I realized that I was voiding differently because of my shelf. When I was not pregnant, I had always leaned forward, spread my legs, and let the urine stream wash off the perineum. But now I was sitting back on the toilet seat because with the extra bulk it was more comfortable that way. I also had my legs together in front of me to offset the imbalance from leaning back.

When I voided in this position, I was allowing urine to flow back up into the vagina. Later, the urine seeped out, causing the wet underpants. Such intravaginal reflux of urine, I thought, must be very common in pregnant women. We all get these shelves and we all probably like to lean back when we urinate.

The problem, of course, is that urine draining out of the vagina will easily be contaminated with bacteria. Therefore pregnant women who re-flux urine into their vaginas might be misdiagnosed as having bladder infections.

I asked Miriam if she had damp underpants.

"Why, yes I do," she said. "Most of the time. But I thought it was just excess secretions from my vagina with pregnancy and all."

"Do you sit back when you void?"

"Yes, I do," she said. "I have trouble leaning forward because I'm too big." And thus, using a commonsense approach, we solved her mystery. Once she understood what she was doing, she learned to lean forward by spreading her legs wide apart to make room for her enlarged uterus. The damp underwear stopped and her urine samples in the future were sterile.

I believe that genuine bladder infections during pregnancy are less common than is thought. Intravaginal reflux of urine, this "shelf syndrome," should be ruled out before antibiotics are prescribed as a result of contaminated urine. The lone finding of bacteria in urine is not satisfactory grounds that you have a bladder infection. The urinalysis is not the only thing to take into consideration.

However, the fact that bacteria-laden urine is constantly present in underwear could lead to bacterial infection of the urethra. When your physician discovers you have infected urine, he or she will sound the alarm and your gynecologist may assume you have a genuine serious bladder infection. He or she may then prescribe suppressive antibiotic therapy to prevent the danger of premature contractions. *But if you don't have a bladder infection, you are taking the drugs unnecessarily.* And, since antibiotics are known to cross the placental barrier, the baby is likewise needlessly exposed to medications.

How to Give a Urine Sample

You should know how to give a urine sample during pregnancy. As part of prenatal care, women routinely give such samples to test for bacteria, glucose, blood, protein, or other factors not present in normal urine.

When you give a sample, be sure that urine does not backflow into your vagina. The best way to go about this is to lean forward and *half stand up* when you void. *Lift your buttocks off the toilet seat and put your weight onto your thighs.* In this position, you can look down and see what you're doing. When you urinate in this half-standing position, the stream will drop down and not wash the perineum. You can catch some in the container, knowing it won't contain bacteria from the vagina.

Don't sit down on the toilet seat and place the container underneath, hoping that the stream will be caught well enough. Your pelvis is tilted in the wrong direction, causing urine to flow back over the perineum. Attempts at catching this will only result in pubic hair and skin contaminating the container and urine.

It is important whenever you void during pregnancy that you don't give in to the shelf. *Always lean forward and spread your legs apart.* After you void, you might also take a piece of toilet tissue and dab it into the vagina. This catches some of the backflowing urine.

Hopefully, by properly catching a urine sample, you can show that you do not have a urinary tract infection just because bacteria showed up in your urine. If your urine tests positive for bacteria and you feel fine, ask to give another sample for culture. This should be done *as a catheterized sample* and compared to your voided one.

You can also monitor your urine at home throughout pregnancy with home test kits, put out by different manufacturers. With these you can test urine for blood, glucose, bacteria, pH, or proteins.

If you have a history of bladder infections, these tests are useful. If you develop sudden feelings of urinary frequency on a Saturday night (and doesn't it always seem to happen then, when physicians are hard to locate?), you can find out right away if there is cause for concern.

But, I want to emphasize, some things that indicate a urologic problem in a nonpregnant woman may turn out to be normal in a pregnant woman. Not every "abnormal" finding in blood or urine is a sure sign of urologic disease during pregnancy. So before considering what to do if you *do* have a genuine infection of the upper or lower urinary tract during pregnancy, you should understand what normal changes your kidneys, ureters, bladder, and urethra undergo during those remarkable nine months.

Water Retention: When Not to Worry

When you are pregnant, you can develop any urologic problem that might also affect a nonpregnant woman. During pregnancy, however, such problems are compounded by profound physiologic changes in your body plus the presence of a rapidly growing fetus. This combination of factors makes it very difficult to diagnose and treat urologic disorders in pregnant women. Conventional techniques such as X rays, cystoscopy, and surgery are used only as a last resort. However, in recent years the new technique of ultrasound is shedding light on what the urinary tract really looks like during pregnancy. As with cystitis, the answers are still evolving; not all the information is in.

It is known that during pregnancy your body undergoes some extraordinary changes. Early on, you produce large amounts of the female hormone estrogen. It elevates a substance in blood plasma called angiotensin, which increases the kidneys' filtration rates. Thus early on blood flow to the kidneys increases so that you can filter more toxins, including those produced by the fetus. This is natural and necessary, and such increased blood flow is maintained at fairly constant levels all through your pregnancy.

Moreover, when you are pregnant, you retain fluids. This is because your kidneys become very adept at reclaiming any sodium, or salt, that passes through them; not much is lost to urine. As a result, some *edema,* or water retention, is normal during pregnancy.

How can you tell if you have edema? Look for the thinnest part of your leg along the shinbone. Press in with your finger, count to three, and release. The degree of impression left by your finger indicates how much edema you have. You have some excess fluid on board if there is a mild depression. If you made a deep cavity, you have excessive fluid retention and should see a physician.

Some women find the edema of pregnancy an upsetting side effect but you should be aware that there is a reason behind it.

First consider what happens when you are not pregnant. Your kidneys must continuously filter blood at a proper, controlled rate. When for various reasons (changes in posture, salt intake, drugs, or other factors) blood pressure falls, so that the blood flow through the kidneys falls below the normal range, your kidneys are stimulated to excrete an enzyme called *renin*. This in turn stimulates your body's smallest blood vessels to constrict, reducing volume of the circulatory system and increasing blood pressure. It also stimulates the adrenal glands to secrete a hormone that promotes reabsorption of salt and water by the kidneys. More fluid stays in the circulatory system and this also elevates blood pressure. The higher blood pressure signals the kidneys to no longer release renin. The whole system operates on a feedback mechanism.

In pregnancy, the same mechanism is present but in much higher levels. You are now filtering the blood of two people. Since the kidneys of the fetus are not yet working, your kidneys serve as the filtration system for both of you.

The increased edema that is so often seen with pregnancy should, in the absence of chronic high blood pressure, be viewed as just a normal physiologic response to pregnancy. You should not have to limit your salt or take diuretics unless the edema is excessive.

Some pregnant women strive to maintain their slim body image by taking diuretic medication during pregnancy, often without the knowledge or approval of their obstetrician. My advice is, don't do it. Edema is a normal response to pregnancy. The state is temporary, and you should not interfere with the natural course of pregnancy for reasons of vanity.

Glucose or Protein in Urine During Pregnancy: When Not to Worry

It used to be thought that finding glucose in urine was a sign of latent diabetes; if glucose showed up in your urine during pregnancy, the doctor might suspect you are diabetic. Recent work, however, has shown this to be untrue.

Remember the kidneys are working overtime during pregnancy. High levels of estrogen can increase the release of insulin from the pancreas. Normally this would result in low blood sugar levels if it weren't for one problem—the higher levels of estrogen in a woman's body during pregnancy cause a delay in the peak level of insulin, so there is a lag period. Excess sugar is then dumped out in urine. It happens only temporarily and usually disappears after the second trimester. So if you are told you have sugar in your urine during pregnancy, don't panic. This does not automatically mean you are diabetic. Ask for a glucose tolerance test to see if your blood sugar levels are remaining in the normal range.

In a similar manner, protein is sometimes found in the urine of pregnant women. This may be caused by the same mechanism of the protein load outstripping the ability of the kidneys to reabsorb all of it.

To repeat: Finding glucose or protein in urine is not an absolute diagnosis that you have a metabolic problem. It can be a normal occurrence during pregnancy.

However, if you are a diabetic and you are pregnant, take very special care to maintain proper glucose metabolism. In the past, women with kidney diseases were generally told never to get pregnant because they would be unable to handle the complex physiologic changes of pregnancy and childbirth. Today, with drugs to control edema and high blood pressure, as well as more aggressive management of pregnancy, many more women are completing pregnancies despite abnormal kidney function.

However, in this situation it is important to find a gynecologist and nephrologist who can deal with high-risk obstetric problems. Before you get pregnant, discuss with them the types of diet and monitoring that may be necessary and the risks to your general health.

Reducing Your Risk of Kidney Stones During Pregnancy

Some women develop kidney stones during pregnancy. This may be related to their high intake of calcium. Some women eat calcium like crazy in their zeal to "give my baby strong bones," but excess calcium in your diet in the absence of extra magnesium can lead to kidney stones.

It happens like this. When you eat certain foods, such as some green leafy vegetables, you increase the amount of the substance *oxalate* in your bloodstream. Oxalate is derived from an acid found in certain plants. It is generally excreted in urine as an unwanted, toxic substance. Oxalate carries a negative charge, and as it passes through the kidneys, it tends to bind electrically to elements that carry a positive charge. Calcium and magnesium are such positively charged elements. They attach to oxalate in the urine.

During pregnancy, the placenta signals the parathyroid glands to decrease their output of parathyroid hormone, which regulates calcium metabolism. At the same time, it produces another hormone, 1,25-dihydroxycholecalciferol, which causes increased calcium excretion in urine. As it happens, calcium is not very soluble in water. When it binds with oxalate, it has the tendency to form crystals. These can grow into what are known as calcium-oxalate kidney stones. Magnesium, however, is more soluble in water. When it binds with oxalate, it tends to carry the substance out of the kidney in urine. It binds to oxalate before calcium has a chance to do so and serves as a protecting agent against stones.

You can see how you might get into trouble by taking in a lot of calcium by eating green leafy vegetables (which are good for you) and not adding magnesium to help rid your kidneys of oxalate.

Many prenatal vitamins contain calcium and magnesium. Others do not. Check your prescription and talk it over with your physician. For best urologic health, both elements should be taken. Another supplement using calcium citrate also inhibits calcium-oxalate crystallization. It contains a component of citrus fruits.

Recent studies conducted in England stress the importance of prenatal vitamins. They found there is an association between not taking vitamins (especially early in pregnancy) and neural tube defects in infants. Such defects involve malformation of the spinal cord and brain. Since neural tube defects occur in about one in every one thousand births, doctors who did the study recommend strongly that women take vitamins even when they are trying to get pregnant.

It is extremely important that you keep yourself hydrated during pregnancy. Some women, in trying to maintain a slim figure, will dehydrate themselves. They forget pregnancy is temporary and not a time for great vanity. This puts them at risk for stones and risks the baby's well-being. Remember, your urinary tract is designed to clear wastes from the fetus as well as from your body. I do not adhere to the drink-eight-glasses-of-water-a-day school but think you should use common sense. Adjust your water intake according to climate and activity: If your urine is so concentrated that you can't read a newspaper through it, you need more fluids.

The rate of incidence of kidney stones in pregnant and nonpregnant women of the same age is really no different. The most common signs of stone disease in pregnancy include pain in the groin and back, with tenderness, fever, nausea and vomiting, blood and pus in the urine, and even frequency or irritation while urinating. However, stones can also be present without any noticeable symptoms. A woman who has had more than one child seems to be more prone to kidney stones than the woman having her first child. This may be because earlier pregnancies alter the urinary tract, allowing changes to the protective layer of the kidneys to occur more readily.

As you can imagine, kidney stones during pregnancy present a problem. An abbreviated X ray can be done to evaluate quickly whether or not a stone is present. Ultrasound may be tried but tends to present a confusing image; it is hard to tell if the swelling of the kidney is caused by the obstruction of a stone or just by the normal changes found in pregnancy.

Several less insoluble substances in urine can abnormally crystallize into kidney stones. Calcium phosphate stones tend to grow quickly. Calcium oxalate stones are slow growing and tend to have sharp jagged edges. Uric acid stones are seen in people with a family history of gout. Exactly what causes these different stones is not known. Nevertheless, these stones can be dissolved by alkalizing urine with sodium bicarbonate tablets and a low uric acid diet. When the pH factor of urine is kept above 8, uric acid stones tend to dissolve away.

Magnesium phosphate stones are a different variety. They cannot be dissolved by altering urinary pH. These stones, which cannot be picked up by a single X ray (called a flat plate) but require other imaging techniques, often get infected (another name for them, in fact, is "infected stones"). Infected stones tend to occur in women who have chronic kidney infections and rarely occur in those without that medical history. They are treated with antibiotics.

Any stone can become lodged in the renal pelvis or in a ureter. When this happens, urine is prevented from flowing into the bladder, and pain and infection can ensue.

Ovarian vein syndrome, which is discussed below, may also be involved with some kidney stone formation during pregnancy. In this syndrome, the right ureter becomes partially blocked. As a result calyxes, the cuplike structures that drain urine from above, become distended by the increasing pressure of urine. As in bladder tissue, this distension, or stretching, alters the protective GAG layer of the calyxes.

Instead of an electrically neutral surface, an electrically charged surface is now exposed. Charged elements in urine are magnetically attracted to damaged surface tissue. Also, urine drainage is not as fast or efficient when a ureter is partially blocked. The renal pelvis therefore turns into a kind of reservoir. Stones may then form. Like the sugar crystals you grow in water, stone crystals begin to aggregate in stagnant urine. Kidney stones are more frequently found late in pregnancy as the ureteral obstruction increases.

In my experience, however, most kidney stones that arise during pregnancy tend to pass about six weeks after delivery. Most women never know they have them until their bodies return to a normal "hydrodynamic" state. That is, once their hormones resume a nonpregnant balance and the ureters become less dilated, the stone dislodges and passes on its own accord.

Postpartum stone disease may be prevented by taking care to eat a balanced diet with special attention to the proper balance of minerals and vitamins and maintaining adequate fluid intake.

Why Your Ureters Will Dilate in Pregnancy

It has been known for over one hundred years that one region of the urinary tract dilates significantly in about 90 percent of all pregnant women: where the ureters, the tubes that carry urine down to your bladder, meet the kidney. This whole upper portion of the urinary tract, called the *renal pelvis,* enlarges when you are pregnant. This is seen to occur as early as the sixth to the tenth week of pregnancy and reaches its peak around twenty-two to twenty-four weeks. It is a normal physiologic change that causes no problem unless there is some complication, such as a urinary tract infection.

Urologists have given this phenomenon some thought and are still coming up with reasons to explain why it occurs. Today there are three main theories. All may be correct.

The first is based on principles of what happens when you obstruct the flow of water. When you step on a garden hose, less water comes through the line. Pressure builds behind the point where you put your foot. Similarly, as your uterus enlarges, it partially obstructs and puts pressure on the ureter. The increased urinary flow coming down the ureter has less of a caliber to get through. Therefore, the ureter expands in response to the partial obstruction.

However, dilation of the upper part of the urinary tract occurs very early in pregnancy, before the uterus is big enough to put pressure on the ureter. Thus a second theory has been proposed. Early in pregnancy, hormones act on smooth muscle in the uterus, permitting it to expand to hold the growing fetus. The nearby ureters are also composed of smooth muscle, which propels urine toward the bladder. And there is a smooth muscle lining in the bladder. Thus hormones that expand the smooth muscle of the uterus probably affect smooth muscles in the urinary tract. The ureters and the bladder enlarge.

Finally, it is theorized that ureters expand because more fluid is draining through the system. You are simply clearing more urine. And, like the system of the diabetic with increased urine flow, your system expands to cope with the volume.

Interestingly, this dilation of the upper part of the urinary tract is not seen in animals that walk on all fours. It is found only in primates and is thought to be a consequence of our upright posture. Because of gravity, the abdominal contents of four-legged animals fall forward, away from the ureters.

Most pregnant women experience some degree of ureteral obstruction throughout most of the day. This is why lying down and putting your feet up feels so good. You are reducing congestion in the veins around your uterus and urinary tract. And you relieve some of that pressure on your lower back. At the same time, this change in position increases the amount of blood flowing through the kidney. Your system is relieved overall.

If you lie on the opposite side from the side that hurts, you may be able to relieve pressure by causing the contents of your abdomen to fall away from the area being obstructed. Our mothers and grandmothers knew this instinctively but now there is a medical explanation for why it helps. The swelling of kidneys during pregnancy often can be managed simply by changing positions. You should sleep and rest on your side.

There is a related condition of pregnancy that you may hear mentioned if you experience a backache in your right side as pregnancy progresses. It is fairly common and usually no cause for concern. It is called *ovarian vein syndrome*. To see what happens, see the illustration on p. 203. A system of veins stems from both the right and left ovaries. The veins from the left ovary enter into the main renal vein. But veins from the right ovary join and drain into the vena cava. This causes the vein to cross over the right ureter. When you are not pregnant, this body architecture has no untoward consequences.

But when you are pregnant, a problem can arise. First, as discussed, the ureters expand. At the same time, the veins expand as they clear more blood from the uterine complex. If the enlarged vein compresses the right ureter, obstruction can ensue. The system gets clogged and you feel pain in your right upper back.

Most of the time this condition is just a nuisance. But sometimes the obstruction becomes so great that a true kidney infection, complete with fever and chills, follows. Then you and your doctor are faced with a real

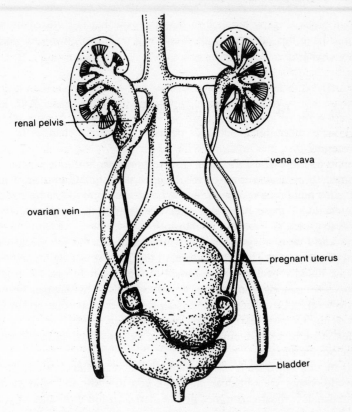

renal pelvis

ovarian vein

vena cava

pregnant uterus

bladder

Figure 8-1, Ovarian Vein Compressing the Ureter

dilemma. The condition itself is self-limiting. Once pregnancy is over, the vein returns to normal size and the ureter functions normally. Women with kidney infection resulting from ovarian vein syndrome may be given antibiotics to save their kidney from damaging bacteria and to prevent premature labor. Once the baby is delivered, however, an IVP is necessary to ensure that no anatomic problem exists that would continue to affect the kidneys.

Some women have an abnormal urinary tract that works fine until they become pregnant. The physiologic changes that ensue serve to unmask a latent kidney or bladder problem. It is not until their systems have to work for two that, say, a mild reflux problem is manifested. If you ever develop a fever during pregnancy along with back pain, urinary frequency, and burning when you urinate, you should seek immediate medical attention. If you have pyelonephritis (an infection of the kidney), the usual treatment is antibiotic therapy targeted to the organism that is cultured from urine. If you have this problem, your doctor will want to follow your pregnancy very closely.

Bladder Changes During Pregnancy

Your bladder, too, undergoes normal physiologic changes in response to pregnancy.

One of the earliest changes is in response to hormone changes. Your trigone, the sensory area of the bladder that signals you have to void, contains numerous receptors for the hormones estrogen and progesterone. Molecules of these hormones affect the trigone, binding or attaching to receptor sites, just as keys fit into locks.

In early pregnancy the body rapidly increases the release of estrogen and progesterone. These hormones, in turn, overstimulate the trigone. Until the bladder becomes accustomed to the higher levels, the trigone responds by making you want to void frequently. This happens around the sixth week after conception and is an early indication that you are indeed pregnant. In those early weeks, many women report they have to void often at night, even though the fetus is too small as yet to be producing much extra waste.

Increased hormone levels also serve to increase the elasticity of smooth muscle within your bladder, allowing you to carry and hold more urine than usual. It must accommodate the increased filtration load of your kidneys, which are now working overtime.

You may in fact notice that you void more often in pregnancy. This is because you are voiding for two. You are probably drinking more fluids as well, to meet the needs of two bodies. Although the uterus is enlarging, it does not—contrary to popular belief—press down on the bladder, so that it has less room and needs to be emptied more often.

As you can see from the illustrations here, the bladder may assume all sorts of shapes and positions during pregnancy. It sits in front of the uterus and it flattens out somewhat as the fetus grows. While the uterus may even push out the inside of your belly button, the bladder only changes shape. It does *not* lose capacity.

Only in the last month or so of pregnancy does the greatly enlarged womb have the effect of truly crowding the bladder. The bladder could still handle a high volume of urine but it just doesn't have the room. You may develop urinary frequency around this time, since there is no space left in your pelvic area for the baby and a full bladder at the same time.

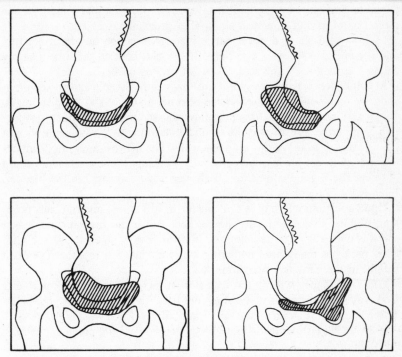

Figure 8-2, Various Positions of the Bladder During Pregnancy

Safely Treating Bladder Infections in Pregnancy

When Melissa came to see me, she was seven and a half months pregnant and frightened. Her gynecologist had found bacteria in her urine. He told her the dangers of cystitis during pregnancy and she was, of course, deeply concerned.

Unlike Miriam, Melissa had symptoms other than a positive urine culture. She felt burning and pain when she voided. Her urine was a smoky color and it contained blood. She had frequency and felt pressure.

Melissa had been given ampicillin to knock out the infection. Penicillin and some of its variations have been used for decades in treating bladder infections during pregnancy with no obvious ill effects in the majority of people. Nevertheless, these drugs are used cautiously and only when indicated, for no drugs are 100-percent safe during pregnancy.

But Melissa was concerned that if she had to take an antibiotic during pregnancy she might need to do the same after she delivered. She came to me to find out why she had an infection in the first place and how she might avoid having it happen again after pregnancy.

Melissa said she had never had a bladder infection before in her life, and it came as a real shock to her. "If I'd had these all the time, like my friend Carole does," she said, "I might be less upset."

My first step was to give her a uroflow exam. Since Melissa was pregnant, we could eliminate mechanical obstruction caused by the diaphragm.

Just as I suspected, Melissa's uroflow showed primary bladder dysfunction. Her urine stream was weak and intermittent. It was certainly not strong enough to move dirt on a sidewalk. The nerves stemming from her lower back to her bladder were not fully working. Melissa's bladder could not generate a good contraction. Leftover urine stagnated in her bladder. Eventually, she got an infection.

Upon questioning, Melissa said she never had an out-and-out back problem, nothing that ever landed her in bed. But it did hurt at times when she was overzealous in gardening or in lifting heavy objects. But, she said, "My back has really been bothering me in the last few months. The extra weight of the baby is a real strain."

Often pregnancy will tip the scales of an incipient lower back problem. You may stand differently, swaying your back, to accommodate your belly. This lordosis puts strain on the back, particularly if you wear high heels.

If lower back strain leads to cystitis when you are not pregnant, bethanechol chloride helps to correct the problem while strengthening your back and correcting your posture. Unfortunately, this drug should not be taken in pregnancy. It can cause uterine contractions and therefore lead to miscarriage or premature delivery.

Melissa began special back exercises, recommended by her obstetrician, to strengthen her abdominal and lower back muscles. She also wore a maternity girdle to maintain firm back support. She avoided that duck waddle walk favored by pregnant women and straightened up as much as possible.

After she delivered her baby, her lower back problem was resolved. A uroflow now demonstrated a good flow. Melissa was happy. And she also knew that should she ever develop another bladder infection, pregnant or not pregnant, she could likely trace the problem to her lower back.

More often than not, women who develop bladder infections during pregnancy have a previous history of recurrent urinary tract infections. There is something not right in the way their bladders work. Thus, if you have recurrent urinary tract infections, I urge you to have your situation evaluated before you get pregnant. Pregnancy puts an enormous stress on your body and it is prudent to be as healthy as you can before going through it.

Beware of Exercising for Two

During this age of physical fitness, many women are tempted to continue vigorous exercise throughout their pregnancy. It is certainly possible to do so—with some modifications. You don't want to exercise in a way that could injure your lower back and possibly promote bladder infections during pregnancy.

Some exercise books and videotapes—even those designed for pregnant women—contain harmful exercises. Check with your obstetrician before undertaking such a regimen. You might bring the books or tapes to your doctor's office so you can review the steps together.

Use your better judgment before putting yourself in contorted positions. Pregnancy is a time to forget that slim self-image. You cannot deliver your baby and wear your tightest-fitting jeans home afterward.

Having been pregnant, I understand the vanity of wanting to maintain your former self-image. In my case, there was a great concern not to show that I was pregnant. I was in residency training. This meant that I was treating patients, and my professors worried that a pregnant female surgeon would disturb some people. But, as I soon learned, it is senseless to try to hide pregnancy. You can only cause harm to yourself and the unborn baby.

Use common sense and take good care of yourself during pregnancy. Your body will return to its former self soon enough.

Solving Postpartum Urologic Problems

The final moment arrives. You've made it through nine months and, at last, that little package you've been waiting for is placed in your arms. You count your blessings. But later on that day, you realize you can't urinate.

Don't panic. This is a fairly common problem. It is temporary. As the baby came through the birth canal, its head pressed against the nerves that go into your bladder and urethra. These nerves may become temporarily paralyzed. There may be some swelling in the tissue. Usually this problem resolves itself in twenty-four hours. It is nothing to worry about.

Pat experienced this problem briefly and was then fine. She went home the day after her baby was born. Everything was going along smoothly until about one month after delivery. She and her husband resumed active intercourse. Then Pat developed her very first bladder infection.

She went to her gynecologist, who reassured Pat that bladder infections are sometimes seen in postpartum women and it is nothing to worry about. Pat took an antibiotic and the infection cleared up—but for only two days.

Then she developed a second infection. She took more antibiotics, followed by another infection. At this point, Pat was very concerned. There had been nothing wrong with her before the baby was born. She feared that maybe everything falls apart after childbirth.

Pat came to my office for a urologic workup. She looked healthy. Her uroflow, IVP, and cystrometrogram were normal. What could be her problem?

Pat had an infected Skene's gland. Skene's glands are located at the opening of the urethra and secrete wetting agents that help keep tissue healthy. After delivery, one of her glands became clogged, probably from the swelling that followed the birth. The opening to the gland was closed down and the gland itself became infected. When Pat and her husband had sexual intercourse, bacteria from the infected gland were being deposited into her urethra. The bacteria could then work their way into the bladder and cause infections.

A Tratner urethrogram study confirmed the diagnosis. We were able to demonstrate the track along which the bacteria moved from the gland into the urethra. Pat was treated in the office. I anesthetized the outer portion of her urethra where the gland opening could be seen. Then I opened the gland and let it drain. Within a few days, it healed naturally.

As proof this was Pat's problem, she never had another bladder infection. She has since delivered two more children.

Meredith is another patient with a similar story but who had a different problem. The mother of three children, she never had a bladder infection in her life until after the last child was born. Then she had chronic infections. She got them whether or not she had intercourse. Moreover, different organisms were cultured from her bladder each time.

Like Pat's, Meredith's uroflow and cystometrogram were normal. But her IVP—which reveals anatomic details of the urinary tract—showed a little pocket or pouch situated in the area of the urethra. A Tratner urethrogram then confirmed the presence of a urethral diverticulum.

After delivery, a small gland within Meredith's urethra had distended. Called a diverticulum, the sac was big enough to hold a stone (I actually saw this in one patient). Like a pouch or a mini-bladder, the diverticulum filled with urine. And the urine provided a stagnant breeding ground for bacteria. Meredith developed many infections as the bacteria migrated into her bladder. Each time an infection was eradicated, a new one, usually caused by a different organism, appeared.

Once Meredith's urethral diverticulum was surgically repaired, her infections stopped for good.

Sometimes women are born with diverticula. A very small number of women who have not had a child have this problem, but almost all diverticula appear in women who have had children.

Medicine in recent years has made great advances. Not long ago a woman with severe kidney disease could not bear children. Kidney transplant patients were sometimes even given a hysterectomy so they would not accidentally become pregnant.

Now, however, even transplant patients can have children because of improved management of pregnancy and kidney rejection. This was brought home to me when I was a resident in training at UCLA. During one month, I was apprenticed to the former chief of the department, a physician who had done pioneering work in kidney transplantation.

When I asked, "Can kidney transplant patients bear children?" he turned and looked at me, all the while chewing on his pipe. He then reached into his hip pocket and withdrew his wallet. I had absolutely no idea what he was up to. He took out a photograph that showed a woman, a man, and four children. He said with evident pride, "Look at this picture." I thought maybe it was his daughter and his grandchildren. Instead, to my surprise, this was one of his kidney transplant patients. After her operation, she had all those children—each named in part after the distinguished doctor. This photograph was a constant reminder to him of why urology is such a satisfying profession. It was a reminder to me of what medicine, at its best, can do to maintain and promote life.

NINE

❦

Like Mother, Like Daughter: Safeguarding Your Child's Urologic Health

THERE are some agonizing moments in motherhood and one of them goes like this:

You put your two-year-old daughter on the toilet to urinate. Instantly, she puts her hand between her legs and starts to cry. You get that sudden clutch at the throat. She has been doing well in toilet training. Yet now she is in pain, saying her pee-pee hurts. It is almost impossible to get really useful information out of her. She's too young to tell you if it hurts when she urinates or after she urinates, if it hurts on the outside or inside. And she may be faking it, in an effort to escape the socialization of toilet training.

But there isn't any mother who doesn't panic when her child cries out in pain. It is not unusual for a mother to call my office at any hour of the day or night in great concern over the agony of her daughter's possible bladder infection.

Children are subject to the same laws of nature as adults. What gets in must get out. When, for any reason, bacteria are not flushed from the bladder in the normal course of urinating, an infection can ensue.

It is not normal for a child to have a bladder infection. The idea that it's "no big deal" to have three or four infections a year is as unacceptable in girls as it is for their mothers. Moreover, bladder infections in children should not be taken lightly. We are born with two kidneys that have to last a lifetime. If there is damage to these organs, a person must compensate for that damage for the rest of her life.

A few children suffer neurologic damage that results in urinary tract problems. Others are born with anatomic problems that affect the function of the urinary tract. Some defects are quite severe and get diagnosed early, while others are mild and may go on for years before a physician detects the problem. Some are never picked up.

Most often, though, bladder infections in children are the result of a functional problem. That is, the urinary tract is not working properly even though all the parts are in the right place. With a little detective work, the cause can be tracked down and treated.

What would make you suspect your child has a urinary problem? She may complain that it hurts when she urinates. Or she may experience nausea, vomiting, and pain. Children with urinary dysfunction can have as many diverse symptoms as adults do. Usually, a child with a more serious problem becomes lethargic. She does not run around as usual, driving Mom crazy; she may sit quietly, hugging a favorite toy. Abdominal pain is a sign that something is wrong and you should take her to a pediatrician whenever such symptoms occur.

Amy

Amy's pediatrician diagnosed her as having a bladder infection. Since even one infection in a young child can be a sign of serious trouble, the doctor referred Amy to a urologist. If her anatomy was abnormal or there was a neurologic problem, this would be the time to pick it up. If not, at least her mother could rest assured.

At age two years and eleven months, Amy was one of those bright, determined little souls who could chatter your ear off. She flopped herself down in a chair in my office and began to swing her legs in the air. Amy's mother shushed her and then began to talk.

She poured out a great deal of emotion and very few facts. Since Amy was too young to give me facts, I had to rely on her mother for them.

I really wanted to know about Amy's voiding habits. Was she in the process of being toilet trained? Has she achieved nighttime control or does she wet her bed at night? How high was her fever? Was there blood in her urine? What happened in the twenty-four hours before her symptoms occurred? Does she ever come home from nursery school with wet pants? What foods does she like best? Is there a family history of urinary problems? Did Amy have any medical problems in the first year of her life? And so on.

Amy's mother said her daughter was completely toilet trained. She looked at her daughter and said, ''Amy knows how to wipe from front to back, don't you?'' The mother was quite adamant about this. She seemed to think that I was questioning her competency as a parent in asking how Amy was taught to wipe herself.

After the interview, I took Amy into the bathroom and asked her to urinate. She cheerfully cooperated. And as we chatted about nursery school, sure enough, she wiped herself back to front.

Because Amy so fiercely wanted to be independent, she decided she could manage her own toilet habits. Her mother had indeed told her how to wipe herself properly. And Amy steadfastly maintained—to Mommy—that she was following orders.

But alone with me, Amy admitted otherwise. She used the same piece of toilet tissue on her rectum and vagina, rubbing back to front. After all, she was her own boss. Like active youngsters everywhere, she was always in a hurry to get back outside to play. Amy would sit for hours with her friends and hold in urine so as not to give up the game or a toy. She even wet her pants at such times. This is a commonplace problem in nursery schools.

I explained to Amy that she was only hurting herself. She literally rubbed bacteria from her perineum into her urethra. By sitting on wet pants, the bacteria count to her urethra increased. The result: a painful bladder infection.

In assessing children's bladder infections, hygiene becomes extremely important. How many kids wash their hands after they urinate? As many of us note, the hand towels are always dry and the soap seems to last a long time in the kids' bathroom.

One way to orient children to the importance of hygiene is to follow what I did with my own daughter. She uses two pieces of paper, one to wipe from the front which is discarded into the toilet. A second piece is then used to wipe between the buttocks. She never uses the same piece of paper twice. This two-paper technique helps many children to get dry and stay clean at the same time.

Teach your little girl about her body. Use a mirror and don't be afraid to give her the correct words for her vagina and urethra.

Vaginitis is another problem in children related to hygiene. Even though children are not sexually active, vaginal secretions or urine on underpants can lead to urethritis and bladder infections.

Then there is the bubble bath syndrome. Chemicals in many bubble bath solutions will irritate the protective lining on a child's vagina and urethra creating a chemical burn. This irritated tissue no longer has a way to keep bacteria from adhering. Inflammation and infection may follow.

Foreign objects lodged in the vagina can also lead to vaginitis and recurrent bladder infections in young children. When a child has infections and no obvious cause can be found, she is often given a general anesthetic so that a cystoscopic examination can be done. The examination may include the vagina too. It is not possible to explore the vagina of young girls by any other means, and the cystoscope can take a look inside without traumatizing the child. You wouldn't believe what turns up. In naturally exploring their bodies, some young girls put pieces of toys, springs, chalk, or other foreign objects into their vaginas. This leads to recurrent vaginitis, which can promote chronic cystitis.

Pinworms are another hygiene issue. Young children playing in the dirt easily pick up bowel pinworms. You might notice that she has a scratchy bottom and seems to pick at herself. Careless wiping can spread pinworm infection from the perineum and give rise to chronic irritation of the urethra.

In terms of body hygiene, do not worry about repeating yourself if you think your daughter has not gotten the message. The effort you make is worthwhile. Good habits will last a lifetime.

Rebecca

At age eight going on nine, Rebecca was in the fourth grade at a new school. Like any new kid on the block, she was nervous. But for Rebecca, there was reason for extra apprehension. All her life, she had had the problem that she needed to urinate frequently. Sometimes at her old school she could make it to recess. Often she could not. In first, second, and third grades she probably had five to six accidents a week. These mortified her. Yet her parents told her she would one day outgrow the problem. She must try to control her bladder. If she tried harder, she could improve.

Of course, the worst happened. On the first day of class, ten minutes before recess, Rebecca knew she had to go. She raised her hand. The teacher did not respond. Then, to her shame, the boy next to her yelled, "Mrs. Smith! She has to go because she wet her pants!"

Rebecca's parents finally brought her to see a urologist. They knew something was wrong but had hoped it would pass. Rebecca did occasionally wet her bed at night but her main problem was with frequency during the daytime. The new teacher was the type who did not excuse children from class without a good reason. In her book, going to the bathroom frequently was not one of them.

My first step was to write a note to Rebecca's teacher. She needed to know that this student had bladder dysfunction. The second was to see, through questioning, if Rebecca might have severe emotional problems causing her frequency. In my experience, this is rare. Like Rebecca, most children with this problem are intelligent, emotionally stable children who happen to have true urinary problems.

So we hunted for facts. Rebecca told me that her symptoms of frequency often worsened after she came home from school in the afternoon. I asked her what she liked to eat. She said her favorite snacks were chocolate-covered bananas with nuts on top. And yogurt. Or cheese on toast.

As I made a list of the foods she liked best, it soon became clear that Rebecca ate many foods containing tryptophan and tyramine. These amino acids promote the production of serotonin, a brain chemical that transmits along nerves found in the brain, heart, gut, and bladder. As described in Chapter Two, this nerve pathway responds to a limited number of neurotransmitters. Serotonin is one.

Rebecca's problem came into focus. She is a member of the teeny-weeny bladder club. Some children (and even some adults) have immature bladder membranes. They are born that way. In essence the final coating layer of their bladders has not fully developed. It is missing some components. This may be caused by hormonal factors with a genetic basis. No one really knows as yet.

But the consequences are predictable. If you recall from Chapter Four, a normal bladder does not respond to small amounts of urine. The GAG layer is impervious to the charged ions in urine. But as the bladder expands, the GAG layer becomes less intact. A miniature leak of urinary ions crosses the GAG layer and tickles the nerves intermeshed below. This is the signal to void. It takes place only when a relatively high volume of urine is in the bladder, generating that tickle.

But a member of the teeny-weeny bladder club does not have a normal GAG layer. Her bladder does not have to expand to the same ratio to feel the signal to void. Indeed, relatively small amounts of urine are enough to stimulate the neural receptor systems telling them that it is time to void.

In treating Rebecca, I decided to first try some simple steps involving her diet. If changes in diet improve bladder function, drugs may not be needed, and as much as possible, I like to avoid medicating children. Some drugs have side effects such as dry mouth, dizziness, light-headedness, and even fainting.

The body breaks down certain foods and uses the products to make neurotransmitters. Some foods—chocolate, bananas, nuts, and yogurt—promote the synthesis of the neurotransmitter serotonin. (For a full list of these foods see Chapter Eleven.) Rebecca went on a low-tryptophan diet. With the by-products of this amino acid kept out of her urine, her symptoms improved. In just four days she experienced less frequency. Indeed, for some children, such dietary changes are enough to control urinary frequency completely.

When Rebecca came back to see me after one week on her new diet, she was better but still not comfortable with herself. She still could not "make it to recess" on some days, and her goal was to last that long every day.

The second step was to give her a urodynamic workup. Did she have a neural problem? A normal uroflow shows a nice smooth curve as urine leaves the body. But Rebecca's uroflow indicated a high, quick voiding pattern. Her urine volume was small, but it left her body in a rapid, forceful manner. This indicated she had neurologic immaturity.

In this instance, children can be given an antispasmodic medication. The drug inhibits the response of the bladder muscle to neurotransmitters. The muscle is slowed down. It cannot contract or respond as quickly as before.

Many times, a combination of diet and medication will be enough to prevent urinary frequency in members of the teeny-weeny bladder club. But each child must also be followed closely. After some time, she may need less medicine. Her dietary restrictions may be eased up. She may be able to tolerate a food once on the forbidden list. This same pattern can be seen in some interstitial cystitis patients; I suspect a subset of those patients have always been members of the club. Diet tends to improve their symptoms of frequency although they still experience the symptoms of burn and pressure.

When I saw Rebecca three years after her first visit, she was off medication but still watched her diet. And, she exclaimed, "I'm fine. I can make it to lunch nearly every day without having to go. And I haven't had an accident in a long time."

Prolonged Bed-wetting May Point to a Urologic Problem—and What to Do About It

Children with daytime urinary frequency may also be bed-wetters. The scientific term for this problem is *enuresis*. It is defined as the involuntary passage of urine, usually occurring at night when the person is asleep. When bed-wetting continues after age five, parents often seek help.

Patty was eleven when she came to see me. She had been to other doctors and had tried different treatments. She never drank fluids in the four hours preceding bedtime. She slept on her back. Then on her stomach. She slept on a hard surface, with and without covers. Her parents bought a moisture-sensitive pad with a special buzzer that activated when she wet the bed.

But such interventions did not work. Patty continued to wet her bed, on average, three times a week. She did not dare spend the night at a friend's house. It was her deep dark secret; only her parents and her little brother knew.

In evaluating Patty, I first made sure that the obvious causes of bed-wetting had been ruled out. In checking over her medical records, I saw that complete urologic workups had been done on her in the past. There were no anatomic or neurologic explanations for her problems. If she had an anatomic problem, we could correct it with surgery; if she had a functional problem, we could treat it with medications. Her mind and body, however, were sound.

Patty's case, like those of many children, fell between the cracks. Her symptom of bed-wetting was real and, in a way, incapacitating. How to deal with it?

At the time of my training (1974–1980) there were two theories in vogue to help explain why children wet the bed. One postulated a sleep disorder and the other had to do with maturation of the bladder tissue itself.

Many children who wet at night are heavy sleepers. They do not wake up to the sense that they need to void. To help keep the sheets dry, many parents get up in the middle of the night to take their children to the bathroom. I remember my own mother doing this with me and my sisters and brothers.

Sleep occurs in cycles. During the night we follow a kind of roller coaster of sleep states. Stage one is light sleep that we can be easily aroused from. Stage four is the deepest, heaviest sleep, when our bodies are virtually paralyzed. Stages two and three are in between. During the night we move up and down through these stages. We dream when rapid eye movement (REM) occurs.

Bed-wetting seems to arise in the oblivion of the first stage four sleep of the night. At this time, body movements and autonomic activity are intense. Nearly all children are difficult to rouse at this stage. It can take several minutes to arouse them to awareness, if they can be aroused at all.

It may be that some children are particularly heavy stage four sleepers, says the first theory about bed-wetting. That is, they are more affected by this deep, sedated state than others. They are even more difficult to arouse and awaken. And they do not respond to internal bodily signals such as the need to urinate when they are sleeping.

British urologist Commander Richard Turner-Warwick has tried an interesting technique for bed wetters who are primarily heavy sleepers. He uses an egg timer. Each time the child has to void during the day, she must first turn over an egg timer and hold it until the grains of sand run out. She holds the timer longer each time until she builds up enough control to inhibit voiding for ten minutes.

Parents find that children tend to imagine that they turn the egg timer over unconsciously in their sleep, giving them enough time to come out of a deep sleep cycle and get to the bathroom. I have found this technique useful in getting children to awaken at night to go to the bathroom.

Recent research, related to what I have learned about cystitis, indicates the second theory—that some bed wetters may suffer from an immature urinary system. If the bladder's GAG layer is immature then certain neurotransmitters derived from food may trigger the bladder. The child wets without forewarning. Hence bed-wetting in some children is primarily physiological. They too are members of the teeny-weeny bladder club.

Fortunately, most children outgrow the problem. The sex hormones estrogen and testosterone affect components of the GAG layer. They aid in cellular maturation. With maturation, especially when the sex hormones begin to circulate around puberty, the GAG layer matures and bed-wetting disappears.

The reverse is true in older people. As discussed in Chapter Seven, when women lose estrogen they are prone to bladder infections, in part because their GAG layers become less mature. Immature cells do not make good GAG layers because loss of the GAG layer in the vagina allows more bacteria to latch on to tissue.

Bed wetters urinate frequently, perhaps fifteen or twenty times a day. But during the day, no one cares how often they go. At night, it matters because the sheets get wet. Many children in the club outgrow the problem at puberty when their systems mature.

Nevertheless, parents can get pretty desperate in the years between toilet training and puberty. Disciplines and rewards never seem to work.

One approach is to try various dietary restrictions, as I did with Rebecca. If your child has an immature bladder, certain foods would tend to exacerbate the problem. One of the major offenders is chocolate. It is high in the amino acid that is a precursor to the neurotransmitter serotonin. White chocolate, which contains no serotonin precursor, is okay. Children with enuresis probably should not eat corned beef, hard cheese, nuts, pineapple, raisins, bananas, or carbonated beverages. (See Chapter Eleven.) Restricting these foods for a while to see if it helps reduce bed-wetting is certainly worth a try to most families.

A few medications have been tried on bed wetters with some success. One is the antispasmodic drug oxybutynin chloride, also known by the trademark Ditropan, which seems to relieve symptoms of bladder spasm. The drug works by inhibiting the contractability of bladder muscle.

Another is the antidepressant imipramine hydrochloride, also known by the trademark Tofranil. It works by decreasing bladder tone—basic muscle response—and thereby increasing capacity. The bladder holds more with the hope the child can make it through the night. This drug inhibits another neurotransmitter, norepinephrine, that is responsible for muscle tone (the tension present in resting muscle) in the smooth muscle of the bladder.

Ironically, antidepressants induce sleep. The child may be able to hold more urine but she may also fall into a deeper sleep and not be able to respond to her full bladder.

Newer research, however, has revealed that some children experience a nighttime change in the hormone levels of vasopressin (antidiuretic hormone, or ADH), which regulates the clearance of water from the kidneys. As you recline, the change in renal blood flow blocks the release of the hormone vasopressin, causing the kidneys to increase their clearance of water to the bladder. By using the new drug, DDAVP nasal spray, a synthetic hormone is delivered directly to the pituitary, causing the kidneys to hold on to more water. This decreases the amount of urine made overnight and the child remains dry.

Given a choice, I prefer not to use antidepressant medications such as imipramine to treat bed-wetting children. The drug may compensate for the immaturity of bladder membranes by altering tone, but we can do the same thing for children by altering the foods they eat. (We can't, however, compensate for spasticity problems with diet.) Dietary and other environmental management help many children until their systems mature naturally and should be tried first. The addition of DDAVP spray should be the second choice of therapy. The combination of dietary management and hormone stimulation should handle the majority of bed-wetting problems.

In taking a close look at bed wetters, in fact, I found they have much in common with certain interstitial cystitis patients. Their urinary pH is alkaline and they show all the symptoms of a leaky cell membrane disease.

If you have a bed wetter, do not restrict his or her fluid intake all day long in hopes of keeping him or her drier. Less fluid means more concentrated urine, which might affect the chemical exchange gradients between urine and bladder tissue and might serve to make the bed-wetting more frequent. You may, however, restrict fluid intake in the two to three hours before bedtime.

Bed wetters, I would like to emphasize, do not usually have primary psychological problems. In fact, these children are usually very capable and bright. Bed-wetting is not, in my opinion, an early sign of aggression, rebellion, or "getting back" at parents. These children do not need psychotherapists.

Desiree

Sometimes bed-wetting appears suddenly. Desiree was seven and had been dry (continent) for four and a half years. Then she began wetting her bed two to three times a week. Her mother was puzzled. Desiree was going through one of those stages in that she seemed very self-centered and demanding. Was this bed-wetting a sign of anger?

In my office, Desiree seemed like a normal kid. She did not report any symptoms of pain or burning but I suspected that she might have a low-grade bladder infection. A urine culture proved this hunch to be correct.

Some children develop urethritis without obvious symptoms. The bacteria get into their bladders but don't alter the surface enough for painful infection to occur. They experience—and usually ignore—some urethral irritation. During the day they may have to void more frequently but then they think nothing of it. Parents often do not notice.

Such urinary tract infections can first show up in children as bed-wetting. After years of total continence, they lose control at night. So if your daughter suddenly starts wetting the bed, she might have cystitis. Such infections, of course, can be treated with an antibiotic.

Other Problems That Undermine a Child's Well-being

Whenever urologists examine children, a primary concern is to find out if any anatomic defects are causing the child's symptoms. It is important to diagnose them as early as possible.

In some children, there is an obstruction at the *ureteropelvic junction* (UPJ), the place where the ureter enters the kidney. Called *hydronephrosis,* the defect causes the renal pelvis above the construction to balloon out from back pressure (see illustration page 220). Urine still gets through the ureter but is greatly impeded. The renal pelvis then starts to hold urine in pools. It becomes a holding area for urine instead of a conduit for urine. The balance of the urinary tract is altered.

As a reservoir, the renal pelvis encounters the same problems of a bladder that does not empty. Pain and infection are not uncommon.

Hydronephrosis is dangerous because the increased pressure against kidney tissue can damage the kidney's glomeruli, the delicate little filtering units. The filtration mechanism may be thrown off balance, dumping protein into the urine. Permanent kidney damage can result. Hydronephrosis can be picked up with ultrasound devices even in utero, or it may not be picked up until the child is older. Sometimes the renal pelvis is as large as the child's own bladder.

The problem is corrected surgically. The doctor fashions a new ureteropelvic junction, or ''funnel,'' so that urine drains properly, the ultimate idea being to save the kidney from damage.

Errors in the genetic code can lead to duplicated organs of the urinary tract. The most exotic in my experience was a man with six kidneys. Most duplications, however, involve a lesser degree of redundancy of the upper

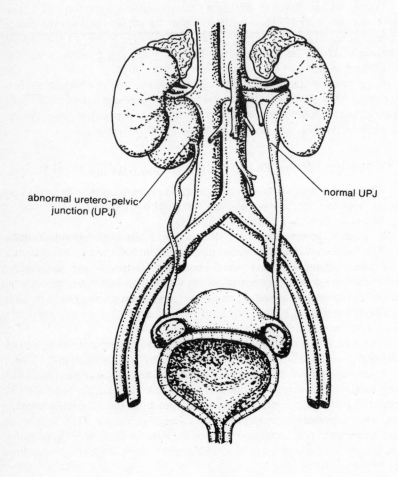

abnormal uretero-pelvic
junction (UPJ)

normal UPJ

**Figure 9-1, Swelling of the Right Kidney from an Obstruction
of the UPJ**

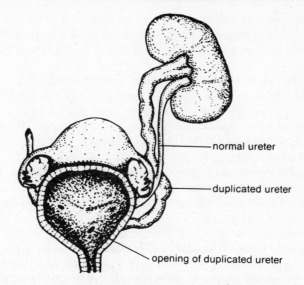

normal ureter

duplicated ureter

opening of duplicated ureter

Figure 9-2, Complete Duplication of the Left Ureter

urinary tract. A common manifestation is multiple ureters (see illustration above). Normally there are two ureters, one from each kidney. But there can be three or more ureters, all going to the bladder below. They can join together on one side anywhere along the tract and enter as one ureter. Or they can remain separate, creating multiple openings anywhere in the bladder or beyond.

A normal ureter enters the bladder at the muscular area called the trigone. The trigone has room for two ureters, one from each kidney. Extra ureters tend to enter the bladder elsewhere, away from the trigone. This creates problems. The trigone contracts when the bladder voids so that urine is prevented from flowing back up the ureters. But an abnormal ureter has no such stopper mechanism. Each time the bladder empties, urine may be forced back up into the kidney.

When an extra ureter empties beyond the bladder neck or into the urethra, the child will have wet underpants almost all the time. The tiny extra ureter drips urine all day and all night long. I once saw a twenty-three-year-old woman who continuously had damp underwear. No one had ever evaluated her problem. She did indeed have a duplicated system, with an extra ureter draining into her urethra.

But anytime urine is forced back into a kidney—a condition called reflux—an infection is likely to occur. It can happen with multiple ureters or with the right number of parts. Infants with this disorder frequently have high fevers of unknown origin. The baby cries a lot and is called "fussy." Then when she is old enough to talk or at least point to the part of her body that hurts, the doctor may suspect an infection and take a urine culture.

Urine cultures of very young children are difficult to obtain. An adult or an older child can catch a urine sample in midstream, the best way to test whether or not bacteria are in voided urine. A young child, however, needs help to give a clean urine sample. Have her sit on the toilet with her legs spread wide apart. As she starts to urinate, put the cup underneath and catch a urine sample for her.

Refluxed urine washes back into the kidney like waves hitting the shore. And as waves erode the shore, the urine begins to erode delicate tissues that filter wastes from the body. If the problem goes undetected, serious kidney damage may result.

The problem of an abnormal ureter can be corrected surgically. It can be moved into a correct position and reshaped so that it closes when the bladder muscle contracts. The idea is to reconstruct what nature did not do right. A newer approach, using collagen, has also been successful. Through the cystoscope, the urologist injects collagen into the tissue just under the opening of the ureter, reducing the size of the enlarged opening. I would recommend this approach first because it leaves no scar and the child can go home the same or next day.

Much kidney damage in adults can be traced back to a presumed reflux problem in childhood. Some women recall having one or two kidney infections as children. But the problems cleared up. Children can have a mild amount of reflux that may affect only the lower part of the ureter. Such mild or low-grade reflux does not present a problem unless an infection develops and tends to disappear when girls reach puberty. Estrogen then affects the tone of the bladder base by thickening tissue. The ureter then closes completely and the reflux stops spontaneously. In fact, many children are not suspected of having reflux because it becomes obvious only if they develop a kidney infection. If they make it to puberty without an infection, the reflux is never diagnosed.

I mention these conditions as examples of what can go wrong anatomically with the upper urinary tract. As many ways as the body forms itself correctly, there are ways it can do so incorrectly. Fortunately, most of these conditions can be corrected with surgery.

No Strictures, Please

There is one anatomic malformation of the lower urinary tract that, while extremely rare, has caused much confusion in urology. It is called a *Lyon's ring.* Named after the French physician who discovered it, this congenital defect consists of a fibrous band of tissue in the urethra. When a girl who has this voids, her urethra takes on the characteristic shape of a spinning top. The urethra is essentially blocked by the fibrous tissue. Urine backs up and balloons the urethra. Reflux is a common complication. The Lyon's ring shows up clearly on X rays and is not difficult to diagnose.

As a real stricture, the condition is corrected surgically. Under anesthesia, the urethra is dilated. The fibrous tissue is broken open and normal voiding follows.

Unfortunately, this rare condition has been used to justify urethral dilations in many children. When no cause can be found for recurrent urinary tract problems, physicians will sometimes dilate a child's urethra— that is, force it open with instruments—to "make urine flow more easily." The child is said to have a stricture in her urethra, even though there is no evidence of a Lyon's ring. As discussed in Chapter Four, strictures rarely exist in healthy women or in young children. External sphincters, a normal part of female anatomy, are mistaken for strictures. Urethral dilations are done on children as well as women, all because of misunderstanding the female anatomy.

As expressed in Chapter One, I feel very strongly that urethral dilation is a procedure *that rarely, if ever, should be performed.* In my practice I have only one patient who requires her urethra to be dilated and that is because, as a child, she had surgery done on her urethra that left internal scar tissue. She was not born with that scar, but today it interferes with her normal bladder function.

There is a handful of extremely rare neurologic conditions that can give rise to urethral spasms or other urinary tract problems. If your child is born with obvious birth defects, you need a urologist who is well trained in urodynamics to sort out the problems. *Urodynamics* is a relatively new field that examines the urinary tract as it functions, according to principles of fluid mechanics. You also need a good pediatric urologist. As has happened in most areas of medicine, urology is breaking up into subspecialties.

What's a Mother to Do?

If your little girl says it hurts when she urinates, there are things you can do to help her.

Have her drink lots of fluids. If the pain persists, don't wait more than a day to take her to a doctor for a urine culture. If she has a true infection, treatment should start as soon as possible.

If she has a high fever, you know she's really ill. If she's under two, you should use Tylenol instead of aspirin to reduce fever. Aspirin has been associated with Reye's syndrome, a fatal liver disease, in children and young adolescents.

Put her in a tub of tepid bathwater to bring down the fever. The lukewarm water will conduct heat out of her body. This is a good quick way to reduce high fevers in young children. Many parents are tempted to bundle up a child, thinking she will get chills. But to bring the fever down, you should leave her uncovered, with only a diaper, after taking her out of the tub. The air will continue to pull heat from her body.

If the child has to give a urine sample, be sure she does it correctly, as described in this chapter. Do not let her contaminate the urine sample, which would lead to the diagnosis of a bladder infection when none is present.

If she hurts and has no fever, try cutting back on bubble baths. Bubble bath does not carry infection. Rather, as noted, it alters the GAG layer and affects the way bacteria adhere to tissue.

For the child who has accidents but would rather play than go to the bathroom, you might try to develop a system that will reward her and make her responsible for keeping dry. You might give her stars or stickers each day that she stays dry. She should be aware of her bodily functions and how to control them.

Be on the lookout for yeast infections, which children do get, especially if they have been taking antibiotics for any condition. For children who have inborn metabolic disorders that prevent normal digestion of sugars, yeast infections are common.

Check for pinworms by looking for tiny white worms coming from the rectum or in the stool.

Even diaper rash can cause infections. If a child scratches diaper rash, ammonium in urine affects sensitive tissue. A way to combat this problem is to dilute the urine by giving the child plenty of fluids.

Bear in mind that if a child complains of urinary pain and then runs out to play minutes later, the condition is not yet serious. Irritations usually resolve quickly, and children are very resilient little critters. But be sure they are not so stoic that they are hiding a serious problem from your attention.

A final word of advice. If your child has chronic fevers of unknown origin, ask your pediatrician to do a urine culture. If there is a problem with her urinary tract, the sooner you know, the better.

TEN

A Special Challenge: Facing the Changes Wrought by Cancer

I F you have been diagnosed as having cancer, you should not let that overwhelm you. Your illness is something that you can cope with, given knowledge and support!

If you have cancer, you may feel angry, hurt, and sorrowful but you need not lose hope. There are certain strategies you can use to keep your spirit intact. And you have the power to make choices over which therapies to use, considering your lifestyle and what type of disease you have.

The Misunderstanding of Cure

When people are sick, they want to be cured of their diseases. But, in my opinion, medicine does not cure diseases. When we treat you for a disease, we might arrest its progress or alter its symptoms. We may extend your life expectancy. But every treatment for a disease involves trade-offs that can generate new sets of problems.

You need to discuss the many cancer therapies with your physician to find how they apply to you. Armed with information, you can make a conscious decision of how you want to proceed.

You can't make your cancer go away by thinking happy thoughts. A positive attitude will not cure you, but it will make a *tremendous* difference in how you live out the rest of your life.

This is an important point. When you are diagnosed as having cancer, no matter what the eventual outcome, you are forced to face up to your own mortality. Each of us has a life left to us, whether it be days, weeks, or years.

If you can accept the fact that one day you will die, you will begin to live.

Take a Week to React, Reflect, and Regroup

If you are diagnosed as having cancer, you should not discuss therapies and treatments right away. This is not a time when you are able to comprehend all the choices and make a decision.

No cancer grows so rapidly that you cannot delay a decision about what treatment to use. Instead you should take a week to orient yourself psychologically to the fact that you have cancer. You need time to go through several stages of coping with the information.

- The first stage is one of denial. You may feel isolated from everyone around you.
- The second stage is anger. You are furious, asking, "Why me?"
- The third step is to start bargaining. "Please, God," you may say, "if I do such and such, this problem will go away. I'll be good. I'll change, if only you make it go away."
- Fourth is a stage of depression. You may eat more or less, sleep more or less. It is a quiet time and a period of withdrawal. You feel helpless, thinking, "I'm now out of control. I can't take charge of my body."
- The fifth and last stage is acceptance. At this point, you may think to yourself, "Okay. I have cancer. That's it. I must deal with it as sensibly as possible."

These stages, drawn from research on death and dying by Elisabeth Kübler-Ross, apply to serious diseases such as cancer. You may not go through these stages in this exact order; you may feel anger before bargaining or depression before anger. In general, however, denial and isolation are the first feelings most people have after hearing the shocking news that they have cancer. And, given time, most come to accept the fact.

The best way to get through these stages is to let them happen naturally. If you are feeling temporary denial, it is not a time to have to face facts. Allow yourself to experience your full range of feelings. It will take more than a week to ten days to go through these emotional stages, of course, but the important thing is that you allow yourself that time to get the process started. You need to begin to feel those emotions and internalize the fact that you have cancer, before you go back to the doctor's office.

This week is also a time to bring near and dear friends to your side.

Being told that you have cancer is like coming home one day to find that your whole family has disappeared. Imagine you find an empty house and are immediately faced with a plumber who says, "Ma'am, you have a broken faucet and I have to replumb the entire house. Tell me this instant whether or not you want me to go ahead." Being forced to make that kind of decision at that time is unfair. No one could handle it without time to prepare emotionally and mentally.

By the time you return to the doctor, you should be at the stage of having made a conscious decision not to roll into a ball and hide. You are taking one day at a time and concentrating your efforts on making each day worthwhile.

What Are My Options, Please?

When you go back to the doctor, about a week after you learn of your cancer, take someone to be another "set of ears" for what the doctor tells you. Someone who lives with you day in and day out might not be the best choice at this time; like you, he or she may be overcome by emotion. Rather, it should be someone who is not so emotionally involved with you that he or she would have trouble hearing what the doctor says. You need someone with you in that office visit who will say, "Right. What exactly are our choices here to help my friend?"

On this visit, the doctor will tell you what therapies or treatments are available for the type of cancer you have. Your laboratory tests will be complete and you will have solid information to go on. Each therapy has something to offer different people. What you choose must be tailored to your needs—your age, the stage of your disease, your outlook on the rest of your life.

This is the critical time to find a physician who will allow you to be a partner in the decision-making process. Many people tend to worship physicians, thinking them to be somehow wiser than everybody else. How can I choose what treatment is best for me, I hear you saying, when I'm not trained in medicine? But you do know what's best for you. You can make intelligent choices. It is terribly important that you make an informed decision on what therapy to undergo. And then stick to it; don't look back once you've made a decision with a disease like this.

And please don't abdicate your responsibility in the matter. Some people let themselves be pushed into treatments. It is important that you have a physician who supports you wholeheartedly in your decisions, who will do for you what you want done.

Some physicians are not sensitive to individual needs. When one patient questioned her need for surgery, her surgeon said, "I'm sorry. There is nothing I can do to help you. Good-bye and good luck." He tried to make her feel guilty for wanting to try a nonsurgical approach.

If you do not like any of the choices offered to you, or if the doctor is pushing you in a direction you don't like, this is the time to seek a second opinion. You may want to hunt down an oncologist—a cancer specialist— who may be better versed in treatment choices. You should begin treatment as soon as possible, but only if you feel it is in your best interest.

In my own office, I discuss with patients the pros and cons of each treatment. I give them my opinion based on what I know about them as individuals, what makes sense to me. Then they decide if it makes sense to them. They choose. This way, I've never had a patient regret the way a tumor was handled.

Are You at Risk?

There are many kinds of cancers found in the urinary tract and I discuss some of the treatments now being used to combat them later in this chapter.

But who gets cancer, anyway? What are the risk factors in this disease?

Bladder cancer is the second most common malignancy of the combined genital and urinary tract. Only cancer of the prostate is more prevalent. In 1985 an estimated 40,000 new cases of bladder cancer were diagnosed. Approximately 10,800 people died. This cancer occurs most often after age fifty. Men are two to three times more prone to bladder cancer than women.

Bladder cancer is caused by many things. The disease affects people in every nation, but its rate of incidence varies from country to country, which makes us think that different environmental exposures are involved. People in Argentina are exposed to different chemicals, foods, and environments from people in Zaire, for example. As a result, their occurrence rates of bladder cancer are different.

As you can imagine, your bladder sees numerous toxic substances over a lifetime. It is a reservoir for temporarily storing the body's wastes, some of which are poisons. By and large, the bladder does an extraordinary job of removing these poisons from our systems without harm. Bladder tissue is fast growing and cells are continuously sloughed off in an attempt to rid the bladder of damage. Chances are good that you won't get bladder cancer.

But you certainly stack the odds against yourself if you smoke. Cigarette smokers develop bladder cancer two to five times more frequently than nonsmokers. The more you smoke, the greater your chances are of getting cancer. Cigarettes contain numerous potent carcinogens. When you inhale smoke, these poisons are filtered by your lungs and excreted into the bloodstream. The kidney then removes them and they pass in urine into your bladder. Cancer-causing agents in cigarette smoke are known to favor the lung and bladder as sites in which to initiate disease.

According to toxicologist Bruce Ames of the University of California at Berkeley, a two-pack-a-day smoker, on average, takes eight years off his or her life. The amount of burned material inhaled from badly polluted city air, on the other hand, is relatively small. You would have to breathe smoggy Los Angeles air for one to two weeks to equal the soluble organic matter of particulates or mutagens (agents that cause healthy cells to mutate) from one cigarette. The air in the house of smokers is far more polluted and dangerous to everyone who lives there than city air outside.

Other environmental carcinogens—things we breathe and eat over a lifetime—are also implicated with some kinds of bladder cancer. Common chemical cleaners (benzidine, naphthylamine, and 4-aminobiphenyl) induce bladder cancer in animals. People who handle these chemicals in factories are also more prone to develop bladder cancer than the general population.

People who work with leather, dye, rubber, printing industry chemicals, electric cable, paint, and metallurgic products have a higher risk of developing bladder cancer.

Recently, it was found that heavy use of phenacetin (found in the aspirin-phenacetin-caffeine compound called APC), once one of the nation's most popular over-the-counter painkillers used for menstrual cramps and migraine headaches, is linked to rare bladder cancers in young women. The research showed that young women with bladder cancer were seven times more likely than other women to have taken phenacetin at least a year before their disease was discovered. (Bladder cancer is most common in older men and rarely occurs in younger women.)

Heavy coffee drinking has been associated with cancer of the ovary, pancreas, and large bowel.

Artificial sweeteners such as cyclamates and saccharine have been associated with bladder cancers in animals. Although study results have not proven a link between such chemicals and cancer, you should probably ingest these substances in limited quantities. As with everything you eat and drink, moderation is the key to good health.

Many of these environmental agents are believed to be cofactors in bladder cancer. The theory holds that carcinogenesis (the rise of cancer) is a two-step process. In the first step, called *initiation,* something irreversibly alters the cell. The cell becomes abnormal or sensitized. The biochemistry of initiation is still a mystery. These changes remain unex-

Stages of Bladder Tumor Growth

Bladder cancers are classified according to how deeply they penetrate the tissue. Each stage (see illustration) is associated with decreasing survival rates.

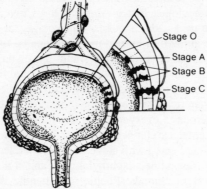

Stage O
Stage A
Stage B
Stage C

Figure 10-1, Stages of Bladder Cancer

• A stage O tumor is confined to the urothelium, the bladder lining. It only involves the cells of the top layer of the lining, just below the GAG layer, and it resembles a mossy carpet.

• A stage A tumor infiltrates other layers of urothelial cells down to (but not including) the bladder's superficial smooth muscle layer, the lamina propria. This layer contains a very thin muscle and should not be confused with the bladder's main muscle.

• A stage B tumor is one that has broken through the lamina propria and invaded the interstitium beneath. This is where capillaries and lymphatic cells reside and communicate with other parts of the body. Therefore, stage B tumors have the potential of traveling to other body sites.

• A stage C tumor invades deep muscle such as the detrusor.

• At stage D, the tumor extends to adjacent tissues such as the uterus, vagina, or lymph nodes. It may spread into more distant lymph nodes and distant sites in the body.

pressed until the second step, *promotion*—when a second agent, called a *promoter,* comes along to stimulate the abnormal cells into proliferating. Any number of carcinogens in the environment can cause initiation. But it takes a second influence, known as a co-carcinogen, to cause promotion.

Many suspected co-carcinogens, such as cyclamates, may be harmless when they encounter healthy tissue. But they can promote cancer in tissue that is previously sensitized, or initiated, by something else. Thus, even if we do not know the full story behind what causes cancer, we can as individuals limit our exposure to known cofactors in the disease. That's plain common sense.

Bladder cancer is insidious because generally there are no overt symptoms—no pain, no irritation—until the disease is well progressed. The most common early warning sign is blood in the urine. Since this is also a symptom of common cystitis, you should always get a urine culture done to determine if bacteria are present.

Women over fifty, particularly if they smoke, should get a yearly physical to check the early warning signs of bladder cancer. Some indications are bladder irritability, urinary frequency, pain with voiding, or urgency. Sometimes lower abdominal pain and pain around the pubic bone are symptoms in later stages of bladder cancer.

Cancers of the urinary tract can be mild or severe. Some involve superficial lesions in the bladder that look like little fronds of seaweed. These *papillary cancers* can be surgically removed, sometimes in the doctor's office. Like warts, they may or may not recur. They involve what are called *transitional cells* on the bladder surface.

Most bladder cancers involve transitional cells. But about 12 percent involve two other cell types, *squamous cells* and *glandular cells.* Cancers involving these cells, squamous carcinoma and adenocarcinoma, tend to be more malignant and difficult to diagnose in their early stages.

Getting a Diagnosis

Because she is over fifty, June gets an annual checkup from her gynecologist. She has a family history of cancer and is prudent about seeing her doctor.

On one visit, June's doctor found minute amounts of blood in her urine. The blood could be seen only under a microscope but it was enough to wave a warning flag. June had nary a symptom of bladder distress. There was no pain, no urinary frequency, nothing unusual to the eye about the appearance of her urine. With a lot of convincing, she agreed to see a urologist.

In my office, we proceeded to find out what might be wrong. I soon learned that June was a heavy smoker. This put her at risk for having true bladder cancer. But what type? Where was it located? What are all the possibilities?

First, June underwent an IVP. This test outlined her urinary tract so we could look for abnormal tissue. Sometimes a tumor will show up as an irregular shape inside the bladder. Irregular shapes in the renal pelvis or ureter could also be tumors. A dilated ureter could indicate a tumor outside the bladder that is obstructing the ureter.

Second, we ran June's urine through a cytology test. Since tumor cells are shed into urine, it is possible to inspect urine for abnormal cells. A cytologist looks at the first voided specimen obtained early in the morning and stains the cells. Abnormal nuclei containing different DNA can be noted by their unusual appearance. Some hospitals today use a special device called a *flow cytometer* that automatically identifies and counts tumor cells. Like an automated Pap test of the bladder, it is 98 percent accurate in detecting hard-to-find cancers.

Third, I looked inside June's bladder with the cystoscope. I was looking for papillary tumors, little growths that resemble warts. These are the most easily treated cancers and, indeed, June had one in her bladder. The size and location of tumors can often be determined through a cystoscope. If small, they can be removed in the office. If larger, they must be removed under anesthesia so that more tissue can be cleared away.

Treatments depend on how cancer is diagnosed and staged according to the classifications given in the box on page 230. There is no single definitive treatment that works against any particular cancer. A plethora of choices is available to you. Only you can decide what quality of life you want to maintain during any treatment.

Treatments for Superficial Bladder Tumors

June had a superficial stage A tumor, the type found in the mucous membrane and epithelial lining of the bladder. These tumors are unlike warts. Though not life-threatening at this stage, if left untreated they may become more invasive and gain access to the rest of the body, but like warts, these lesions can return again and again.

June's tumor was on a stalk but did not appear to have invaded more deeply into her bladder. I was able to snip it off, right in the office, by using a biopsy forcep or tweezer put through the cystoscope. The pathologist confirmed that she had a stage A, papillary transitional cell carcinoma. June then returned for periodic checkups—first every three months, then six months, and then yearly—for three years. If new tumors appeared, we could remove them before they had a chance to become invasive.

Superficial tumors recur in 50 to 70 percent of patients. There are many theories about why. Superficial bladder tumors may recur because a carcinogen has initiated changes in many cells, not just one. A carcinogen in the bladder would be likely to affect the entire lining. After all, the bladder is a reservoir for liquid toxins, and the carcinogen would bathe the bladder. Many sites would potentially undergo the two-step process of carcinogenesis. Or many cells would be initiated, waiting for a cofactor to come along and promote a new cancer.

Another theory holds that tumor cells slough off the tumor, float in the urine, and then "re-seed" at other sites, causing initiation of new cancer sites. It is one cancer showing up in multiple sites. For this reason, we biopsy what appears to be normal tissue in your bladder. That is, we take pieces of tissue from areas with no apparent tumor growth. Indeed, when other areas of the bladder are biopsied in patients, abnormal cells are frequently found under the microscope.

Maryann is also a heavy smoker who was found to have blood in her urine. She had several large wartlike tumors, which required general anesthesia and the removal of large amounts of tissue from her bladder in the hospital.

I find it odd that Maryann has continued to smoke heavily. For one year now she has had six new bladder tumors occur and removed. Fortunately, they were not invasive; they did not gain access to routes outside the bladder. It is her choice to continue smoking but she is willing to accept the responsibility for her addiction, which means more to her than her health. Although I strongly disapprove of her behavior, my role as a physician is to try to help patients as best I can. So I offered her another form of therapy to try to control, or slow down, the rate of her recurrences.

Recent work by Dr. Gregory Cook has shown that bladder tumors invade tissue through the production of prostaglandin E_2. Ibuprofen (Advil, Motrin), which is an antiprostaglandin, prevents bladder tumor cells from invading the tissue in cell cultures by inhibiting an enzyme, *cyclooxygenase,* a potent free radical. Although the dose of ibuprofen that is effective in humans has not yet been calculated, I have recommended that she take 400 milligrams twice a day as long as she continues smoking.

Chemotherapy—that is, giving drugs that kill cells—used topically in the bladder has been moderately successful in controlling the rate of recurrence of low-grade bladder tumors. The most popular drug is triethylenethiophosphoramide, also known as thiotepa. It is not used as a means of shrinking tumors that already exist; rather, its purpose is to slow down the process of recurrence. Since the drug is used directly on bladder tissue, side effects on the rest of the body are minimal. Some people respond well to changes in diet, cessation of smoking, and chemotherapy; that is, they do not go on to develop more serious lesions. The drug is often given as a prophylactic, a guard against recurrence, after initial tumors are surgically removed.

Other drugs have been tried in patients with recurring tumors. Mitomycin C, instilled through a catheter to the bladder, has helped people who have frequent relapses despite surgery and other drugs. An agent called HCG (bacille Calmette-Guérin) is sometimes given to prevent new tumors. As of today, surgery is the only proven way to eliminate a lesion. Once the lesion is gone, the goal is to prevent early tumor cells elsewhere in the bladder from developing into abnormal tissue.

Keep in mind that no single treatment has been found to work even 90 percent of the time. If there were one, everybody would use it.

Radiation therapy is rarely used to treat superficial tumors. It does not appear to prevent recurrences of tumors and is no more effective than surgical and drug treatments now available. But it has a significant benefit in a different stage of the disease, described next.

Treatment for Invasive Bladder Tumors

What happens to the patient whose tumor has spread to the interstitium and may soon be traveling through the circulatory system? A superficial tumor is like a carpet that can be taken up; an invasive tumor has gone through the floor and possibly broken up the foundation.

When tumors become invasive, the potential for a cure is greatly reduced. About one-third of patients who have bladder cancer show up in the doctor's office with invasive tumors. In other words, often by the time the symptoms prompt them to see a physician, their cancer is no longer superficial and may be severe. (Lung cancer is similar. The cancer is often advanced by the time the symptoms lead the patient to seek medical attention.)

If the tumor has broken into your bladder's communication center, which is the interstitium, you run a higher risk of your cancer going out of control. It may no longer be contained in the bladder. The deeper it is, the less chance that it can be handled by simply removing the cancer. At this point, chemotherapy is less effective. We have not yet found a medication or combination of drugs that will guarantee suppression of tumor cell growth.

However, there is hope. Over the years, urologists have been able to obtain the best cure rates for stage B and C tumors by totally removing the bladder. Called a *cystectomy*, the operation is done in hopes of removing the cancer before it spreads beyond the bladder to a significant degree.

* * *

Ruth sold real estate for twenty-five years and smoked as a way of appearing more businesslike. Five years ago her children got on her case and persuaded her to stop smoking. Nevertheless last year she was diagnosed as having invasive bladder cancer. It appeared to be a stage B tumor that had broken through the lamina propria and into the interstitium.

A series of tests was performed to see if the cancer had spread. These included a CAT scan (see Appendix E) of the lymph nodes in her abdomen, a liver and spleen scan, and a bone scan. If the cancer had spread, those were the most likely sites it would turn up. Happily, all the results of these tests were negative. Ruth was otherwise healthy. This meant she had good odds of surviving the cancer if her bladder was removed.

Cystectomy involves removing the bladder, uterus, and ovaries. Because these organs are interconnected, they must all come out together. Once these organs are removed, the pathologist checks over all the lymph nodes removed with them. If the nodes are clear of cancer cells, the patient stands a good chance of surviving five years after her operation. If cancer has spread to the nodes, her odds are reduced.

In Ruth's case there was no evidence of tumor cells anywhere else in her body. Hers had been a true stage B tumor.

"I have a lot of living to do," Ruth told me. "I want to see my grandchildren grow up." Ruth took a very positive attitude about her situation. She knew she would have problems but planned to cope with them as they arrived.

Her first hurdle was to face the need for a urinary diversion. With her bladder removed, she needed a way to drain urine from her body. Various methods have been developed to divert urine and, as with other aspects of urology, surgeons differ in their approach of how to do it.

Most common is the Bricker urinary diversion. In this procedure, a small portion of bowel is disconnected from the stream of stool. Then the bowel is rejoined so that stool continues to come out at the rectum (see Figure 10–2).

This borrowed piece of bowel is then used as a conduit to get urine from the ureters to outside the body. It is simply a piece of "pipe" borrowed from another part of your body. The two ureters are attached to this piece of bowel, which is then brought out to the skin where it forms a *stoma,* or opening on the skin. The stoma, which resembles a rosebudlike nipple, is placed below the waist. Urine drains passively from the hole and is collected in a small bag that serves as an external bladder. The bag is emptied as needed through a stopper.

Ruth chose this standard procedure over a newer one, the *Koch pouch* (it also goes by the names Indiana pouch and Mainz pouch), in which a

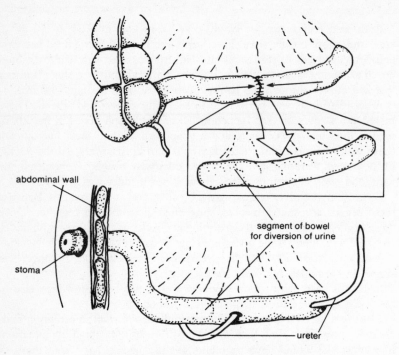

abdominal wall

stoma

segment of bowel
for diversion of urine

ureter

Figure 10-2, A Bricker Urinary Diversion

piece of bowel is fashioned into an internal reservoir—essentially a new mini-bladder. Instead of having a bag on the skin, this piece of bowel forms a bag inside the abdominal cavity. A stoma is made through the skin, and to drain urine, the patient simply places a catheter through the hole and the urine comes out. With this relatively new technique, the urine is not collected outside the body. Long-term statistics on its advantages and disadvantages are only recently becoming available. However, it is an alternative for those who have serious problems with body image.

As you know, outlook is important in coping with cancer and its aftermath. At her follow-up visit, Ruth laughingly explained that her urinary diversion had given her an unexpected benefit: "I can sit through an entire Dodger game, drinking all the beer I want. My friends all have to get up to go to the bathroom, and they always seem to miss the home runs. I can outlast them all. I even bought a sexy cover for it and my boyfriend gave me a red lacy cover for Valentine's Day."

Some patients, however, balk at the idea of losing their bladders. Body image is paramount to them. In fact, I know of a woman who refused every argument her doctor made in an effort to persuade her that her bladder had to come out. To her, it was unthinkable. She said if that happened to her, she would never leave her house again. She would rather die than have a cystectomy and urinary diversion.

It is a physician's task to help every patient by taking her lifestyle into consideration. Like the woman who won't stop smoking, the woman who can't accept cystectomy must still be helped. Human beings are fallible. Doctors need to work around them.

For this patient, the only alternative was radiation therapy alone. It is sometimes recommended to someone who cannot accept the loss of her body image. It may not be the best approach, but it was best for this woman. And it is better than doing nothing.

Proponents of radiation therapy point out that the five-year survival rates of their patients match those of patients who have their bladders surgically removed; others challenge these statistics. Your physician will advise you on choices of therapy and palliation. For example, an eighty-five-year-old with stage C bladder cancer is not a good risk for surgery; but radiation or another approach could provide some benefit. Each patient's needs and prognosis are different.

Urologists often combine radiation and surgery. The patient is irradiated to kill small tumor cells that may have spread beyond the bladder, then the bladder is surgically removed.

Chemotherapy is also used in conjunction with surgery. What if you are found to have a stage D tumor? Perhaps cancer cells have shown up in your lymph nodes but there are no tumor masses elsewhere in your body. This is when chemotherapy can be helpful. The physician may surgically "debulk" the tumor mass. Chemotherapy then has a better chance of killing tumor cells that have spread to other parts of the body.

Chemotherapeutic drugs are delivered via routes. They have different potentialities and affect different systems. No single agent of chemotherapy has been found to treat all aspects of metastatic (spreading) cancer.

One of the most successful drugs now used is cisplatin. It is delivered intravenously over a course of therapy lasting several weeks. Complete remission or shrinkage of invasive tumors is extremely rare when not coupled with cystectomy. But about a third of the patients treated with this drug partially respond. Another third find that their cancer is stabilized for six months.

If you have cancer, you need a specialist in urologic oncology. The field is changing rapidly and it is the expert who has access to the newest treatments.

Treating Cancers of the Ureter and Kidney

Cancerous tumors also occur in the upper portions of the urinary tract. They are less common and are usually picked up by an IVP exam. There is also a new instrument, the ureteroscope, that feeds into the ureters to view the interior directly.

When a cancerous lesion is found in a ureter, generally the ureter and the healthy kidney above it are removed. The remaining kidney takes over the job previously done by both kidneys. We cannot yet make a substitute ureter and calyx system, so the whole unit must come out. Also, cancers of the ureter tend to occur in multiple sites, so it seems prudent to remove the whole system, and the best cure rates are seen when this is done.

Unfortunately, cancer of one ureter can later crop up in the remaining ureter. Then the patient and physician are faced with a dilemma. You can't take out the only remaining kidney. The best approach is excising the lesions in the second ureter. The ureter can be hooked back up or a piece of bowel can be patched in to make up for the portion of the ureter that was lost.

Cancer can also strike the kidneys.

Vicky is a university professor of economics. She was healthy all her life. But on a routine physical, her gynecologist found blood in Vicky's urine. The physician did not waste any time. She ordered an IVP for Vicky and sent me the results.

Vicky had a kidney cancer, more properly called *renal cell carcinoma.* A massive lesion in her right kidney showed up on the IVP and was confirmed on a second test, called an *arteriogram.* The only cure we have at this time for this type of cancer is removal of the entire kidney.

This was the best course for Vicky. Her left kidney is healthy and is able to do all the work in filtering wastes from her bloodstream. There was no evidence that the tumor spread. For the past five years she has been fine and is back at work.

Vicky is followed closely, however, for such tumors can recur in the other kidney. As you can imagine, this has had an enormous emotional impact on her. She lives with the fear that a second tumor will grow as silently and asymptomatically as the first. It has not been easy for her to resume a normal life. As she said one day, "I've had to learn to accept my mortality. I don't take things for granted. I'm happy to be alive."

Exciting New Methods Promise Future Breakthroughs

Because our current methods have drawbacks, cancer researchers worldwide are looking at new ways to diagnose and treat bladder cancer.

One new treatment involves lasers. When I was trained, I learned to remove tumors using electrocautery. Today I remove them with a laser. The proponents of laser therapy believe it promotes less tissue damage and may be a factor in preventing the spread of tumors. We don't know if that is correct, but lasers are a new method of treatment that shows promise.

Conventional cystoscopes can easily miss certain lesions that could be cancerous. An experimental technique called *HPD* (hematoporphyrin derivative phototherapy) makes cancer cells "light up." HPD, a derivative of a natural pigment in blood, is injected into the patient and later concentrates in bladder cancer cells. When a cystoscope with ultraviolet light is inserted into the bladder, the areas with cancer cells stand out. The side effects of this treatment have not been fully evaluated and it is not widely available.

A whole new strategy for fighting disease using *monoclonal antibodies* will one day be tried against bladder cancer. Monoclonal antibodies are like "magic bullets," substances that selectively seek out and attach to cancer cells. If such bullets are attached to anticancer drugs, the drugs would be delivered only to cancer cells, and healthy cells would be unaffected. This would be a big improvement, since all of the cancer drugs used today kill healthy cells as well as cancerous ones.

In other studies, new ideas about carcinogenesis are suggesting new treatments. Damaged and dying cells sometimes release oxygen atoms that are extraordinarily reactive. Called *free radicals,* these atoms tend to damage cells with which they come into contact. Like meteors, they bombard healthy cells and knock through their protective surfaces. Free radicals are also introduced into the body by certain foods, tobacco smoke, air, and water. They are a part of the environment and may be co-carcinogens in some cancers.

However, there are ways to reduce free radicals in the human body. One involves taking in substances that are "traps" for free radicals. Their molecular configuration is such that it attracts free radicals and takes them out of action. Vitamin A compounds, known as *retinoids,* are effective free radical traps. Studies have shown that synthetic vitamin A inhibits cancer growth in animals. It is hoped such agents can be used to prevent cancer from recurring in people after initial treatment.

It will take a generation before we know if diet or vitamins can protect against cancer. The problem is, you are alive now; you can't wait for the final proof to come in. Also, we live in a world with numerous man-made carcinogens and co-carcinogens. It seems prudent to eat a healthy diet, taking into account the latest information on dietary factors in cancer.

You can maintain your body as you maintain other possessions. You repaint your home as it is exposed to weather, you change the oil in your car when it gets dirty, and you clean and repair appliances. Your diet is basic body maintenance. Just as well-cared-for property increases in value, your body will similarly benefit from proper care and nutrition. The next chapter is devoted to the important relationship between diet and urologic health.

Remember this commonsense advice:

• Do not smoke.
• Eat a diet with plenty of fresh fruits and vegetables.
• Reduce your exposure to known carcinogens in the workplace and elsewhere.
• Get regular checkups.

ELEVEN

~─✦─~

The Right Diet
Can Help

Nearly one hundred years ago Thomas Edison made a prediction. "The doctor of the future will not give medicine," he said, "but will interest his patient in the care of the human frame, in diet, and in the cause and prevention of disease."

The doctors of the future have not yet arrived in great number, but there are signs that Edison will prove correct. As never before, today's physicians are looking at the complex relationships between diet and disease. Dietary elements once thought inconsequential are turning out to be important factors in widespread ailments such as cancer and hardening of the arteries and in orphan diseases such as interstitial cystitis.

The problem is that most physicians are not well trained in nutrition. The subject is virtually ignored in medical schools. When I studied at UCLA there was not a single class on nutrition!

From the standpoint of urology, diet rarely has been considered important. But from the viewpoint of someone with bladder problems, diet can make the difference between a normal life and a life in constant pain.

Women with cystitis may notice that certain foods and beverages accentuate their symptoms of pain and burning. Alcohol and acid foods, for example, tend to increase discomfort. Men with nonspecific urethritis may feel better when they eliminate the very same foods that have been found to trouble women with interstitial cystitis.

It was these female patients, in fact, who prompted the first detailed look at how diet affects bladder function. They noticed that they could virtually turn their pain on or off by ingesting certain foods. Every time

Janet drank orange juice, for example, she felt pronounced discomfort within twenty minutes.

An Old Wives' Tale Debunked

Unfortunately for many women, both with common cystitis and interstitial cystitis, the old wives' tale that says, "Drink cranberry juice to acidify your urine and combat cystitis," is about the worst advice you could follow.

The rationale probably stems from the fact that women with cystitis tend to have alkaline urines, whereas normal urine is acid. Thus, drinking acid fluids such as cranberry juice presumably would make your urine more "normal" and less hospitable to any bacteria.

This makes about as much sense as putting out a fire with gasoline.

In actuality, the more you acidify your urine, the better bacteria like it. This is because bacteria use a component of acidic urine, called urea, to help them multiply and thrive. When the bacteria of common cystitis are present, they tend to make your urine more alkaline as they split molecules of urea in the process of multiplying. In other words, your alkaline urine is *the result* of a bacterial infection, not *the cause* of it.

When you acidify your urine in the course of a bacterial infection, you are helping the bacteria by giving them more fuel! And, of course, when you acidify your urine because your bladder is inflamed from interstitial cystitis, you fan the flames and increase burn to the tissue.

The Five-Minute Cystitis Checklist

You can take immediate steps to help reduce your symptoms of pain and burning. For common cystitis, they are as follows:

1. Take ¼ teaspoon of baking soda in water. This will alkalinize your urine and help deprive bacteria of what they need to grow. (Do not take more than ¼ teaspoon, or you might suffer bowel problems.) One-quarter teaspoon of baking soda will work for about eight hours.
2. Drink a lot of fluids over the next couple of hours. This will help rid your bladder of bacteria. The more you can void with efficient volumes of urine, the better.
3. Consult your doctor and *get a urine culture*. You need to know if bacteria are present to know whether an antibiotic will help rather than hurt you.

4. You can take Re-Azo or Azo-Standard, both over-the-counter bladder analgesics, or the prescription drug Pyridium, to reduce pain.
5. Immediately eliminate all foods that have been found to bother interstitial cystitis patients (see list that follows). You do not want to do anything that might further irritate your bladder. In a few days, when your infection has cleared up after proper medical treatment, you may resume your normal diet.

The Twenty-Four-Hour Interstitial Cystitis Checklist

If you have the symptoms of cystitis but no bacteria are found in your urine or you have been diagnosed as having interstitial cystitis, you should do the following when symptoms flare up:

1. Take ¼ teaspoon of baking soda in water. This will alkalinize your urine and help prevent the acids in urine from interacting with sore and damaged tissue. The action is rapid.
2. A few hours later, take four Tums or another form of calcium carbonate. Repeat the dose twelve hours later. This will slowly release bicarbonate into your bladder tissue.
3. Take the bladder analgesic Pyridium (available with a doctor's prescription) or over the-counter analgesics Re-Azo or Azo-Standard.
4. Drink a lot of clear fluids. You want to dilute your urine. Remember concentrated urine contains more harmful elements that can interact with damaged tissue.
5. Experiment with ice packs or heating pads to see which helps best. Put those refreezable blue ice packs or a heating pad between your legs, pressing the pad against your pubic bone and clitoris.
6. Avoid all foods on the Pain Control Diet below:

ACID FOODS TO BE AVOIDED

All alcoholic beverages, except for the wines listed later in this chapter

apple juice	citrus fruits (lemons, limes,
apples	oranges, etc. and their
apricots	juices)
cantaloupes	coffee
carbonated drinks	cranberries
cayenne	ginger
chilies/spicy foods	grapes

ACID FOODS TO BE AVOIDED (cont'd.)

guava	strawberries
lemon juice	tea
peaches	tomatoes
pineapple	vinegar
plums	watermelon
rhubarb	

FOODS HIGH IN TYROSINE, TYRAMINE, TRYPTOPHAN, AND ASPARTATE TO BE AVOIDED

anchovies	mayonnaise
avocado	NutraSweet (aspartame)
bananas	nuts
beer	onions
brewer's yeast	papaya
canned figs	pickled herring
caviar	pickles
champagne	pineapple
cheeses (hard and soft such as brie, camembert, and tome)	pork
	prunes
chicken livers	raisins
chocolate	rye bread
cold cuts	saccharine
corned beef	sour cream
cranberries	soy sauce
fava beans	wines, except for those listed later
lentils	yogurt
lima beans	vitamins buffered with aspartate

You will feel better in twenty-four hours if you follow the regimen just described. All six points must be observed for you to get relief and to control your symptoms. If you smoke, stop! Smoking causes damaged blood vessels to narrow and decreases the amount of oxygen to sensitive bladder tissue.

When I first show this list to women diagnosed as having interstitial cystitis, most of them shake their heads in utter disbelief. Often these are the very foods they love and crave. "You don't seriously expect me to give up chocolate for the rest of my life?" exclaimed Stacey. "You've got to be kidding!"

I told her firmly, "It's your bladder. I can only advise you. But, like a diabetic, you can genuinely hurt yourself with certain foods. The decision is yours.'' Two weeks later, Stacey was back. ''I was good for ten days,'' she said, ''and then I cheated. I thought how could one little old avocado be harmful? Within twenty minutes my bladder started hurting. It was incredible. I knew oranges did that but never before associated avocados with the pain. What a surprise.''

Mimi was hiking and, without thinking, ate a sandwich her friend had made. It contained aged cheese. ''Within twenty minutes I felt pain,'' she said. ''It took me a minute to figure out what had happened.''

It is clear that if you have an attack of interstitial cystitis, you may have been exposed to or ingested something within the past twenty minutes that is likely to be the agent that promoted the attack. It may be the banana you ate or the chemical fumes you inhaled. In either case, you feel the intense discomfort of your bladder disease.

Since diet plays such a major role in interstitial cystitis, it is important that you understand how your stomach works.

A Trip Through Your Digestive Tract

Imagine your stomach is like a washing machine. You first ''load'' it with food that has not yet been carefully sorted; that is, proteins, carbohydrates, and fat all get tossed in together. Your stomach next adds the ''pretreatment enzymes'' and hormones, including gastrin, which stimulates the release of serotonin and histamine, and hydrochloric acid and acetylcholine, which cause the stomach to contract. The enzyme pepsin efficiently seeks out any of the aromatic amino acids in your food, that is tryptophan, tyrosine, and phenylalanine, and chops them off from the rest of the proteins. The ''cycle'' changes and the emulsified food is now spun into the duodenum where chymotrypsin acts like a ''bleach,'' removing any residual ''stains'' or pieces of these same amino acids. Carbohydrates and fats are broken down with the help of bile, which is released from the gallbladder. Finally, the pancreas ejects bicarbonate and ''rinses'' the food, stopping all the action of the stomach's enzymes while it performs the last cycle before sending it to the ''dryer,'' your small bowel, where any excess water and tiny nutrients are absorbed into the bloodstream. The entire cycle normally takes one hour.

How Stress Affects Digestion

Stress, either physical or psychological, changes the timing of the cycle. Instead of taking one hour, the stomach rapidly dumps its contents into the small bowel in twenty minutes, which is not enough time to metabolize the aromatic amino acids efficiently. Instead, the stomach is left with excess amounts of hydrochloric acid, which begins to dissolve the protective lining of the stomach, and the pancreas doesn't have enough time to release sufficient amounts of bicarb to neutralize the acid. Excess water, nutrients, and amino acids are delivered to the small bowel in a wet, undigested state. As a result, your "washing machine" ends up eating a sock! An ulcer develops.

Stress causes changes in blood flow in the stomach, and this results in less oxygen getting to the tissue. Like a problematic bladder, the stomach tissue begins to swell and leak fluid. The lining becomes "leaky," allowing the entrance of food proteins into the mucosa that cause immune reactions to occur.

How can you slow down your stomach? Unbelievably, fat is the answer. By eating some fat, your stomach automatically decreases its contractions, and this slows down the metabolism of the biogenic amines. Epileptics have been placed on a high-fat diet for the same purpose. That is, by using fat to slow down the stomach's ability to excite nerves in the autonomic nervous system, seizures can be controlled. This same principle can decrease the excitement to the nerves that go to your bladder's blood vessels. You want to use monounsaturated fats such as olive oil, but even a small amount of unsalted butter on bread will do in a pinch. Baking soda has the same effect, but it carries the side effect of fluid retention and diarrhea if too much is taken.

Diet Matters!

Let's explore why the foods just listed can be harmful or irritating to sufferers of interstitial cystitis.

Two major groups of food are implicated in bladder pain. One is acid foods such as alcohol, citrus fruits, and carbonated drinks. They intensify a burning feeling in the bladders of patients. The other group is foods containing certain amino acids, the building blocks of proteins. Four amino acids are of particular interest to urology—tyrosine, tryptophan, tyramine, and phenylalanine.

In order to understand why foods high in these particular amino acids would cause problems for interstitial cystitis patients, I did a metabolic study of their digestion. The results of this study were published in the *British Journal of Urology* in 1993.

Two hundred fifty patients ate the foods on The Pain-Control Diet and collected their urine for twenty-four hours. The blood levels of serotonin and other neurotransmitters were evaluated as well. The results were surprising.

Normal people who ate the same diet had normal levels of all neurotransmitters and hormones studied, confirming that a normal digestive tract can handle any amount of "laundry" you put in it. However, patients with interstitial cystitis could not.

They demonstrated low levels of serotonin in the blood along with high levels of histamine and ammonia. No wonder so many of the patients felt "groggy" after following the diet—they were feeling like people after a New Year's Eve blowout! Their urine, however, contained higher than normal amounts of highly charged chemicals that are abnormal metabolites of tryptophan—kynurenic and xanthurenic acid. These chemicals have the ability to inactivate the "perimeter alarm" of your bladder, the GAG layer.

More surprising was the discovery that the normal metabolite of norepinephrine, the "zip in your do-dah," was very low. It is well-known that low serotonin and low norepinephrine are related to depression, so it was now clear that interstitial cystitis patients had both a physiological and psychological reason for depression.

When I looked at another factor, genetic predisposition, I discovered that 38 percent of the patients had red hair or a redheaded relative. Now this is important because red hair has six thousand times the amount of an enzyme, tyrosinase, that is important in the conversion of DOPA to melanin and tyrosine to DOPA. It now made sense why the highest incidence of interstitial cystitis was in countries with redheads or very light blonds, such as Ireland and the Scandinavian countries.

The source of the "dead mouse" odor was also discovered, since very high levels of *indicans,* which smells like "rancid pineapple," was found in their urine. Indicans is the final by-product of tryptophan metabolism, and when there is too much tryptophan presented to the bowel, it is reabsorbed and excreted in the urine as indicans.

As food ages, tyrosine (which is formed from phenylalanine) is converted into a special substance called tyramine. Foods high in tyramine are wine, cheese, yogurt, beer, and pickled herring—all to be avoided if you have interstitial cystitis. Tyramine and tyrosine are problematic to damaged bladders because once ingested they help build the proteins called norepinephrine and serotonin. These substances are neurotransmitters, which means they carry messages in the brain as well as throughout the body. When these neurotransmitters are produced, a normal bladder feels nothing; the bladder membrane is competent and acts as an insulator. But the bladder of an interstitial cystitis patient is incompetent. It leaks. The neurotransmitters become active across the membrane and produce discomfort.

For example, if you have a bowel-absorption problem and you eat foods high in the precursors to serotonin, excess abnormal metabolites may be excreted in urine. Again, in a normal bladder this has no effect. But in a bladder with surface damage, these by-products in the wrong spots can cause burning and swelling.

Appetite suppressants and diet pills work by raising the level of norepinephrine in your brain. The neurotransmitter dampens your appetite control centers. But the extra norepinephrine can torture the bladder of someone with interstitial cystitis.

Incidentally, when the brain levels of serotonin increase, you feel sleepy and calm. This may be why chocolate is the food of lovers. It contains high levels of the amino acid that helps make serotonin. When you are in pain or nervous, you may find that you crave foods that help produce serotonin, since it calms you down.

A second amino acid, tryptophan, is very often improperly metabolized by interstitial cystitis patients. An abnormal breakdown product of tryptophan ends up in their urine. As a charged molecule, it interacts with tissue to increase symptoms of cystitis. Thus these patients should avoid foods high in tryptophan, such as bananas, plums, pineapple, chocolate, and nuts.

The amino acid aspartate is found in meats and milk. It is also a major ingredient in NutraSweet, the trademark for the artificial sweetener aspartame. Aspartate is turned into phenylalanine, which is converted into serotonin, norepinephrine, and another neurotransmitter known as dopamine. Thus intake of NutraSweet causes extreme discomfort to damaged bladders in patients with abnormal digestion. Again, those individuals with normal digestion do not have a problem, which is why some patients feel the diet does not help with their pain.

How to Cope

Despite these problem foods, interstitial cystitis patients can eat a varied, delicious diet. All it takes is some imagination and willingness to experiment. Here are some guidelines to follow in making dietary substitutions:

• You may eat cooked onions in small quantities. Raw onions, on the other hand, are not allowed. Green onions are permissible, if you keep the amounts down. A tablespoon of onions will give flavor, whereas two cups of onions will cause pain.

• You can use alcohol or wines for flavoring. Just be sure to reduce the liquids through cooking so that the volatile elements in alcohol (the part that harms your bladder) are removed.

• You may eat a small amount of certain "forbidden fruits" if taken raw and in small amounts. One small yellow apple should not cause a problem. But if you make apple pie using a lot of green apples and lemon juice, you will have a problem.

• You may substitute white chocolate or carob for chocolate in any recipe.

• Use the zest of orange or limes—that is, a little scraping of the peel—for flavor. Do not use the white part of the rind.

• You may use processed cheeses, such as American cheese, ricotta, cottage cheese, or cream cheese. These are not aged.

• Sugar substitutes can be a problem. NutraSweet contains aspartate, an amino acid that is related to the production of neurotransmitters. Saccharine contains elements that prevent the resecretion of the protective layer on the bladder surface. Fructose, as found in Superose, is a safe sugar substitute and may be used freely.

• To make tea, dunk the bag in water only four times, quickly, just to color the water. By not steeping it, you will avoid tannic acid buildup. So-called sun tea is permissible. (Put three teabags into a gallon jar of cold water and let it sit in the sun for several hours.) Steeping in cold water reduces the acid content of the tea. Many herbal teas are fine for your bladder, provided they do not contain large amounts of citrus fruits.

• You may drink coffee that has had the acid removed. (Caffeine is not the problem for patients with interstitial cystitis, acid is.)

• You can buy a Toddy Maker, a coffee-making device that uses cold water to extract coffee flavor from coffee beans without caffeine or acid. You merely add hot water to the homemade extract. Look for one in shops that specialize in coffee and tea.

• Wines? Originally my patients found that only French sauternes and late-harvest Johannesburg Riesling wines were okay to drink. However, there has been a significant change in the California wine industry's methods for making several wines. Craig Williams, the winemaker at Joseph Phelps Vineyards, noted that wines that did not undergo a process called secondary malolactic fermentation would not produce the acetic acid and aldehydes in wine that were the problems for my patients. This process is used in winemaking to prevent the formation of reductive compounds and alters the amino acid and the nitrogen content of wine. The longer wine is in contact with the yeast, the more opportunity for protein breakdown, resulting in amino acids that can penetrate the cell wall and pass into the wine.

Most California sauternes and savignon blanc wines do not undergo this process. As a result, they are usually "bladder safe." Among the red wines, Nouveau Beaujolais is also safe. However, if you should drink a wine that you suspect is the cause for your bladder pain, take ¼ teaspoon of baking soda in water. One enterprising patient informed me that on New Year's Eve she prevented a problem by taking two Tums before she drank any wine. This is another approach that can help keep your bladder as happy as the rest of you!

• You may drink carbonated beverages if you first get rid of the bubbles. Just sprinkle a little salt on your favorite nondiet soft drink and it will go flat.

• Home-grown tomatoes labeled as low acid may be used in virtually any amounts. Try Burpee's Ace VF55. Grocery stores now carry yellow tomatoes, which are fine to use in unlimited quantities.

• You may freely use extracts (brandy, rum, etc.) for flavoring.

• Check the labels of drink mixes carefully to make sure citric acid is not present in high levels as a preservative.

• Imitation sour cream may be substituted for sour cream or *crème fraîche.*

• Pine nuts will not hurt your bladder. Use them instead of your other favorite nutmeats.

• You can make freezer jams and jellies without using lemon juice to set the pectin. This works with boysenberries, loganberries, and other young berries.

• You can eat Gala apples, yellow apples, and any of the other low-acid apples.

Some patients, unfortunately, say to themselves, "Well, I just won't eat anything much. I can always stand to lose more weight." I strongly advise against that course. I have noticed that many interstitial cystitis patients develop the disease after going on repeated anorexic and bulimic swings. To lose just one more pound, they cut out foods that were beneficial for them and eventually altered their gastric and pancreatic function. The food they ate then was improperly digested, causing harmful elements to end up in their bladders and bowels. Indeed, I consider women who are ano-rexic and bulimic to be women looking for another disease to happen to them.

A Diet for More than Interstitial Cystitis

When I first began to prescribe these dietary restrictions, an interesting thing happened to many patients. Alexian, for example, had classic inter-stitial cystitis symptoms and was easily diagnosed. In addition to bladder pain, she had joint pains and terrible problems with her bowels. She complained, "If it isn't my bladder doing me in, it's my bowel. I can tell when everything falls apart. I get headaches and my joints ache." Having been to numerous doctors, Alexian was convinced that her headaches were psychological and that her associated symptoms were probably imagined. Then she went on the diet. After the first week, she swept into my office as excited as a teenager. "I can't believe it!" she said. "My headaches are gone. I'm not bloated. My bowel movements are regular. I don't have leg cramps or hand spasms. This diet is fantastic. Talk about biofeedback!"

The next time Alexian came to my office she reported that her husband was also feeling better. His symptoms of prostatitis were completely gone. "He's even adapting his favorite recipes. He wouldn't dream of cheating on the diet."

Other patients said that when they cooked these recipes for the whole family, children with bed-wetting problems improved. Since many bed wetters have immature protective layers on their bladders, they do better when not exposed to certain foods that produce harmful elements in urine.

After a while, it became clear that these dietary restrictions were helpful to people with cystitis, migraines, nonspecific urethritis, early prostatitis, and enuresis. These disorders involve similar principles of how dietary factors affect cell membranes and neurotransmitter function. By following the same guidelines, patients of all ages and with very different backgrounds dramatically improved.

Intracellular Warfare

While putting patients on the diet, I began to prescribe vitamin supplements to make sure that each person received enough vitamins and minerals. Many taboo foods are extremely nutritious, and supplements can make up for what might be lost in following the restrictions.

Are supplements good for you? They may be better than you think. In looking at how diseases work at the cellular level, researchers in recent years have focused on a voracious type of molecule called the oxygen free radical. Free radicals are inherently unstable molecules. They have an odd number of electrons, which causes them to react savagely with other compounds. The ammonium ion in urine, for example, is a very potent free radical.

As free radicals roam through tissue, they bind to and change the structure of cell membranes, making them more permeable or "leaky." They can, for example, damage tiny air spaces so that lungs fill with fluid. In the bladder, free radicals can attack the protective layer and create leaks. This is the basic hypothesis for the cause of interstitial cystitis.

Free radicals can be generated from food, tobacco smoke, air, and water. They are found in all biologic systems and may be a factor in aging.

Imagine, if you will, that your bladder lining is like one of those electronic bug zappers that kill insects on contact. Molecules in urine, in general, are like the bugs. They can't get past the zapper. But free radicals are different. They can explode the bug zapper and then allow other elements to get inside.

Fortunately, we can counteract these "superbugs" before they have a chance to penetrate the bladder's barrier through the intervention of antioxidants, which you get in your diet. Like scavengers, or little Venus flytraps, they envelop, gobble up, and inactivate free radicals.

What you eat and the supplements you take play an important part in this intracellular warfare. Many researchers think that if you are careful to take in adequate antioxidants you can help protect yourself against certain diseases. That is, you increase the number of Venus flytraps as opposed to the number of superbugs in your body.

The Role of Free Radicals in Disease

Research has now shown that free radicals are capable of controlling your blood flow by changing the tone of the tissue lining your vessels. The primary means by which free radicals cause cancer is by launching an attack on the nucleus of cells and damaging the DNA, which can lead to cellular mutations. In the same way, free radicals can damage blood vessels so that atherosclerotic plaque builds up on the ragged surface. Cataracts can be formed in a similar way, as a result of damage to the protective lining of the lens of your eye. Our environment is full of these rogue molecules.

The Natural "Poisons" in Foods

Many good foods, it turns out, are loaded with carcinogens, agents that may cause cancer in man and animals. If this surprises you, think for a moment about how plants in nature ward off bacteria, fungus, insects, and even animals. They contain natural pesticides or, if you will, poisons. Foods with built-in carcinogens are black pepper, celery, parsnips, figs, parsley, potatoes, coffee, cocoa, honey, fava beans, mustard, horseradish, cottonseed oil, and even that health-food favorite, alfalfa sprouts.

As surprising as it may seem, the dietary intake of nature's pesticides can be ten thousand times higher than the dietary intake of man-made pesticides.

What, then, is our risk of getting cancer from these foods? Haven't people eaten them for centuries and stayed healthy? Isn't anything safe?

Before you panic, rest assured that most of these plant toxins are not new to humans. We have been eating them for a long time, and we have developed protective mechanisms to defend ourselves against mutagens and carcinogens. For one thing, we continuously shed the surface layers of our skin, stomach, cornea, intestines, colon, and bladder.

We also have an impressive arsenal of enzymes that protects cells from oxidative damage. They are our built-in Venus flytraps.

Furthermore, some protective factors are also found in foods. Several vitamins and minerals are now being labeled anticarcinogens. Research in the field of nutritional therapy has exploded this past decade. Where physicians once considered vitamin supplements unnecessary and foolish, they are now trying to find ways to make the results of this research a part of their lives.

The most important antioxidants from the standpoint of urologic health are discussed below. I cannot, of course, give you precise dosages or recommendations on how much of any given supplement to take. Every person's biochemistry, lifestyle, environment, emotional state, and body weight are different. Thus I can only give a suggested range for supplements, with the caveat that you do not adopt a new supplementation program without the advice of your physician. Self-treatment can be harmful. For example, an excess of the supplement methionine can result in a higher risk of arteriosclerosis.

Medical Dietary Intervention Supplements

Vitamins, minerals, and amino acids work synergistically. You might think of your body as being a walking laboratory. The nutrients you put into the laboratory interact in extraordinarily complex ways—many of which are still poorly understood. However, research has shown that tyrosine works best with copper, vitamin C, vitamin B_6, magnesium, and manganese, while methionine, cystine, and cysteine require B_6, vitamin C, magnesium, B_{12}, and folate for optimal utilization by your body.

Interstitial cystitis patients should not take multi-B complex supplements: B_{12} is derived through a fermentation process; B_5 goes into the neurotransmitter cycle; and niacin is produced from tryptophan. The B complex in general works to increase serotonin, norepinephrine, and acetylcholine, which cause spasms, cramping, and burning. B_6 (also called pyridoxine), however, prevents undesirable degradation of excreted tryptophan in urine and is helpful to interstitial cystitis patients. Other antioxidants that are also of benefit include:

VITAMINS

Beta carotene

Found in the yellow pigment in dark green and dark yellow vegetables (broccoli, spinach, cauliflower, squash, etc.) and deep-yellow fruits (nectarines, peaches, apricots, etc.).

Turns into an amazingly efficient quencher of singlet oxygen and other free radicals.

As it is water soluble, it is not stored in the liver, but can be stored elsewhere and should be taken in the morning and evening, either before meals or in between meals.

Suggested dosage up to 30,000 international units a day.

Vitamin B$_6$

This is the only B vitamin that interstitial cystitis patients should use to supplement their diet.

B$_6$ helps prevent tryptophan metabolites in urine from being used as free radicals. It may convert other amino acids into scavengers of free radicals. The active form of B$_6$ is called pyridoxal-5-phosphate.

As it is water soluble, excess is excreted in urine. Take it at night.

Suggested dosage should not exceed 50 to 100 milligrams a day.

Vitamin C

An important synergist in many nutrients.

Harmful for interstitial cystitis patients if taken as ascorbic acid and should be buffered with calcium carbonate. Calcium ascorbate is more easily absorbed. Vitamin C without calcium is like a gun without a trigger—you need both for maximum effectiveness.

It replenishes the calcium that is excreted in urine and helps store potassium ascorbate in cells.

It is a natural antihistamine.

Take in a corn-free base.

Water soluble. Divide daily dose into morning and evening.

Suggested dosage up to 2,000 milligrams a day as calcium ascorbate co-buffered with 500 milligrams a day of calcium carbonate.

Vitamin D

Helps calcium metabolism; aids in assimilation of vitamin A.

Fat soluble, so take with meals.

Suggested dosage up to 100 international units a day as cholecalciferol (vitamin D$_3$).

Vitamin E

Works to dilate blood vessels and helps prevent bladder spasms.

A natural antihistamine.

Helps absorb vitamin F. Prevents oxidation of fat compounds. Increases activity of vitamin A.

Fat soluble, stored in liver only for a short time, so take with meals.

Take in powder form instead of oil capsules (including oil of evening primrose). Oil capsules can go rancid, counteracting effectiveness of vitamin E as an antioxidant.

Suggested dosage 500 to 800 international units a day. (Doses over 800 milligrams can raise blood pressure.)

Vitamin F

Also known as EPA (eicosapentaenoic acid) and DHA (docosahexaenoic acid), a natural trigylceride marine lipid concentrate providing a dietary source of omega 3 fatty acid.

Makes calcium available to cells.

Is important for restoration of lipid membrane function.

Fat soluble; take with meals.

Suggested dosage up to 180 milligrams as EPA and 120 milligrams as DHA.

MINERALS

Calcium

It prevents buildup of toxic heavy metals such as lead and cadmium.

Important synergist for vitamin C.

Suggested dosage up to 500 milligrams twice a day.

Magnesium

This mineral is more soluble in urine than calcium is.

When increasing calcium, you should increase magnesium so as to help prevent stones.

Magnesium plays a role in the synergy between calcium and vitamin C.

Suggested dosage up to 1,000 milligrams twice a day.

Selenium

Like vitamin E, selenium is a potent antioxidant.

Protects the membrane of scavenger cells called macrophages.

Take as selenium dioxide (an inorganic form) rather than as the organic compound selenocystine or selenomethionine.

Suggested dosage 75 to 250 micrograms a day.

AMINO ACIDS

Cystine and Cysteine (levo)

These amino acids act as antioxidants and scavengers of free radicals. They are converted into one another with cystine as the stable form of cysteine.

Promotes healing from burns.

Stabilizes cellular membranes.

Promotes formation of carotene.

Involved in synergies with vitamins C and B_6.

Binds heavy metals such as mercury, cadmium, and copper.

Suggested dosage 60 to 180 milligrams a day.

Glutathione Peroxidase

Protects cell membranes from damage by free radicals.

Maintains integrity of membranes of red blood cells.

Assists white blood cells in destruction of bacteria.

Suggested dosage 40 to 120 milligrams a day

Methionine (levo)

A sulfur-containing antioxidant and free radical deactivator.

If you eat meat, you probably do not need to supplement methionine.

If you are a vegetarian, suggested maximum dosage is 25 milligrams a day.

PABA (para-aminobenzoic acid)

Important for utilization of protein.

Promotes wound healing.

Water soluble.

Suggested dosage from 30 to 100 milligrams a day.

DHEA Sulfate

There is another antioxidant that should be considered. *Dehydroepiandrosterone* and its precursor, *DHEA sulfate,* is produced by the adrenal gland and is the most dominant steroid hormone in the body. It is the only hormone that declines with age in a linear fashion in both men and women. At age eighty, blood levels decline to 5 percent of what they were at age twenty. However, I found that pain patients of all ages had levels of this hormone almost as low as that of an eighty-year-old. This hormone also elevates estrogen in women and stimulates the release of other pain-relieving neurochemicals. Although researchers are hard at work investigating this chemical, a minimal dosage of 5 to 10 milligrams is currently being used by physicians for lowering cholesterol.

It is important to find supplements formulated without yeast, wheat, corn, soy, dairy products, salt, sugar, flavors, colors, starch, or preservatives. Look for the purest ingredients available. When selecting dietary supplements, ask the manufacturer for its stabilization studies. How do they assure that the product lasts? Is there some type of moisture protection in the product? How pure are their compounds and what is their bioactivity? It is all too easy to buy supplements that are worthless because of poor manufacturing processes. However, as most supplements are manufactured by the same processing plants that make your pharmaceutical over-the-counter drugs, this is becoming less of a concern.

It is gratifying to see interstitial cystitis patients who have found that they can hold urine longer and experience less burning, pain, and pressure while taking antioxidants. Antioxidants end up in your urine and help wage the war against interstitial cystitis and bladder cancer. When food is improperly digested, however, extra free radicals dump out in urine, causing a kind of "bubbling pot" reaction. The radicals release charges, which then result in leaky membranes and the flow of electrons in the bladder that are the "little electric shocks" felt by many patients. But when antioxidants are excreted in urine, they may prevent further damage to bladder tissue.

But How Do I Cook?

While vitamin and mineral supplements have helped patients feel better physically, dietary restrictions have shattered the self-confidence of many good cooks. As I have led women out of my office, they have turned and said things like, "My husband is Italian. How am I going to make pasta?" When I observed carefully and prepared my own family's meals, I began to realize how difficult it is to cook for a household when *only you* have a dietary problem. I saw that in every dish I prepared there was at least one, if not many, of the forbidden ingredients. Obviously, you need to be very creative to readapt cooking styles learned over a lifetime.

With that in mind, I called upon friends who are cookbook authors, restaurant chefs, and patients. We collected recipes that make it easier for women to follow dietary restrictions. These recipes have been collected into a cookbook called *The New My Body My Diet*. You can obtain a copy of this cookbook by contacting me through Healthy Life Publications (see Appendix A).

In bladder proofing their favorite recipes, patients were helped in many ways. Of course, their families appreciate the tasty foods, but more important is that women who take positive action in dealing with their disease are much happier and healthier than women who feel stymied and helpless. The knowledge that you are helping yourself is extremely therapeutic. The knowledge that you are helping others is ever rewarding.

Epilogue

A patient recently came to my office saying that all her bladder problems had recurred. The reason was quickly apparent. She had decided a week earlier that she simply did not like taking many pills. "I didn't want to be a pill druggy," she said. "So I stopped all my medications." She hung her head, waiting for me to say something, when she knew quite well what was wrong. Then she said, "Well, I guess every doctor's greatest difficulty is the noncompliant patient."

The story illustrates a quandary. For a doctor-patient relationship to work, both sides have to cooperate. The doctor's job is to educate, to advise, to counsel. The patient's job is to accept responsibility to tell the physician what works and what does not work.

The woman in my office was on an emotional seesaw. One part of her wanted to be well. The medications had stabilized her bladder for many months. But part of her thought, "Damn it all, my body should work after all this time. It should be well on its own without these pills." Within days of stopping her medication, she was right back into being a victim. She had abdicated responsibility for her own wellness. She wanted someone else to be responsible.

Unlike many physicians, I have no interest in power games of this sort. Instead I expect to relinquish control to you and merely serve as your adviser in helping you regain control of your urinary tract. But to give you this gift, you must listen to my advice, weigh it, and do what you think is right.

If, like the woman in my office, you choose not to take the required medications or follow my advice, it does not reflect on me. It is your choice. It is your body, your health. Only you can choose how you wish to live and manage your illness.

I use this story to illustrate an important theme of this book: Every woman should be an equal partner with her doctor. Medicine should not mystify and frighten you. It is mostly common sense!

It is possible to work with your physician in managing your health, but you cannot remain a victim. Victims are self-made. It is a self-defeating attitude that leads to fear and depression.

This book should persuade you that knowledge and self-confidence are tools for forging a doctor-patient partnership. You now have the knowledge to avoid the victim mentality. But with this knowledge comes the responsibility to act sensibly. You certainly should not turn around and reject the medical profession because you think someone once hurt you. Urologic problems, as you have seen, are enormously complex. This book does not contain all the answers about urogynecologic disease. It is not a handbook for treating diseases at home. Rather it is a foundation that gives you an idea of how difficult and complicated these diseases are. It is a starting point for you to use in taking charge of your life. It should give you the knowledge base to use in finding an appropriate physician/partner.

You need to trust your physician and your physician needs to trust your observations. Medicine is an art, not a science. It is a continuously evolving process in which there are no edicts. If you don't tell your physician how you are responding to any given treatment, no one will. Without that feedback, your physician will not know how to help you.

I hope this book has met the three goals that I initially set out to achieve:

First, to teach you about your body. By knowing how it works, you can help assess how it goes awry.

Second, to persuade you to take responsibility for your own health. You are a smart consumer of medical care as well as other goods and services.

Third, I hope that by giving you knowledge, I have given you the power to find that sense of self that will sustain you through all of life's challenges.

APPENDIX A

Resources

T HE following is a list of self-help and resource organizations, some of which may prove useful to my readers. The information contained in this list is current as of this printing. I have found input from my readers invaluable and invite you to share your personal experiences or helpful tips by contacting me at:

Dr. Larrian Gillespie
c/o Healthy Life Publications
505 S. Beverly Drive, Suite 1233
Beverly Hills, CA. 90212
310-471-7532
800-554-3335   e-mail: lgille01@interserv.com
310-471-9041 fax

The cookbook *The New My Body, My Diet* contains more than 170 pages of recipes "bladder-proofed" by my patients. To order it or other products (including books on women's health issues, audio tapes, booklets, and my nutritional supplements) call the toll free number above. My web site (http://www.ReadersNdex.com/DrGillespie) will be updated frequently with current medical news along with links to other relevant medical sites. You will be able to view sample chapters from my other books and participate in a women's health forum.

Search Tips

Digital Equipment Corporation has a search engine located at http://www.altavista.digital.com that claims to index 8 billion words in more than 16 million World Wide Web pages, as well as 13,000 news groups. Searches are surprisingly fast and reasonably accurate, and search results are presented quite coherently. Since the Web keeps changing every moment, use this search engine to look up key words for any medical topics.

The most useful online library catalog is that of the University of California, which has brought together its holdings in the huge Melvyl system. To get directly to it, telnet melvyl.ucop.edu. When asked, tell the computer your terminal type (vt100 will usually work) and follow the directions on screen. You can access both periodicals and books. This system goes back more than ten years. Accessing library catalogs is relatively simple if you use a gopher, which will offer you a choice called "Libraries." Examples are gopher.micro.umn.edu for the University of Minnesota or libgopher.yale.edu, which offers a choice of continents from which to search libraries. Pick one and you will get submenus until, eventually, you can choose the library you want.

Dr. Tom Ferguson, founder of *Medical Self-Care Magazine,* provides a primer to the online world in his book *Health Online: How to Find Health Information, Support Groups, and Self-Help Communities in Cyberspace,* published by Addison-Wesley. With this guide, anyone with access to a computer can become a more informed and successful medical consumer.

Back Pain

The Texas Back Institute has a hotline that can be reached at:

The Texas Back Institute
3801 W. 15th Street
Plano, TX 75075
800 247-BACK (2225)

This institute is familiar with spinal instability as well as scoliosis.

The Back Stores is a nationwide chain with over 500 neck- and back-care products. You can reach them on the Web or by phone at:

http://www.backstore.com
800-971-BACK (2225)

The Self-Care Catalogue carries many useful items including the BetterBack© Portable Seat, which I have recommended to my patients. You can reach them at 800-345-3371.

Cancer

ECaP (Exceptional Cancer Patients) is the not-for-profit organization founded by Dr. Bernie Siegel in 1978. I have personally worked with a few of his patients and strongly recommend that anyone with cancer contact this valuable organization. ECaP publishes a resource directory with self-help information and has a free catalogue of books and tapes.

ECaP
300 Plaza Middlesex
Middletown, CT 06457
860-343-5950

Chronic Fatigue Syndrome

CFIDS Association of America
P.O. Box 220398
Charlotte, NC 28222-0398
800-442-3437
900 896-2343 information line

National Chronic Fatigue Syndrome and Fibromyalgia Association
33521 Broadway, #222
Kansas City, KS 66111
816-931-4777

Endometriosis

Endometriosis Association
8585 N. 76th Place
Milwaukee, WI 53223-2600
800 992-3636
414-355-6065 fax

The Endometriosis Alliance of Greater New York
Old Chelsea Station
P.O. Box 634
New York, NY 10113-0634

Fibromyalgia

American Fibromyalgia Syndrome Association
P.O. Box 9699
Bakersfield, CA 93389-9699
805-633-1137

Fibromyalgia Network
P.O. Box 31750
Tucson, AZ 85751-1750
602-290-5508

The Fibromyalgia Network publishes a very informative newsletter.

Government Sources

The National Library of Medicine has specialized information services that can be reached in a number of ways. Their database of publications can be reached through DIRLINE. To search DIRLINE call: 800-553-6847.

To access the MEDLARS search, call this number for a users' code: 800-638-8480.

National Library of Medicine
8600 Rockville Pike
Bethesda, MD 20894
301-496-3147

National Technical Information
Services
U.S. Department of Commerce
5285 Port Royal Road
Springfield, VA 22161
703-487-4650

To find other national health groups contact:

National Health Council Inc.
1730 M Street, N.W., Suite 500
Washington, DC 20036

The Library of Congress can be accessed by opening your URL and pointing it to: http://www.loc.gov. You can perform online searches on the spot.

Holistic Treatment Referral Sources

The Health Resource Newsletter
209 Katherine Drive
Conway, AR 72032
501-329-5272
501-329-8700 fax

World Research Foundation
15300 Ventura Boulevard, Suite 405
Sherman Oaks, CA 91403
818-907-5483

Hormone Replacement Therapy

Dr. C. Alan Sevener has written a thoughtful book entitled, *It's Okay to Take Estrogen* ($14.95 + $1.17 CA tax + $3 s/h). He addresses real-life concerns and exposes the myths and misconceptions that have long accompanied the treatment.

Eclectic Publishing Inc.
P.O. Box 28340
Fresno, CA 93729-8340
209-434-3549
209-434-0448 fax

Women's International Pharmacy
5708 Monona Drive
Madison, WI 53719-3152
800-279-5708
608-221-7819

This pharmacy specializes in natural progesterone, DHEA, and estriol, which is available by prescription. They also have a time-release progesterone.

Delk Pharmacy
1602 Hatcher Lane
Columbia, TN 38401
615-388-3952

This company has developed natural estradiol (0.5 milligrams) and progesterone (100 milligrams) capsules that stop periods and do not cause bladder problems. Available only by prescription.

Incontinence

Help for Incontinent People (HIP)
2650 E. Main Street
Spartanburg, SC 29307-2425
800-252-3337
803-579-7900

The Simon Foundation for Continence
P.O. Box 835
Wilmette, IL 60091
800-237-4666 (SIMON)

Interstitial Cystitis

The Interstitial Cystitis Association
P.O. Box 1553
Madison Square Station
New York, NY 10159
212-979-6057
800-422-0696
http://www.sonic.net/~jill/icnet/
icnet.html

Irritable Bowel Syndrome

*IBS: A Doctor's Plan for Chronic
Digestive Troubles*
Gerard Guillory M.D., Hartley &
Marks Publishing, Inc.
P.O. Box 147
Point Roberts, WA 98281
$14.95 plus $3.50 shipping

Kidney Stones

Gail Golomb has written an informative, first-person account of what it is like to pass a kidney stone. Her book tells you about preventive measures and explains the current technology involved with treating stones. *The Kidney Stones Handbook: A Patient's Guide to Hope, Cure and Prevention* ($12.95 plus $3.00 shipping, California residents add $.94 sales tax).

Four Geez Press
1911 Douglass Boulevard, Suite 85
Roseville, CA 95661
916-781-3440
http://www.readersNdex.com/FourGeez

Osteoporosis

National Osteoporosis Foundation
1150 17th Street N.W.
Washington, DC 20036-4603 Suite 500
202-223-2226

Pregnancy

I highly recommend the quarterly issues of *Fit Pregnancy,* 800-998-0731, published by *Shape* magazine. It contains practical, well-researched information on exercise, breast-feeding, diet, and mental well-being. Available at newsstands or by subscription.

Seasonal Affective Disorder

These companies provide quality full-spectrum light bulbs and accurate information on the therapeutic use of light.

The SunBox Company
19217 Orbit Drive
Gaithersburg, MD 20879
800-548-3968

The Whole-Life Products Catalogue
1334 Pacific Avenue
Forest Grove, OR 97116
800-634-9057

APPENDIX B

The Pelvic Pain Questionnaire

T AKE a few moments to recall when your symptoms began and how they change in relation to changes in treatment approaches, diet and medication, activities, etc. Use the following questions as a guide to help you record the specific details. Remember, a complete and accurate history of your symptoms can greatly assist your physician in making a swift and exact diagnosis and truly effective treatment plan.

1. History of pain:

2. Brief history of present pain to point of origin: (You were perfectly fine until . . .)

3. Use of medication:

4. Description of things that increase pain:

5. Description of things that decrease pain:

6. Prior treatment:

Pain Description

Label each pain by number on the body grid on page 271.

1. Describe typical pain:

2. Rate average pain (1 to 10, with 10 the worst):

3. Rate lowest degree of pain (1 to 10):

4. Rate highest degree of pain (1 to 10):

5. Overall interference of pain with life (1 to 10):

Related History

1. Any history of sexual abuse?

2. Any history of mental or emotional disorders?

Adjective Checklist of Pain

Some of the words below describe your present pain. Circle *only* those words that best describe it. Leave out any category that is not suitable. Use only a single word in each appropriate category—the one that applies the best.

1. flickering, quivering, throbbing, pounding, beating, pulsating

2. shooting, jumping, flashing

3. pricking, stabbing, boring, drilling, lancinating

4. sharp, cutting, lacerating

5. pinching, pressing, gnawing, cramping, crushing

6. tugging, pulling, wrenching

7. hot, burning, scalding, searing

8. tingling, itchy, smarting, stinging

9. dull, sore, hurting, aching, heavy

10. tender, taut, rasping, splitting

11. tiring, exhausting

12. sickening, suffocating

13. fearful, frightful, terrifying

14. punishing, grueling, cruel, vicious, biting

15. wretched, blinding

16. annoying, troublesome, miserable, intense, unbearable

17. spreading, radiating, penetrating, piercing

18. tight, numb, drawing, squeezing, leering

19. cool, cold, freezing

20. nagging, nauseating, agonizing, dreadful, torturing

Other Symptoms

Indicate below whether you experience the following symptoms by rating your discomfort on a scale of 1 to 4, with 4 indicating the most intense discomfort.

Cramps—pelvic———
Cramps—other———
Backache———
Leg aches (R or L)———
Pelvic pain—left———
Pelvic pain—right———
Pelvic pain—low middle———
Pelvic pain—Other———
Clitoral pain———

Painful bowel movement

1. Before———
2. During———
3. After———

Painful intercourse

1. During———
2. After———

Urinary problems

1. Pain before, during, after———
2. Burn, pressure, cramp———
3. Frequency———
4. Urgency———
5. Getting up at night (number of times)———

General aches and pains———
Muscle aches———
Headaches———
Feeling the blues———
Fatigue———

Where Does It Hurt?

Use the illustrations on this page and opposite to indicate exactly where it hurts. Some women find it easier to indicate the spot on the body grid, while others can locate the spot more precisely on one of the two illustrations of the pelvic region.

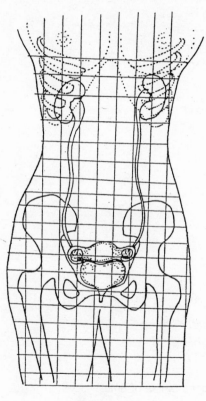

Body Grid

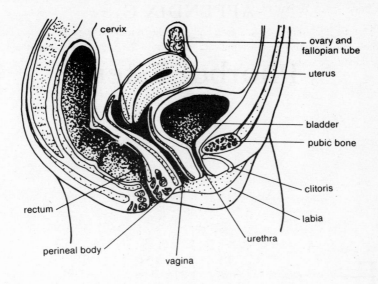

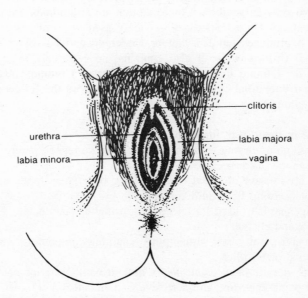

Anatomy of the Female Pelvis

APPENDIX C

Phorbol Esters

TUNG oil is extracted from seeds of the tung oil tree, *Aleurites fordii*, grown only in southern China, though small amounts are produced in the southern United States. It is widely used in varnishes and paints because it produces rapid drying or hardening and has other desirable properties. Unfortunately, it also contains the extremely toxic phorbol esters. I have found that patients suffering from Chronic Fatigue Syndrome and interstitial cystitis improve if they avoid the following products containing tung oil:

Wood oil or wood wax for furniture
Varnishes, quick-drying varnishes, most spar varnishes, many polyurethanes, some lacquers, and some shellacs
Coating for interior of metal cans used for beverages, food, and water, and for proofing fiberboard containers
Insulating varnish, used in electrical insulating laminates, insulating masses, and enamel
Anticorrosives, putty, self-setting putty, caulking compounds, wood filler, and wood panel filler
Oil paints, acrylic-latex paint, ship's bottom paint, exterior house paint, bridge paint, car paint, anti-corrosive iron and steel paint, marine paint, anti-fouling paint, quick-drying house paint, highway traffic line paint, concrete paint, waterproof concrete paint, plaster paint; in lead, tungsten, and other paint driers in resins and plastics, elastic film resistant to chemical agents, India rubber substitutes, and in synthetic rubber

Coating aluminum, aluminum paint, and anodes for brine electrolysis

Manufacture of fiberboard, press board, hardboard, wallboard in paper laminates, in photocopying paper coating and lamination of printed circuit boards, and in resins for making circuit boards

Artificial leather, shrink-proofing wool, glossy coating on rubber, linoleum manufacture, floor tile, gaskets, ground cork binder, sandpaper binder, and brake shoes

Printing ink, lithography ink, photo-curable printing inks, photo-hardenable printing inks, lithography sensitizing solution, rapid-drying printing inks, printing ink binder, photo image formation dye, and photo-sensitive paper coating

For permanent-press coating on garments

Patented in United States as cigarette tobacco additive

Stabilizer for pentachlorophenol, binder and coating for herbicide granules

Self-hardening sand molds

Used in China for polishing, preserving, and waterproofing woods, for waterproofing paper, cloth, umbrellas, bamboo hats, and nets, and occasionally to adulterate edible oils and machine oils

Soaps made in Japan

Polyurethane nail polishes, hair spray, deck seal, swamp cooler anticorrosive or caulking, and many other products requiring drying oil

APPENDIX D

Pill Guide

What follows is a pill guide of commonly prescribed medications that affect the urinary system. It is not all-encompassing and it does not cover every brand name of medicine in a given category. Drugs are listed by types of medication, generic names, and by brand names. You will learn what each drug is, whether it is important to take it with food or without, its known interactions with other drugs, and what to expect it to do for you. In addition, medications that should not be taken by patients with interstitial cystitis are marked by an asterisk (*). These drugs will increase gastric motility or affect the metabolism of serotonin, norepinephrine, or epinephrine and cause pain. I recommend that you purchase a guide to prescription drugs if you have any questions about your medication.

This guide is intended to augment the information given by your doctor. It should not take the place of your physician in prescribing medicine. If you have any questions about a drug you are taking, call and discuss them with your physician. *Never* change medication you have been prescribed based solely on information in this pill guide. Remember, in order to maintain a working partnership with your doctor you must keep him or her informed of any side effects or possible drug interactions.

Antibiotics

Antibiotics are used to treat infections that may be caused by hundreds of microorganisms known as bacteria. A urine culture identifies the specific offending "bug" and determines which antibiotics will destroy the organism. This is called sensitivity testing.

In general, antibiotics are considered either bacteriocidal or bacteriostatic.

Bacteriocidal antibiotics kill the microorganisms they affect by interfering with natural processes in cellular growth, such as the development of the cell wall or normal chemical reactions. Examples of this type of antibiotic include penicillin, ampicillin, cephalexin, nystatin, and bacitracin.

Bacteriostatic antibiotics work by disturbing chemical processes (usually stages in protein production) required by the bacteria for their reproduction. Tetracycline, doxycycline, minocycline, and erythromycin are examples of bacteriostatic antibiotics.

Finally, there is a select group of urinary antiseptics that destroy bacteria by interfering with enzymes. Macrodantin, nitrofurantoin, noroxin, and ciprofloxin are examples of this category of bacteriocidal drugs.

THE PENICILLIN FAMILY

Generic Name
Penicillin G, penicillin V, ampicillin, amoxicillin, dicloxacillin, cephalexin, cefaclor

Brand Name
SK-Penicillin G, Pfizerpen G, Pen-Vee K, Penicillin VK, Suspen, Robicillin, Omnipen, Polycillin, Amoxil, Trimox, Wymox, Dynapen, Veracillin, Keflex, Celcor, Duricef

General Information
All the members of the penicillin family are manufactured in the laboratory by fermentation and by general chemical reactions and are therefore classified as semisynthetic antibiotics. These drugs work by affecting the cell wall of the invading bacteria. The medication should be taken on an empty stomach one to two hours after meals.

Cautions and Warnings
If you have a known history of allergy to penicillin you should avoid taking any of the drugs in this category, as they are chemically very similar. The most common allergic reaction is a hivelike rash over the body with itching and redness. Occasionally there may be difficulty breathing. If so, discontinue the medication immediately and contact your physician.

Possible Side Effects
Stomach upset, nausea, vomiting, diarrhea, yeast infections, itching around the anus, fever, chills, changes in one or more components of blood, headache.

Drug Interactions
Aspirin or phenylbutazone will increase the level of free penicillin in the blood by making it more available to blood proteins. Probenecid will slow down the excretion rate in urine. The effectiveness of the penicillin family may be greatly reduced when taken with other oral antibiotics, such as tetracycline or erythromycin, which do not kill organisms but simply stop their growth.

Storage
Ampicillin and cefaclor *should be stored at room temperature,* while penicillin *should be refrigerated.*

THE SULFA FAMILY

Generic Name
azosulfisoxazole, sulfamethizole, sulfamethoxazole, sulfisoxazole

Brand Name
Azo-Gantrisin, Bactrim, Septra, Gantrisin, Sulfasox, Gantanol, Thiosulfil

General Information
Sulfa drugs have several uses. Some are used as diuretics, others to treat high blood pressure or diabetes mellitus. As antibiotics, they are most useful in treating urinary tract infections. Azo-Gantrisin contains phenazopyridine, an orange-red dye that acts as a urinary analgesic. It may interfere with urinary testing for glucose if you are a diabetic.

Cautions and Warnings
Do not take sulfa-based medications if you are allergic to them, salicylates (aspirinlike drugs), or similar agents, or if you have the disease called porphyria. Do not take a drug in this family of medications if you are pregnant or nursing, as it will be passed to the child. If you have kidney disease, do not take this medication, as toxic levels may be produced owing to lack of excretion by the damaged kidneys. Always take this medication with a large amount of water to prevent crystal formation in the kidney.

Possible Side Effects

Headache, itching, swelling around the eyes and soles of the feet, sensitivity to strong sunlight, stomach cramps, yellowing of the skin, arthritis-type pain, alterations in blood components, tiredness, dizziness, general feeling of ill health, sore throat, fever, unusual bruising, or bleeding.

Drug Interactions

When sulfa medication is taken with an anticoagulant (blood thinner), any drug used to treat diabetes, methotrexate (chemotherapy drug), phenylbutazone, salicylates (aspirinlike drugs), phenytoin, or probenecid, it causes unusually large amounts of these drugs to be released into the bloodstream and produces symptoms of overdosage. Avoid large doses of vitamin C, as the drug becomes less soluble in highly acidic urine. Also avoid large doses of para-aminobenzoic acid (PABA), as it is a competitive antagonist to sulfonamides.

THE TETRACYCLINE FAMILY

Generic Name

*tetracycline, *demeclocycline, *doxycycline, *minocycline

Brand Name

Achromycin, Deltamycin, Sumycin, Tetracyn, Tetra-B D, Declomycin, Vibramycin, Vibra Tabs, Minocin

General Information

The tetracycline family works by interfering with the normal growth cycle of the invading bacteria, preventing them from reproducing and thus allowing the body's normal defense mechanisms to fight off infection.

Cautions and Warnings

You should not use any member of the tetracycline family if you are pregnant. Children under the age of eight should also avoid this family of medication, as it has been shown to produce serious discoloration in developing permanent teeth. It may also interfere with long bone development, resulting in retarded growth. Avoid this medication if you have liver disease. The tetracycline family may interfere with your body's normal sun-screening mechanism, causing severe sunburn. This family of medication should be avoided by patients with interstitial cystitis, as it affects the bladder. Do not take these medications after the expiration date, as the decomposing drug may cause serious kidney damage. Do not take these medications with milk, antacids, or dairy products, as they will cause inactivation of the medication. Doxycycline, however, may be taken with dairy products.

Possible Side Effects
Stomach upset, nausea, vomiting, diarrhea, rash, hairy tongue, irritation of the anal or vaginal region, anemia, possible brown spotting of the skin, fever, chills, and peeling of the skin.

Drug Interactions
The tetracycline family may interfere with the action of bacteriocidal agents such as the penicillin family. Do not take multivitamin products, which contain minerals, at the same time, as they will reduce the effectiveness of the antibiotics. Space them at least two hours apart.

Storage
The tetracycline family may be stored at room temperature.

ERYTHROMYCIN

Generic Name
*erythromycin

Brand Name
E-Mycin, Erythrocin, Wyamycin, Robimycin, Eramycin, E.E.S.

General Information
Erythromycin is absorbed from the gastrointestinal tract but is deactivated by the acid content of the stomach. Because of this, the tablet form is coated in such a way as to bypass the stomach and dissolve in the intestine. It is effective against streptococcus, staphylococcus, and gonococcus.

Cautions and Warnings
Erythromycin is excreted primarily through the liver and should be used with caution by those with liver problems. This drug should be avoided by patients with interstitial cystitis, as it may interfere with the bladder.

Possible Side Effects
Nausea, vomiting, stomach cramps, hairy tongue, itching, irritation of the anal or vaginal areas, yellowing of the skin and eyes.

Drug Interactions

Erythromycin interferes with the excretion of theophylline—an asthma drug—from the body, resulting in toxic levels.

NITROFURANTOIN

Generic Name
*nitrofurantoin

Brand Name
Furadantin, Macrodantin, Nitrex, Furalan, Furan

General Information

This medication is a urinary antiseptic that affects enzymes important to bacteria for growth. It may give your urine a brownish color, which is not dangerous.

Cautions and Warnings

Nitrofurantoin should be avoided by patients with interstitial cystitis, as it may interfere with the bladder. Do not take this medication if you have kidney disease or if you are pregnant or near term.

Possible Side Effects

Fever, chills, nausea, vomiting, rash, difficulty breathing, development of fluid in the lungs, arthritislike pains, jaundice, effects on the blood components, thinning of the hair, drowsiness, loss of appetite, stomach pain, and diarrhea.

Antidepressants

Psychotropic drugs are used to alleviate anxiety. These medications affect brain chemicals called neurotransmitters, which cause such basic functions as sleep, wakefulness, and memory by altering the uptake of the transmitter at its receptor site. Each medication is designed to alter acetylcholine, norepinephrine, or serotonin uptake. As a result, some medications have anticholinergic side effects; that is, they prevent acetylcholine from being taken up at its receptor site. This causes the bladder to lose its ability to contract and empty efficiently, making it difficult to void. The tricyclic antidepressants are used by interstitial cystitis patients in low doses to prevent abnormal response to serotonin, a neurotransmitter that causes burning. Monoamine oxidase (MAO) inhibitors make you lose the ability to destroy tyramine in foods such as bananas, nuts, yogurt, wine, cheese, raisins, figs, soy sauce, chocolate, pineapple, and chicken livers rapidly, and as such should be avoided by patients with interstitial cystitis.

TRICYCLIC ANTIDEPRESSANTS

Generic Name
desipramine, amitriptyline, nortriptyline, imipramine, protriptyline

Brand Name
Norpramin, Elavil, Triavil, Aventyl, Tofranil, Limbitrol, Vivactil, Pamelor

General Information
These medications are effective in treating symptoms of depression and are useful in blocking the peptide-containing nerves in the interstitium of the bladder. These drugs are mild sedatives and may affect alertness. Appetite and sleep patterns may also be improved. Imipramine has been used to treat nighttime bed-wetting in children but it does not produce long-lasting relief.

Cautions and Warnings
You need to inform your doctor if you have a history of seizure disorders, kidney or liver problems, Parkinson's or suicidal thoughts, since these medications can worsen such conditions or precipitate an attack.

Possible Side Effects
Headache, seizures, altered taste, insomnia, nervousness, hair loss, loss of sexual function, low blood pressure, nausea, vomiting, diarrhea, and excessive sweating. Because of damage to the lining of the blood vessels, these medications cause increased vasospasming of small capillaries in the bladder.

Drug Interactions
These drugs may increase the effects of diazepam (Valium), digitalis, and phenytoin (Dilantin). When taken with insulin or oral hypoglycemics, they can cause hypoglycemia. These drugs should not be taken with any tricyclic antidepressant. Buspar (buspirone), which is used to control hot flashes, may cause increased anxiety and sweating if combined with this family of drugs.

Antihistamines

Antihistamines block the effects of histamine, a naturally occurring chemical in the body, which is released into the bloodstream in response to a foreign, irritating element. This response is sometimes called an allergic response. Antihistamines can only block the release of histamine after histamine is in the bloodstream; they cannot prevent histamine from being released. Decongestants are often added to antihistamines in order to increase shrinkage of the tissue. Common decongestants include ephedrine, phenylephrine, pseudoephedrine, and phenylpropanolamine. Decongestants work by acting on the swollen vessels and tissues, causing them to return to normal size by vasoconstriction. Decongestants should be avoided by patients with interstitial cystitis, as they will increase bladder pain by increasing the vasoconstriction already present.

ANTIHISTAMINES

Generic Name
chlorpheniramine maleate

Brand Name
Alermine, Chlorophen, Chlor-Trimeton, Chlor Tab, Histaspan, Histex, Isoclor, Phenetron, Teldrin Spansules

Generic Name
Crypoheptadine hydrochloride

Brand Name
Periactin

General Information
Antihistamines generally, and chlorpheniramine maleate specifically, act by blocking the release of the chemical substance histamine from the cell. Antihistamines work by drying up the secretions of the nose, throat, and eyes. Crypoheptadine works by competing for the serotonin and histamine receptors on a cell. This medication also has some antagonistic effect on the action of acetylcholine, a neurotransmitter.

Cautions and Warnings
These drugs should be used with extreme care if you have narrow-angle glaucoma, stomach ulcers, or problems urinating. This medicine *should not* be used by people with asthma.

Possible Side Effects

Sensitivity to light, lowering of blood pressure, confusion, tingling of the hands and feet, blurred vision, nausea, vomiting, wheezing, nasal stuffiness. Use with care if you have a history of thyroid disease, high blood pressure, heart disease, glaucoma, or diabetes.

Drug Interactions

Chlorpheniramine maleate should not be taken with MAO inhibitors. Interaction with tranquilizers, sedatives, and sleeping medication will increase the effect of these drugs. This medication will enhance the intoxicating effect of alcohol.

ANTIHISTAMINES WITH DECONGESTANTS

Brand Names

*Actifed, *Sudafed, *Tuss-Ornade, *Ornade, *Dimetane Expectorant DC, *Drixoral, *Novahistamine Elixir, *Afrin, *Sinubid

General Information

These products are marketed to help relieve the symptoms of congestion from the common cold, such as a runny nose, scratchy throat, or cough. These products are good only for the relief of symptoms and do not treat the underlying condition.

Cautions and Warnings

Do not use these medications if you are taking an MAO inhibitor, other antidepressants, or thyroid medication or if you have diabetes, interstitial cystitis, heart disease, glaucoma, or high blood pressure.

Possible Side Effects

Tension, anxiety, restlessness, inability to sleep, loss of appetite, sweating, nausea, constipation, drowsiness, difficulty voiding. The side effects of Ornade are specifically used to help prevent involuntary loss of urine in women with stress incontinence.

Drug Interactions

Do not take these medications with alcohol, tranquilizers, sleeping pills, thyroid medication, or antihypertensive medication such as reserpine and guanethidine. It is unwise to self-medicate with over-the-counter drugs in addition to these medications, as this may aggravate high blood pressure and thyroid disease.

Amphetamines

Generic Name
phendimetrazine, phentermine hydrochloride, benzphetamine hydrochloride

Brand Name
*Anorex, *Dietaps, *Ex-Obese, *Limit, *Fastin, *Parmine, *Wilpowr, *Unifast Unicelles, *Didrex

General Information
These medications are used to aid in loss of appetite and therefore weight loss. These medications are addictive and highly abusable. They should not be used by patients with interstitial cystitis, as they will increase bladder pain.

Cautions and Warnings
Do not use these medications if you have high blood pressure, thyroid disease, heart disease, glaucoma, or interstitial cystitis.

Possible Side Effects
Palpitations, dizziness, overstimulation, increased blood pressure, rapid heartbeat, hallucinations, loss of sex drive, constipation, diarrhea, dryness of the mouth.

Drug Interactions
Do not take these medications if you have taken an MAO inhibitor within the past two weeks. This may cause severe lowering of the blood pressure.

Antispasmodics

Generic Name
probantheline bromide, oxybutynin chloride, flavoxate hydrochloride, isopropamide iodide

Brand Name
Combid, Donnatol, Librax, Pro-banthine, Ditropan, Urispas, Robinul, Trans-derm Scop

General Information
These medications are prescribed for either bowel or bladder spasms. All drugs in this class will provide symptomatic relief only and will not treat the underlying condition. Each uses atropine or an atropinelike substance to prevent smooth muscle from contracting. Medication such as Trans-Derm Scop or Robinul aid in preventing bladder spasms in patients with interstitial cystitis.

Cautions and Warnings
These medications should not be used if you have glaucoma, asthma, or obstructive diseases of the urinary or gastrointestinal tract. These medications reduce your ability to sweat and may cause heat exhaustion in hot climates.

Possible Side Effects
Difficulty in urinating, blurred vision, rapid heartbeat, nasal congestion, constipation, loss of taste, bloating, itching.

Drug Interactions
These medications may interact with antihistamines, phenothiazines, tranquilizers, antidepressants, or some narcotic painkillers. Antacids should not be taken together with oral dosages of these medications, as they will reduce the absorption. Do not use with MAO inhibitors, as they may potentiate the effect of antispasmodics.

Asthma Medications

Brand Name
*Marax, *Quibron Plus, *Tedral, *Asminorel, *E.T.H. Compound, *Hydrophed, *T.E.H. Compound, *Primatene Formula, *Respirol

Ingredients
ephedrine, phenobarbital, theophyllinehydroxyzine hydrochloride

General Information
These medications are generally prescribed for patients with asthma. These products contain drugs that relieve bronchial spasm, as well as a mild tranquilizer. Other medications in this class may contain similar ingredients, which help to eliminate mucus from the respiratory passages. Any medications with ephedrine should be avoided by patients with interstitial cystitis.

Cautions and Warnings
Do not take these medications if you have severe kidney or liver disease.

Possible Side Effects
Shakiness, dizziness, dryness of the mouth, irregular heartbeat, difficulty in urination, stomach upset, diarrhea, chest pains, sweating.

Drug Interactions
These medications will increase the excretion of lithium. They will also neutralize the effect of propranolol. Erythromycin and similar antibiotics cause the body to hold theophylline, leading to possible side effects. Do not take these medications with alcohol or with MAO inhibitors.

Benzodiazepines

Generic Name
alprazolam, clonazepam, lorazepam, diazepam

Brand Name
Xanax, Klonopin, Ativan, Valium

General Information
These drugs are used to treat anxiety disorders. Clonazepam is used in the treatment of epilepsy.

Cautions and Warnings
These drugs can make you drowsy or less alert. If prescribed in high doses, they can become addicting and withdrawal symptoms may occur.

Possible Side Effects
Loss of muscular coordination, drowsiness, confusion, constipation, dry mouth, headache, hallucinations, memory loss, slurred speech, tremors.

Drug Interactions
Do not drink alcohol while taking these medications. The effect of narcotic pain relievers may be enhanced. These drugs should not be used with other tranquilizers, antidepressants or antianxiety medications.

Calcium Channel Blockers

Generic Name
Nifedipine, diltiazem, verapamil

Brand Name
  Procardia, *Cardizem, *Calan

General Information
  These medications are used to treat angina (chest pain) by relaxing the walls of blood vessels. They also affect the release of calcitonin gene-related peptide, which is contained not only in heart muscle but in the annular fibers of disks in the spine. Due to chemical conformation, diltiazem and verapamil may increase bladder pain in IC patients and therefore should be used with caution.

Cautions and Warnings
  These drugs may cause your blood pressure to become too low, making you feel light-headed or dizzy. They may also cause some fluid retention. These drugs should not be used if you have esophageal stenosis or narrowing of the bowel.

Possible Side Effects
  Constipation, nausea, sore throat, flushing, mood changes, headache, tremors, nasal congestion, muscle cramps.

Drug Interactions
  These drugs should not be taken with histamine blockers such as cimetidine (Tagamet) as the effectiveness of these drugs could be increased, decreased, or delayed.

Fluoroquinolones

Generic Name
  ofloxacin, norfloxacin, ciprofloxacin, lomefloxacin

Brand Name
  *Floxin, *Noroxin, *Cipro, *Maxaquin

General Information
  These anti-infectives work by inhibiting essential enzyme systems of bacterial nucleic acids (DNA). They also prevent bacterial reproduction.

Cautions and Warnings
  These medications have been reported to be associated with rare cases of tendon rupture, so exercising should be done with caution while on them. Latent epilepsy may be activated by this drug family.

Possible Side Effects
Vaginitis with discharge, confusion, urinary frequency, headache, rash, lowering of blood glucose, dry mouth, visual disturbances, lowering of white blood cell count, swollen or painful joints.

Drug Interactions
Iron salts will decrease the therapeutic effect of these drugs. Antacids may also decrease their absorption, as well as zinc. Warfarin will cause increased risk of bleeding if used in combination with quinolone derivatives.

Gastrointestinal Drugs

Generic Names
famotidine, nizantidine, metoclopramide, cisapride

Brand Names
*Pepcid, *Axid, *Reglan, *Propulsid

General Information
These medications are used to treat heartburn caused by reflux of acid into the esophagus. They improve esophageal movement of food, increase the lower esophageal sphincter tone, and promote gastric emptying. Interstitial cystitis patients report increased pain with these specific H-2 blockers.

Cautions and Warnings
These medications could mask a stomach ulcer and should not be taken if you have experienced a reaction to other H-2 blockers.

Possible Side Effects
Abdominal pain, diarrhea, dizziness, gas, headache, inflammation of the nose, sore throat, weakness, indigestion.

Drug Interactions
These medications can alter other drug absorption rates (see Histamine Blockers) and should not be combined with aspirin.

Histamine (H-2) Blockers

Generic Name
cimetidine, ranitidine

Brand Name
Tagamet, Zantac

General Information
These medications prevent excess production of histamine by the stomach, which can result in ulcers. They also slow down gastric emptying time. In addition, Tagamet increases the levels of estrogen in tissue and is recommended over Zantac for female patients with interstitial cystitis.

Cautions and Warnings
If you are being treated for kidney or liver problems, you should be sure your doctor is aware of this. Nursing mothers should not take these drugs as they are excreted in breast milk.

Possible Side Effects
Breast development in men, anxiety, diarrhea, dizziness, hair loss, urinary retention, rapid heartrate, sleepiness, headache.

Drug Interactions
Antacids can reduce the effect of these medications when taken at the same time. The effect of other medications can be altered by the change in gastric motility. Consult with your doctor if you take theophylline, aspirin, antiglycemic medications, digoxin, metronidazole, antiseizure medications, or antismoking medications.

Motility Stimulator

Generic Name
bethanechol chloride

Brand Name
Urecholine

General Information
Urecholine is a stimulator to smooth muscle and aids in increasing tone of the urinary and gastrointestinal tracts. By doing so, it also helps to restore rhythmic contractions and aids in evacuation and emptying.

Cautions and Warnings
This medication should not be used if you have hyperthyroidism, peptic ulcer disease, asthma, Parkinson's disease, hypotension, coronary artery disease, or epilepsy.

Possible Side Effects
Sweating, flushing, cramping, diarrhea, nausea, asthmatic attacks, headache.

Drug Interactions
The effects of this medication will be negated by the use of any antispasmodics or antidepressants that have anticholinergic properties, such as Elavil.

Nonsteroidal Anti-inflammatories (NSAIDS)

ACETIC ACIDS

Generic Name
diclofenac sodium, indomethacin, etodolac, ketorolac, nambumetone, sulindac

Brand Name
*Voltaren, *Lodine, *Indocin, *Toradol, *Relafen, *Clinoril

FENAMATES

Generic Name
meclofenamate, mefenamic acid

Brand Name
*Meclomen, *Ponstel

OXICAMS

Generic Name
piroxicam

Brand Name
*Feldene

PROPRIONIC ACIDS

Generic Name
diflunisal, fenorpofen, flurbiprofen, ibuprofen, ketoprofin, naproxen, oxaprozin

Brand Name
   *Dolobid, *Nalfon, *Ansaid, *Motrin, *Advil, *Orudis, *Naprosyn, *Aleve, *Anaprox, *Daypro

General Information
   These medications are aspirin substitutes and work by blocking the production of prostaglandins in tissue. They cause increased gastric irritability and motility and should not be used by patients with interstitial cystitis.

Cautions and Warnings
   Do not use these medications if you have a history of stomach ulcers. These drugs should be used with caution if you have liver or kidney problems. These drugs can also cause water retention and prolong the time necessary to clot blood.

Possible Side Effects
   Abdominal cramps, bloating, gas, constipation, heartburn, headache, ringing in the ears, vomiting.

Drug Interactions
   The effects of drugs, such as anticoagulants, diuretics, blood pressure medications, and medicine such as Lithium, which treats manic-depressive disorders, may be prolonged, decreased, or altered.

Urinary Dyes, Antiseptics, and Analgesics

Generic Name
   phenazopyridine hydrochloride, methylene blue, methenamine hippurate, trimethoprim

Brand Name
   Pyridium, Azo-Standard, Re-Azo, Urised, Trimpex

General Information
   The urinary dyes are often used as analgesics to help with symptomatic relief from a urinary tract infection. With the exception of Trimpex, there is little antiseptic activity. Pyridium, Azo-Standard, and Re-Azo turn urine an orange-red color, while Urised turns it blue. Atropinelike medication is combined with Pyridium and called Pyridium Plus. Urised also utilizes atropine, a medication that helps to stop smooth muscle spasms.

Cautions and Warnings

Do not take these medications if you have a folic acid deficiency, as this will cause changes in your blood. These medications do not treat the underlying problem. Do not operate machinery while taking these medications if they contain atropine or its analog.

Possible Side Effects

Itching, rash, muscle cramps, changes in blood components, nausea, fever, dry mouth, blurred vision, discoloration of the skin.

APPENDIX E

Tests and Procedures

CAT Scan

The CAT scan device gives physicians a "slice by slice" view of human anatomy. The technique (computerized axial tomography) is used in urology to view the interior of the abdomen. With it, physicians can spot cancerous tumors outside the bladder and view the kidneys, adrenal glands, blood vessels, and even stones in the ureters. A urologist might check a female patient with a CAT scan to see if any uterine or ovarian masses are affecting her urinary function.

Cystometrogram

This test measures the bladder's response to filling and voiding. Two catheters are placed in the bladder, one to carry water and one to measure pressures inside. (Some doctors use carbon dioxide rather than water.) The patient sits on a special toilet as a measured amount of water slowly fills the bladder. The pressure line measures the bladder's response to filling. The patient is asked to say when she first feels the urge to urinate. A normal bladder will be one quarter full before the urge is noticed and the pressure gauge will show no response to filling. An abnormal bladder will begin to contract much earlier and the pressure gauge will show inappropriate response to filling. In this test, the bladder is then filled to capacity. When the patient must void, the water catheter is removed and the pressure line records bladder muscle contraction. In many such tests, the patient voids into a special instrument called a uroflow (see p. 298). When a uroflow is measured with a cystometrogram, the physician has a good picture of how the bladder actually fills and empties.

Cystoscopy

This procedure allows urologists to directly view the inside of the bladder. The cystoscope is a long thin device with a series of lenses that refract light along a pathway. It is inserted into the bladder and the bladder is filled with water. Light shone through the instrument is refracted by water and is carried by the lenses back to the physician's eyes. Using cystoscopes, the urologist looks for anatomic abnormalities such as tumors or lesions in the bladder. Are the ureters in the right place? Is there stone debris? Other instruments to biopsy tissue or gain access to the ureters can be attached to the cystoscope.

Cytology

The cytology test is the Pap smear of urine. A patient collects the first urine of the day. Since it has sat in the bladder for at least six to eight hours, it tends to contain cells sloughed off from the urinary tract. The cytology test collects and stains cells taken from urine to look for abnormalities such as cancers of the urinary tract.

Electrodiagnostic Neurological Studies

There are numerous electrodiagnostic nerve conduction studies, each designed to identify specific nerve pathways, testing for any delay in the time it takes the nerve to transmit a signal from the stimulus site to the receptor site, such as the brain or another muscle. The important studies to determine if any nerve damage may be affecting the bladder are the following:

BULBOCAVERNOSUS REFLEX

This study is designed to determine whether there is any injury to the nerves in the pelvis. The stimulus goes through the clitoris, which is innervated by the L5 nerve, and is picked up by contraction of the rectal sphincter. Normal time for this to occur is 43 milliseconds. A delay greater than 45 milliseconds is considered abnormal.

DERMATOMAL CORTICAL EVOKED STUDIES

These studies determine if there is any injury to a specific nerve root in the spine. This test studies only the sensory response, which controls vascular blood flow into the tissue at the level innervated by the nerve. Electrodes are placed on the scalp and at the end sites of each nerve to be studied. Normal reception time in the brain is 43.4 milliseconds for the fourth lumbar nerve and 39.9 milliseconds for the fifth lumbar nerve. Left to right differences greater than 6 milliseconds represent instability.

H REFLEX

This study determines whether there is any damage to the first sacral nerve in the spine. A bipolar electrode is placed on the back of the knee and a jerk of the ankle is elicited within 35 milliseconds. If the difference between both legs is greater than 1.5 milliseconds, there is injury to the first sacral nerve.

PUDENDAL NERVE TERMINAL LATENCY (ST. MARKS STUDY)

This study uses a special electrode that is placed on a finger through the rectum, where it comes in contact with the pudendal nerve, which is coming through the canal on either side of the coccyx, or tailbone. The pudendal nerve controls muscle contractions in the pelvis. Normal values are 2.1 milliseconds with a standard deviation of .08 milliseconds.

IVP (Intravenous Pyelogram)

This is an X-ray study that reveals anatomic features of the urinary tract. Special iodine is injected into the patient's vein, where it quickly travels to the kidneys and on down the urinary tract. The iodine is opaque to an X-ray device. The physician can view the outlines of the kidneys, ureters, and bladder as the iodine moves along. The anatomy of the kidneys and ureters and the position of the bladder are assessed. Obstructions are located. Stones or tumors may be revealed. The test is purely anatomic; it says nothing about urinary function. (Note that people allergic to iodine cannot have this test done. If you are allergic to shellfish, you might be allergic to iodine.)

Lithotriptors

These are new devices aptly nicknamed "stone bangers." They remove stones safely and nonsurgically. The patient sits in a bath of water as the stone banger aims a special energy source onto stones. The stones break apart and small fragments soon pass painlessly from the body.

Magnetic Imaging Study (MRI)

This study uses magnetic fields to provide much more detailed images of your inner structures. The machine vibrates molecules of water in tissue, making it ideal to see soft tissue. You are placed on a table that slides into a cavelike cylinder. The machine makes a lot of banging noises. Some patients with claustrophobia may need sedation. It is best to do this study with your eyes closed before you are placed in the cylinder in order to help prevent panic attacks.

Tratner Urethrogram

This is the "double bubble" test in urology used to assess the urethra. A catheter with two balloons is placed inside the bladder. One balloon is inflated inside the bladder and the other is inflated at the opening of the urethra. Contrast material is injected through holes in the catheter. A special X ray then reveals full anatomic detail of the urethra only. Diverticula, infected Skene's glands, tumors, or other abnormalities may be seen.

Ultrasound

This is sonar of the urinary tract. Sound waves are used to view anatomic features of tissue. The images are less clear than those of other methods, but ultrasound is totally noninvasive and painless. It is safe for use in pregnant women and others at special risk for more invasive techniques. It uses no radiation.

Urinalysis

This is the type of urine test that can be done immediately in the physician's office. A urine sample is collected and screened for blood, pus, stones, pH, glucose, ketones, bile, specific gravity, and other factors. Bacteria are often found but can derive from pubic hair or other external sources. A urinalysis should not be used as an absolute test for cystitis. It is merely a screening test.

Urine Culture

A urine culture is the definitive test for bacterial infection of the urinary tract. The patient must take great care to collect urine voided in midstream to avoid contamination with external bacteria. The sample is cultured for twenty-four hours on special growth media. The type and extent of bacterial infection can then be determined.

Uroflow

This test measures the patient's flow rate. She sits on a special toilet seat and voids with a full bladder. The weight and duration of urinary flow moves an arm on a special graphing device below. This measures the speed and rate at which she voids.

Voiding Cystourethrogram (VCUG)

This is an X-ray study done to determine the anatomic position of the bladder neck and to check the position of the ureters to assess reflux (the backward flow of urine). A catheter is placed in the bladder and contrast material is added. The X ray shows the angle of support to the bladder neck and to the base of the bladder. The catheter is removed and the patient is asked to cough or strain. If urine leaks out, the condition known as stress incontinence can be diagnosed. Urinary stress incontinence results from a lack of support, which prevents the bladder neck from closing strongly enough to keep urine from passing when you suddenly cough, sneeze, or laugh. If the contrast material goes up toward the kidneys, the patient is shown to have reflux.

Index

THE BELL JAR

Sylvia Plath was born in Boston in 1932. She graduated from Smith College in 1955 and went on to Cambridge University on a Fulbright scholarship, where she met and later married Ted Hughes. She began writing poetry as a child and wrote stories from her mid-teens. *The Bell Jar* is her only novel and was originally published under a pseudonym in 1963, a few weeks before her suicide. She published one volume of poetry, *The Colossus*, in her lifetime. Posthumous publications include a collection of prose, *Johnny Panic and the Bible of Dreams*, and *Ariel*, a poetry collection.

by the same author

poetry

Sylvia Plath Poems chosen by Carol Ann Duffy
Ariel
Collected Poems (ed. Ted Hughes)
The Colossus
Crossing the Water
Selected Poems (ed. Ted Hughes)
Winter Trees

fiction
Johnny Panic and the Bible of Dreams
and Other Prose Writings

for children
The Bed Book
(illustrated by Quentin Blake)
The It-Doesn't-Matter Suit
(illustrated by Rotraut Susanne Berner)

biography
Letters Home: Correspondence 1950-1963
(ed. Aurelia Schober Plath)

The Journals of Sylvia Plath 1950-1962
(ed. Karen V. Kukil)

illustrated
Sylvia Plath: Drawings

SYLVIA PLATH

The Bell Jar

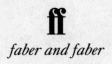

faber and faber

First published in 1963
by William Heinemann Limited
Published in 1966
by Faber and Faber Limited
Bloomsbury House
74–77 Great Russell Street
London WC1B 3DA

This edition first published in 2005

Photoset by Parker Typesetting Service, Leicester
Printed and bound by CPI Group (UK) Ltd, Croydon, CR0 4YY

All rights reserved

© Sylvia Plath, 1963

Sylvia Plath is hereby identified as author of this work in accordance with
Section 77 of the Copyright, Designs and Patents Act 1988

*This book is sold subject to the condition that it shall not, by way of trade
or otherwise, be lent, resold, hired out or otherwise circulated without the
publisher's prior consent in any form of binding or cover other than that
in which it is published and without a similar condition including
this condition being imposed on the subsequent purchaser.*

A CIP record for this book
is available from the British Library

ISBN 978-0-571-22616-0

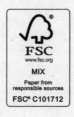

FSC
www.fsc.org
MIX
Paper from
responsible sources
FSC® C101712

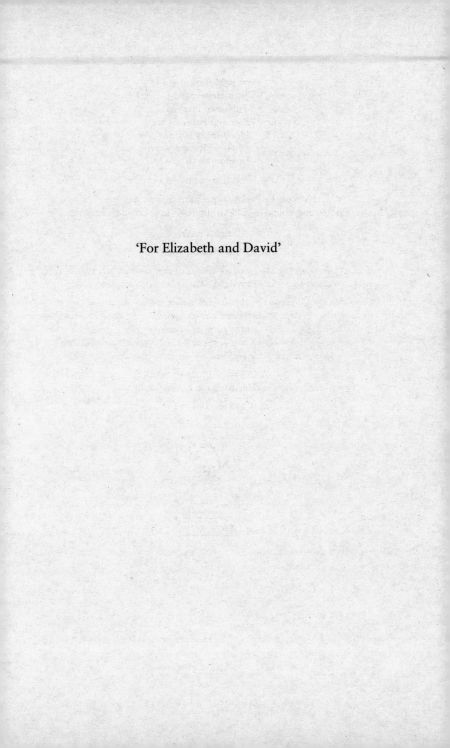

'For Elizabeth and David'

Chapter One

It was a queer, sultry summer, the summer they electrocuted the Rosenbergs, and I didn't know what I was doing in New York. I'm stupid about executions. The idea of being electrocuted makes me sick, and that's all there was to read about in the papers – goggle-eyed headlines staring up at me on every street corner and at the fusty, peanut-smelling mouth of every subway. It had nothing to do with me, but I couldn't help wondering what it would be like, being burned alive all along your nerves.

I thought it must be the worst thing in the world.

New York was bad enough. By nine in the morning the fake, country-wet freshness that somehow seeped in overnight evaporated like the tail end of a sweet dream. Mirage-grey at the bottom of their granite canyons, the hot streets wavered in the sun, the car tops sizzled and glittered, and the dry, cindery dust blew into my eyes and down my throat.

I kept hearing about the Rosenbergs over the radio and at the office till I couldn't get them out of my mind. It was like the first time I saw a cadaver. For weeks afterwards, the cadaver's head – or what there was left of it – floated up behind my eggs and bacon at breakfast and behind the face of Buddy Willard, who was responsible for my seeing it in the first place, and pretty soon I felt as though I were carrying that cadaver's head around with me on a string, like some black, noseless balloon stinking of vinegar.

I knew something was wrong with me that summer, because all I could think about was the Rosenbergs and how stupid I'd been to buy all those uncomfortable, expensive clothes, hanging limp as fish in my closet, and how all the little successes I'd totted up so happily at college fizzled to nothing outside the slick marble and plate-glass fronts along Madison Avenue.

I was supposed to be having the time of my life.

I was supposed to be the envy of thousands of other college girls just like me all over America who wanted nothing more than to be tripping about in those same size seven patent leather shoes I'd bought in Bloomingdale's one lunch hour with a black patent leather belt and black patent leather pocket-book to match. And when my picture came out in the magazine the twelve of us were working on – drinking martinis in a skimpy, imitation silver-lamé bodice stuck on to a big, fat cloud of white tulle, on some Starlight Roof, in the company of several anonymous young men with all-American bone structures hired or loaned for the occasion – everybody would think I must be having a real whirl.

Look what can happen in this country, they'd say. A girl lives in some out-of-the-way town for nineteen years, so poor she can't afford a magazine, and then she gets a scholarship to college and wins a prize here and a prize there and ends up steering New York like her own private car.

Only I wasn't steering anything, not even myself. I just bumped from my hotel to work and to parties and from parties to my hotel and back to work like a numb trolley-bus. I guess I should have been excited the way most of the other girls were, but I couldn't get myself to react. I felt very still and very empty, the way the eye of a tornado must feel, moving dully along in the middle of the surrounding hullabaloo.

There were twelve of us at the hotel.

We had all won a fashion magazine contest, by writing essays and stories and poems and fashion blurbs, and as prizes they gave us jobs in New York for a month, expenses paid, and piles and piles of free bonuses, like ballet tickets and passes to fashion shows and hair stylings at a famous expensive salon and chances to meet successful people in the field of our desire and advice about what to do with our particular complexions.

I still have the make-up kit they gave me, fitted out for a person with brown eyes and brown hair: an oblong of brown mascara with a tiny brush, and a round basin of blue eye-shadow just big enough to dab the tip of your finger in, and three lipsticks ranging from red to pink, all cased in the same little gilt box with a mirror on one side. I also have a white plastic sun-glasses case with coloured shells and sequins and a green plastic starfish sewed on to it.

I realized we kept piling up these presents because it was as good as free advertising for the firms involved, but I couldn't be cynical. I got such a kick out of all those free gifts showering on to us. For a long time afterwards I hid them away, but later, when I was all right again, I brought them out, and I still have them around the house. I use the lipsticks now and then, and last week I cut the plastic starfish off the sun-glasses case for the baby to play with.

So there were twelve of us at the hotel, in the same wing on the same floor in single rooms, one after the other, and it reminded me of my dormitory at college. It wasn't a proper hotel – I mean a hotel where there are both men and women mixed about here and there on the same floor.

3

This hotel – the Amazon – was for women only, and they were mostly girls my age with wealthy parents who wanted to be sure their daughters would be living where men couldn't get at them and deceive them; and they were all going to posh secretarial schools like Katy Gibbs, where they had to wear hats and stockings and gloves to class, or they had just graduated from places like Katy Gibbs and were secretaries to executives and junior executives and simply hanging around in New York waiting to get married to some career man or other.

These girls looked awfully bored to me. I saw them on the sun-roof, yawning and painting their nails and trying to keep up their Bermuda tans, and they seemed bored as hell. I talked with one of them, and she was bored with yachts and bored with flying around in aeroplanes and bored with skiing in Switzerland at Christmas and bored with the men in Brazil.

Girls like that make me sick. I'm so jealous I can't speak. Nineteen years, and I hadn't been out of New England except for this trip to New York. It was my first big chance, but here I was, sitting back and letting it run through my fingers like so much water.

I guess one of my troubles was Doreen.

I'd never known a girl like Doreen before. Doreen came from a society girls' college down South and had bright white hair standing out in a cotton candy fluff round her head and blue eyes like transparent agate marbles, hard and polished and just about indestructible, and a mouth set in a sort of perpetual sneer. I don't mean a nasty sneer, but an amused, mysterious sneer, as if all the people around her were pretty silly and she could tell some good jokes on them if she wanted to.

Doreen singled me out right away. She made me feel I was that much sharper than the others, and she really was wonderfully funny. She used to sit next to me at the conference table, and when the visiting celebrities were talking she'd whisper witty sarcastic remarks to me under her breath.

Her college was so fashion-conscious, she said, that all the girls had pocket-book covers made out of the same material as their dresses, so each time they changed their clothes they had a matching pocket-book. This kind of detail impressed me. It suggested a whole life of marvellous, elaborate decadence that attracted me like a magnet.

The only thing Doreen ever bawled me out about was bothering to get my assignments in by a deadline.

'What are you sweating over that for?' Doreen lounged on my bed in a peach silk dressing-gown, filing her long, nicotine-yellow nails with an emery board, while I typed up the draft of an interview with a best-selling novelist.

That was another thing – the rest of us had starched cotton summer nighties and quilted housecoats, or maybe terry-towel robes that doubled as beachcoats, but Doreen wore these full-length nylon and lace jobs you could half see through, and dressing-gowns the colour of sin, that stuck to her by some kind of electricity. She had an interesting, slightly sweaty smell that reminded me of those scallopy leaves of sweet fern you break off and crush between your fingers for the musk of them.

'You know old Jay Cee won't give a damn if that story's in tomorrow or Monday.' Doreen lit a cigarette and let the smoke flare slowly from her nostrils so her eyes were veiled. 'Jay Cee's ugly as sin,' Doreen went on coolly. 'I bet that old husband of hers turns out all the lights before he gets near her or he'd puke otherwise.'

Jay Cee was my boss, and I liked her a lot, in spite of what Doreen said. She wasn't one of the fashion magazine gushers with fake eyelashes and giddy jewellery. Jay Cee had brains, so her plug-ugly looks didn't seem to matter. She read a couple of languages and knew all the quality writers in the business.

5

I tried to imagine Jay Cee out of her strict office suit and luncheon-duty hat and in bed with her fat husband, but I just couldn't do it. I always had a terribly hard time trying to imagine people in bed together.

Jay Cee wanted to teach me something, all the old ladies I ever knew wanted to teach me something, but I suddenly didn't think they had anything to teach me. I fitted the lid on my typewriter and clicked it shut.

Doreen grinned. 'Smart girl.'

Somebody tapped at the door.

'Who is it?' I didn't bother to get up.

'It's me, Betsy. Are you coming to the party?'

'I guess so.' I still didn't go to the door.

They imported Betsy straight from Kansas with her bouncing blonde ponytail and Sweetheart-of-Sigma-Chi smile. I remember once the two of us were called over to the office of some blue-chinned TV producer in a pin-stripe suit to see if we had any angles he could build up for a programme, and Betsy started to tell about the male and female corn in Kansas. She got so excited about that damn corn even the producer had tears in his eyes, only he couldn't use any of it, unfortunately, he said.

Later on, the Beauty Editor persuaded Betsy to cut her hair and made a cover girl out of her, and I still see her face now and then, smiling out of those 'P.Q.'s wife wears B.H. Wragge' ads.

Betsy was always asking me to do things with her and the other girls as if she were trying to save me in some way. She never asked Doreen. In private, Doreen called her Pollyanna Cowgirl.

'Do you want to come in our cab?' Betsy said through the door.

Doreen shook her head.

'That's all right, Betsy,' I said. 'I'm going with Doreen.'

'Okay.' I could hear Betsy padding off down the hall.

'We'll just go till we get sick of it,' Doreen told me, stubbing out her cigarette in the base of my bedside reading-lamp, 'then we'll go out on the town. Those parties they stage here remind me of the old dances in the school gym. Why do they always round up Yalies? They're so *stoo*-pit!'

Buddy Willard went to Yale, but now I thought of it, what was wrong with him was that he was stupid. Oh, he'd managed to get good marks all right, and to have an affair with some awful waitress on the Cape by the name of Gladys, but he didn't have one speck of intuition. Doreen had intuition. Everything she said was like a secret voice speaking straight out of my own bones.

We were stuck in the theatre-hour rush. Our cab sat wedged in back of Betsy's cab and in front of a cab with four of the other girls, and nothing moved.

Doreen looked terrific. She was wearing a strapless white lace dress zipped up over a snug corset affair that curved her in at the middle and bulged her out again spectacularly above and below, and her skin had a bronzy polish under the pale dusting-powder. She smelled strong as a whole perfume store.

I wore a black shantung sheath that cost me forty dollars. It was part of a buying spree I had with some of my scholarship money when I heard I was one of the lucky ones going to New York. This dress was cut so queerly I couldn't wear any sort of a bra under it, but that didn't matter much as I was skinny as a boy and barely rippled, and I liked feeling almost naked on the hot summer nights.

The city had faded my tan, though. I looked yellow as a Chinaman. Ordinarily, I would have been nervous about my dress and my odd colour, but being with Doreen made me forget my worries. I felt wise and cynical as all hell.

When the man in the blue lumber shirt and black chinos and tooled leather cowboy boots started to stroll over to us from under the striped awning of the bar where he'd been eyeing our cab, I didn't have any illusions. I knew perfectly well he'd come for Doreen. He threaded his way out between the stopped cars and leaned engagingly on the sill of our open window.

'And what, may I ask, are two nice girls like you doing all alone in a cab on a nice night like this?'

He had a big, wide, white tooth-paste-ad smile.

'We're on our way to a party,' I blurted, since Doreen had gone suddenly dumb as a post and was fiddling in a blasé way with her white lace pocket-book cover.

'That sounds boring,' the man said. 'Whyn't you both join me for a couple of drinks in that bar over there? I've some friends waiting as well.'

He nodded in the direction of several informally dressed men slouching around under the awning. They had been following him with their eyes, and when he glanced back at them, they burst out laughing.

The laughter should have warned me. It was a kind of low, know-it-all snicker, but the traffic showed signs of moving again, and I knew that if I sat tight, in two seconds I'd be wishing I'd taken this gift of a chance to see something of New York besides what the people on the magazine had planned out for us so carefully.

'How about it, Doreen?' I said.

'How about it, Doreen?' the man said, smiling his big smile. To this day I can't remember what he looked like when he wasn't smiling. I think he must have been smiling the whole time. It must have been natural for him, smiling like that.

'Well, all right,' Doreen said to me. I opened the door, and we stepped out of the cab just as it was edging ahead again and started to walk over to the bar.

There was a terrible shriek of brakes followed by a dull thump-thump.

'Hey you!' Our cabby was craning out of his window with a furious, purple expression. 'Waddaya think you're doin'?'

He had stopped the cab so abruptly that the cab behind bumped smack into him, and we could see the four girls inside waving and struggling and scrambling up off the floor.

The man laughed and left us on the kerb and went back and handed a bill to the driver in the middle of a great honking and some yelling, and then we saw the girls from the magazine moving off in a row, one cab after another, like a wedding party with nothing but bridesmaids.

'Come on, Frankie,' the man said to one of his friends in the group, and a short, scrunty fellow detached himself and came into the bar with us.

He was the type of fellow I can't stand. I'm five feet ten in my stocking feet, and when I am with little men I stoop over a bit and slouch my hips, one up and one down, so I'll look shorter, and I feel gawky and morbid as somebody in a side-show.

For a minute I had a wild hope we might pair off according to size, which would line me up with the man who had spoken to us in the first place, and he cleared a good six feet, but he went ahead with Doreen and didn't give me a second look. I tried to pretend I didn't see Frankie dogging along at my elbow and sat close by Doreen at the table.

It was so dark in the bar I could hardly make out anything except Doreen. With her white hair and white dress she was so white she looked silver. I think she must have reflected the neons over the bar. I felt myself melting into the shadows like the negative of a person I'd never seen before in my life.

'Well, what'll we have?' the man asked with a large smile.

'I think I'll have an Old-Fashioned,' Doreen said to me.

Ordering drinks always floored me. I didn't know whisky

from gin and never managed to get anything I really liked the taste of. Buddy Willard and the other college boys I knew were usually too poor to buy hard liquor or they scorned drinking altogether. It's amazing how many college boys don't drink or smoke. I seemed to know them all. The farthest Buddy Willard ever went was buying us a bottle of Dubonnet, which he only did because he was trying to prove he could be aesthetic in spite of being a medical student.

'I'll have a vodka,' I said.

The man looked at me more closely. 'With anything?'

'Just plain,' I said. 'I always have it plain.'

I thought I might make a fool of myself by saying I'd have it with ice or soda or gin or anything. I'd seen a vodka ad once, just a glass full of vodka standing in the middle of a snowdrift in a blue light, and the vodka looked clear and pure as water, so I thought having vodka plain must be all right. My dream was some day ordering a drink and finding out it tasted wonderful.

The waiter came up then, and the man ordered drinks for the four of us. He looked so at home in that citified bar in his ranch outfit I thought he might well be somebody famous.

Doreen wasn't saying a word, she only toyed with her cork place-mat and eventually lit a cigarette, but the man didn't seem to mind. He kept staring at her the way people stare at the great white macaw in the zoo, waiting for it to say something human.

The drinks arrived, and mine looked clear and pure, just like the vodka ad.

'What do you do?' I asked the man, to break the silence shooting up around me on all sides, thick as jungle grass. 'I mean what do you do here in New York?'

Slowly and with what seemed a great effort, the man dragged his eyes away from Doreen's shoulder. 'I'm a disc jockey,' he said. 'You prob'ly must have heard of me. The name's Lenny Shepherd.'

'I know you,' Doreen said suddenly.

'I'm glad about that, honey,' the man said, and burst out laughing. 'That'll come in handy. I'm famous as hell.'

Then Lenny Shepherd gave Frankie a long look.

'Say, where do you come from?' Frankie asked, sitting up with a jerk. 'What's your name?'

'This here's Doreen.' Lenny slid his hand around Doreen's bare arm and gave her a squeeze.

What surprised me was that Doreen didn't let on she noticed what he was doing. She just sat there, dusky as a bleached blonde negress in her white dress and sipped daintily at her drink.

'My name's Elly Higginbottom,' I said. 'I come from Chicago.' After that I felt safer. I didn't want anything I said or did that night to be associated with me and my real name and coming from Boston.

'Well, Elly, what do you say we dance some?'

The thought of dancing with that little runt in his orange suede elevator shoes and mingy T-shirt and droopy blue sports coat made me laugh. If there's anything I look down on, it's a man in a blue outfit. Black or grey, or brown, even. Blue just makes me laugh.

'I'm not in the mood,' I said coldly, turning my back on him and hitching my chair over nearer to Doreen and Lenny.

Those two looked as if they'd known each other for years by now. Doreen was spooning up the hunks of fruit at the bottom of her glass with a spindly silver spoon, and Lenny was grunting each time she lifted the spoon to her mouth, and snapping and pretending to be a dog or something, and trying to get the fruit off the spoon. Doreen giggled and kept spooning up the fruit.

I began to think vodka was my drink at last. It didn't taste like anything, but it went straight down into my stomach like a sword-swallower's sword and made me feel powerful and god-like.

'I better go now,' Frankie said, standing up.

I couldn't see him very clearly, the place was so dim, but for the first time I heard what a high, silly voice he had. Nobody paid him any notice.

'Hey, Lenny, you owe me something. Remember, Lenny, you owe me something, don't you, Lenny?'

I thought it odd Frankie should be reminding Lenny he owed him something in front of us, and we being perfect strangers, but Frankie stood there saying the same thing over and over until Lenny dug into his pocket and pulled out a big roll of green bills and peeled one off and handed it to Frankie. I think it was ten dollars.

'Shut up and scram.'

For a minute I thought Lenny was talking to me as well, but then I heard Doreen say 'I won't come unless Elly comes'. I had to hand it to her the way she picked up my fake name.

'Oh, Elly'll come, won't you, Elly?' Lenny said, giving me a wink.

'Sure I'll come,' I said. Frankie had wilted away into the night, so I thought I'd string along with Doreen. I wanted to see as much as I could.

I liked looking on at other people in crucial situations. If there was a road accident or a street fight or a baby pickled in a laboratory jar for me to look at, I'd stop and look so hard I never forgot it.

I certainly learned a lot of things I never would have learned otherwise this way, and even when they surprised me or made me sick I never let on, but pretended that's the way I knew things were all the time.

Chapter Two

I wouldn't have missed Lenny's place for anything.

It was built exactly like the inside of a ranch, only in the middle of a New York apartment house. He'd had a few partitions knocked down to make the place broaden out, he said, and then had them pine-panel the walls and fit up a special pine-panelled bar in the shape of a horseshoe. I think the floor was pine-panelled, too.

Great white bearskins lay about underfoot, and the only furniture was a lot of low beds covered with Indian rugs. Instead of pictures hung up on the walls, he had antlers and buffalo horns and a stuffed rabbit head. Lenny jutted a thumb at the meek little grey muzzle and stiff jackrabbit ears.

'Ran over that in Las Vegas.'

He walked away across the room, his cowboy boots echoing like pistol shots. 'Acoustics,' he said, and grew smaller and smaller until he vanished through a door in the distance.

All at once music started to come out of the air on every side. Then it stopped, and we heard Lenny's voice say 'This is your twelve o'clock disc jock, Lenny Shepherd, with a round-up of the tops in pops. Number Ten in the wagon train this week is none other than that little yaller-haired gal you been hearin' so much about lately . . . the one an' only *Sunflower*!'

I was born in Kansas, I was bred in Kansas,
And when I marry I'll wed in Kansas . . .

'What a card!' Doreen said. 'Isn't he a card?'

'You bet,' I said.

'Listen, Elly, do me a favour.' She seemed to think Elly was who I really was by now.

'Sure,' I said.

'Stick around, will you? I wouldn't have a chance if he tried anything funny. Did you see that muscle?' Doreen giggled.

Lenny popped out of the back room. 'I got twenty grand's worth of recording equipment in there.' He ambled over to the bar and set out three glasses and a silver ice-bucket and a big pitcher and began to mix drinks from several different bottles.

. . . to a true-blue gal who promised she would wait –
She's the sunflower of the Sunflower State.

'Terrific, huh?' Lenny came over, balancing three glasses. Big drops stood out on them like sweat, and the ice-cubes jingled as he passed them round. Then the music twanged to a stop, and we heard Lenny's voice announcing the next number.

'Nothing like listening to yourself talk. Say,' Lenny's eye lingered on me, 'Frankie vamoosed, you ought to have somebody, I'll call up one of the fellers.'

'That's okay,' I said. 'You don't have to do that.' I didn't want to come straight out and ask for somebody several sizes larger than Frankie.

Lenny looked relieved. 'Just so's you don't mind. I wouldn't want to do wrong by a friend of Doreen's.' He gave Doreen a big white smile. 'Would I, honeybun?'

He held out a hand to Doreen, and without a word they both started to jitterbug, still hanging on to their glasses.

I sat cross-legged on one of the beds and tried to look devout and impassive like some businessmen I once saw watching an Algerian belly-dancer, but as soon as I leaned back against the wall under the stuffed rabbit, the bed started to roll out into the room, so I sat down on a bearskin on the floor and leaned back against the bed instead.

My drink was wet and depressing. Each time I took another sip it tasted more and more like dead water. Around the middle of the glass there was painted a pink lasso with yellow polka dots. I drank to about an inch below the lasso and waited a bit, and when I went to take another sip, the drink was up to lasso-level again.

Out of the air Lenny's ghost voice boomed, '*Wye oh wye did I ever leave Wyoming?*'

The two of them didn't even stop jitterbugging during the intervals. I felt myself shrinking to a small black dot against all those red and white rugs and that pine-panelling. I felt like a hole in the ground.

There is something demoralizing about watching two people get more and more crazy about each other, especially when you are the only extra person in the room.

It's like watching Paris from an express caboose heading in the opposite direction – every second the city gets smaller and smaller, only you feel it's really you getting smaller and smaller and lonelier and lonelier, rushing away from all those lights and that excitement at about a million miles an hour.

Every so often Lenny and Doreen would bang into each other and kiss and then swing back to take a long drink and close in on each other again. I thought I might just lie down on the bearskin and go to sleep until Doreen felt ready to go back to the hotel.

Then Lenny gave a terrible roar. I sat up. Doreen was hanging on to Lenny's left earlobe with her teeth.

'Leggo, you bitch!'

Lenny stooped, and Doreen went flying up on to his shoulder, and her glass sailed out of her hand in a long, wide arc and fetched up against the pine-panelling with a silly tinkle. Lenny was still roaring and whirling round so fast I couldn't see Doreen's face.

I noticed, in the routine way you notice the colour of somebody's eyes, that Doreen's breasts had popped out of her dress and were swinging out slightly like full brown melons as she circled belly-down on Lenny's shoulder, thrashing her legs in the air and screeching, and then they both started to laugh and slow up, and Lenny was trying to bite Doreen's hip through her skirt when I let myself out of the door before anything more could happen and managed to get downstairs by leaning with both hands on the banister and half sliding the whole way.

I didn't realize Lenny's place had been air-conditioned until I wavered out on to the pavement. The tropical, stale heat the sidewalks had been sucking up all day hit me in the face like a last insult. I didn't know where in the world I was.

For a minute I entertained the idea of taking a cab to the party after all, but decided against it because the dance might be over by now, and I didn't feel like ending up in an empty barn of a ballroom strewn with confetti and cigarette-butts and crumpled cocktail napkins.

I walked carefully to the nearest street corner, brushing the wall of the buildings on my left with the tip of one finger to steady myself. I looked at the street sign. Then I took my New York street map out of my pocket-book. I was exactly forty-three blocks by five blocks away from my hotel.

Walking has never fazed me. I just set out in the right direction, counting the blocks under my breath, and when I walked into the lobby of the hotel I was perfectly sober and my feet only slightly swollen, but that was my own fault because I hadn't bothered to wear any stockings.

The lobby was empty except for a night clerk dozing in his lit booth among the key-rings and the silent telephones.

I slid into the self-service elevator and pushed the button for my floor. The doors folded shut like a noiseless accordion. Then my ears went funny, and I noticed a big, smudgy-eyed Chinese woman staring idiotically into my face. It was only me, of course. I was appalled to see how wrinkled and used-up I looked.

There wasn't a soul in the hall. I let myself into my room. It was full of smoke. At first I thought the smoke had materialized out of thin air as a sort of judgement, but then I remembered it was Doreen's smoke and pushed the button that opened the window vent. They had the windows fixed so you couldn't really open them and lean out, and for some reason this made me furious.

By standing at the left side of the window and laying my cheek to the woodwork, I could see downtown to where the UN balanced itself in the dark, like a weird, green, Martian honeycomb. I could see the moving red and white lights along the drive and the lights of the bridges whose names I didn't know.

The silence depressed me. It wasn't the silence of silence. It was my own silence.

I knew perfectly well the cars were making a noise, and the people in them and behind the lit windows of the buildings were making a noise, and the river was making a noise, but I couldn't hear a thing. The city hung in my window, flat as a poster, glittering and blinking, but it might just as well not have been there at all, for all the good it did me.

The china-white bedside telephone could have connected me up with things, but there it sat, dumb as a death's head. I tried to think of people I'd given my phone number to, so I could make a list of all the possible calls I might be about to receive, but all I could think of was that I'd given my phone number to Buddy Willard's mother so she could give it to a simultaneous interpreter she knew at the UN.

I let out a small, dry laugh.

I could imagine the sort of simultaneous interpreter Mrs Willard would introduce me to when all the time she wanted me to marry Buddy, who was taking the cure for TB somewhere in upper New York State. Buddy's mother had even arranged for me to be given a job as a waitress at the TB sanatorium that summer so Buddy wouldn't be lonely. She and Buddy couldn't understand why I chose to go to New York City instead.

The mirror over my bureau seemed slightly warped and much too silver. The face in it looked like the reflection in a ball of dentist's mercury. I thought of crawling in between the bed sheets and trying to sleep, but that appealed to me about as much as stuffing a dirty, scrawled-over letter into a fresh, clean envelope. I decided to take a hot bath.

There must be quite a few things a hot bath won't cure, but I don't know many of them. Whenever I'm sad I'm going to die, or so nervous I can't sleep, or in love with somebody I won't be seeing for a week, I slump down just so far and then I say: 'I'll go take a hot bath.'

I meditate in the bath. The water needs to be very hot, so hot you can barely stand putting your foot in it. Then you lower yourself, inch by inch, till the water's up to your neck.

I remember the ceilings over every bathtub I've stretched out in. I remember the texture of the ceilings and the cracks and the colours and the damp spots and the light fixtures. I remember the tubs, too: the antique griffin-legged tubs, and the modern coffin-shaped tubs, and the fancy pink marble tubs overlooking indoor lily ponds, and I remember the shapes and sizes of the water taps and the different sorts of soap-holders.

I never feel so much myself as when I'm in a hot bath.

I lay in that tub on the seventeenth floor of this hotel for-women-only, high up over the jazz and push of New York, for near on to an hour, and I felt myself growing pure again. I don't believe in baptism or the waters of Jordan or anything like that, but I guess I feel about a hot bath the way those religious people feel about holy water.

I said to myself: 'Doreen is dissolving, Lenny Shepherd is dissolving, Frankie is dissolving, New York is dissolving, they are all dissolving away and none of them matter any more. I don't know them, I have never known them and I am very pure. All that liquor and those sticky kisses I saw and the dirt that settled on my skin on the way back is turning into something pure.'

The longer I lay there in the clear hot water the purer I felt, and when I stepped out at last and wrapped myself in one of the big, soft, white, hotel bath towels I felt pure and sweet as a new baby.

I don't know how long I had been asleep when I heard the knocking. I didn't pay any attention at first, because the person knocking kept saying 'Elly, Elly, Elly, let me in', and I didn't know any Elly. Then another kind of knock sounded over the first dull, bumping knock – a sharp tap-tap, and another, much crisper voice said 'Miss Greenwood, your friend wants you,' and I knew it was Doreen.

I swung to my feet and balanced dizzily for a minute in the middle of the dark room. I felt angry with Doreen for waking me up. All I stood a chance of getting out of that sad night was a good sleep, and she had to wake me up and spoil it. I thought if I pretended to be asleep the knocking might go away and leave me in peace, but I waited, and it didn't.

'Elly, Elly, Elly,' the first voice mumbled, while the other voice went on hissing 'Miss Greenwood, Miss Greenwood, Miss Greenwood', as if I had a split personality or something.

I opened the door and blinked out into the bright hall. I had the impression it wasn't night and it wasn't day, but some lurid third interval that had suddenly slipped between them and would never end.

Doreen was slumped against the door-jamb. When I came out, she toppled into my arms. I couldn't see her face because her head was hanging down on her chest and her stiff blonde hair fell from its dark roots like a hula fringe.

I recognized the short, squat, moustached woman in the black uniform as the night maid who ironed day-dresses and party-frocks in a crowded cubicle on our floor. I couldn't understand how she came to know Doreen or why she should want to help Doreen wake me up instead of leading her quietly back to her own room.

Seeing Doreen supported in my arms and silent except for a few wet hiccups, the woman strode away down the hall to her cubicle with its ancient Singer sewing-machine and white ironing-board. I wanted to run after her and tell her I had nothing to do with Doreen, because she looked stern and hard-working and moral as an old-style European immigrant and reminded me of my Austrian grandmother.

'Lemme lie down, lemme lie down,' Doreen was muttering. 'Lemme lie down, lemme lie down.'

I felt if I carried Doreen across the threshold into my room and helped her on to my bed I would never get rid of her again.

Her body was warm and soft as a pile of pillows against my arm where she leaned her weight, and her feet, in their high, spiked heels, dragged foolishly. She was much too heavy for me to budge down the long hall.

I decided the only thing to do was to dump her on the carpet and shut and lock my door and go back to bed. When Doreen woke up she wouldn't remember what had happened and would think she must have passed out in front of my door while I slept, and she would get up of her own accord and go sensibly back to her room.

I started to lower Doreen gently on to the green hall carpet, but she gave a low moan and pitched forward out of my arms. A jet of brown vomit flew from her mouth and spread in a large puddle at my feet.

Suddenly Doreen grew even heavier. Her head drooped forward into the puddle, the wisps of her blonde hair dabbling in it like tree roots in a bog, and I realized she was asleep. I drew back. I felt half-asleep myself.

I made a decision about Doreen that night. I decided I would watch her and listen to what she said, but deep down I would have nothing at all to do with her. Deep down, I would be loyal to Betsy and her innocent friends. It was Betsy I resembled at heart.

Quietly, I stepped back into my room and shut the door. On second thoughts, I didn't lock it. I couldn't quite bring myself to do that.

When I woke up in the dull, sunless heat the next morning, I dressed and splashed my face with cold water and put on some lipstick and opened the door slowly. I think I still expected to see Doreen's body lying there in the pool of vomit like an ugly, concrete testimony to my own dirty nature.

There was nobody in the hall. The carpet stretched from one end of the hall to the other, clean and eternally verdant except for a faint, irregular dark stain before my door as if somebody had by accident spilled a glass of water there, but dabbed it dry again.

Chapter Three

Arrayed on the *Ladies' Day* banquet table were yellow-green avocado pear halves stuffed with crabmeat and mayonnaise, and platters of rare roast beef and cold chicken, and every so often a cut-glass bowl heaped with black caviar. I hadn't had time to eat any breakfast at the hotel cafeteria that morning, except for a cup of over-stewed coffee so bitter it made my nose curl, and I was starving.

Before I came to New York I'd never eaten out in a proper restaurant. I don't count Howard Johnson's, where I only had French fries and cheeseburgers and vanilla frappes with people like Buddy Willard. I'm not sure why it is, but I love food more than just about anything else. No matter how much I eat, I never put on weight. With one exception I've been the same weight for ten years.

My favourite dishes are full of butter and cheese and sour cream. In New York we had so many free luncheons with people on the magazine and various visiting celebrities I developed the habit of running my eye down those huge, handwritten menus, where a tiny side-dish of peas costs fifty or sixty cents, until I'd picked the richest, most expensive dishes and ordered a string of them.

We were always taken out on expense accounts, so I never felt guilty. I made a point of eating so fast I never kept the other people waiting who generally ordered only chef's salad and grapefruit juice because they were trying to reduce. Almost everybody I met in New York was trying to reduce.

'I want to welcome the prettiest, smartest bunch of young ladies our staff has yet had the good luck to meet,' the plump, bald master-of-ceremonies wheezed into his lapel microphone. 'This banquet is just a small sample of the hospitality our Food Testing Kitchens here on *Ladies' Day* would like to offer in appreciation for your visit.'

A delicate, ladylike spatter of applause, and we all sat down at the enormous linen-draped table.

There were eleven of us girls from the magazine, together with most of our supervising editors, and the whole staff of the *Ladies' Day* Food Testing Kitchens in hygienic white smocks, neat hair-nets and flawless make-up of a uniform peach-pie colour.

There were only eleven of us, because Doreen was missing. They had set her place next to mine for some reason, and the chair stayed empty. I saved her place-card for her – a pocket mirror with 'Doreen' painted along the top of it in lacy script and a wreath of frosted daisies around the edge, framing the silver hole where her face would show.

Doreen was spending the day with Lenny Shepherd. She spent most of her free time with Lenny Shepherd now.

In the hour before our luncheon at *Ladies' Day* – the big women's magazine that features lush double-page spreads of technicolour meals, with a different theme and locale each month – we had been shown around the endless glossy kitchens and seen how difficult it is to photograph apple pie *à la mode* under bright lights because the ice-cream keeps melting and has to be propped up from behind with tooth-picks and changed every time it starts looking too soppy.

The sight of all the food stacked in those kitchens made me

dizzy. It's not that we hadn't enough to eat at home, it's just that my grandmother always cooked economy joints and economy meat-loafs and had the habit of saying, the minute you lifted the first forkful to your mouth, 'I hope you enjoy that, it cost forty-one cents a pound,' which always made me feel I was somehow eating pennies instead of Sunday roast.

While we were standing up behind our chairs listening to the welcome speech, I had bowed my head and secretly eyed the position of the bowls of caviar. One bowl was set strategically between me and Doreen's empty chair.

I figured the girl across from me couldn't reach it because of the mountainous centrepiece of marzipan fruit, and Betsy, on my right, would be too nice to ask me to share it with her if I just kept it out of the way at my elbow by my bread-and-butter plate. Besides, another bowl of caviar sat a little way to the right of the girl next to Betsy, and she could eat that.

My grandfather and I had a standing joke. He was the head waiter at a country club near my home town, and every Sunday my grandmother drove in to bring him home for his Monday off. My brother and I alternated going with her, and my grandfather always served Sunday supper to my grandmother and whichever of us was along as if we were regular club guests. He loved introducing me to special titbits, and by the age of nine I had developed a passionate taste for cold vichyssoise and caviar and anchovy paste.

The joke was that at my wedding my grandfather would see I had all the caviar I could eat. It was a joke because I never intended to get married, and even if I did, my grandfather couldn't have afforded enough caviar unless he robbed the country club kitchen and carried it off in a suitcase.

Under cover of the clinking of water goblets and silverware and bone china, I paved my plate with chicken slices. Then I covered the chicken slices with caviar thickly as if I were

24

spreading peanut-butter on a piece of bread. Then I picked up the chicken slices in my fingers one by one, rolled them so the caviar wouldn't ooze off and ate them.

I'd discovered, after a lot of extreme apprehension about what spoons to use, that if you do something incorrect at table with a certain arrogance, as if you knew perfectly well you were doing it properly, you can get away with it and nobody will think you are bad-mannered or poorly brought up. They will think you are original and very witty.

I learned this trick the day Jay Cee took me to lunch with a famous poet. He wore a horrible, lumpy, speckled brown tweed jacket and grey pants and a red-and-blue checked open-throated jersey in a very formal restaurant full of fountains and chandeliers, where all the other men were dressed in dark suits and immaculate white shirts.

This poet ate his salad with his fingers, leaf by leaf, while talking to me about the antithesis of nature and art. I couldn't take my eyes off the pale, stubby white fingers travelling back and forth from the poet's salad bowl to the poet's mouth with one dripping lettuce leaf after another. Nobody giggled or whispered rude remarks. The poet made eating salad with your fingers seem to be the only natural and sensible thing to do.

None of our magazine editors or the *Ladies' Day* staff members sat anywhere near me, and Betsy seemed sweet and friendly, she didn't even seem to like caviar, so I grew more and more confident. When I finished my first plate of cold chicken and caviar, I laid out another. Then I tackled the avocado and crabmeat salad.

Avocados are my favourite fruit. Every Sunday my grandfather used to bring me an avocado pear hidden at the bottom of his briefcase under six soiled shirts and the Sunday comics. He taught me how to eat avocados by melting grape jelly and

French dressing together in a saucepan and filling the cup of the pear with the garnet sauce. I felt homesick for that sauce. The crabmeat tasted bland in comparison.

'How was the fur show?' I asked Betsy, when I was no longer worried about competition over my caviar. I scraped the last few salty black eggs from the dish with my soup spoon and licked it clean.

'It was wonderful,' Betsy smiled. 'They showed us how to make an all-purpose neckerchief out of mink tails and a gold chain, the sort of chain you can get an exact copy of at Woolworth's for a dollar ninety-eight, and Hilda nipped down to the wholesale fur warehouses right afterwards and bought a bunch of mink tails at a big discount and dropped in at Woolworth's and then stitched the whole thing together coming up on the bus.'

I peered over at Hilda, who sat on the other side of Betsy. Sure enough, she was wearing an expensive-looking scarf of furry tails fastened on one side by a dangling gilt chain.

I never really understood Hilda. She was six feet tall, with huge, slanted, green eyes and thick red lips and a vacant, Slavic expression. She made hats. She was apprenticed to the Fashion Editor, which set her apart from the more literary ones among us like Doreen and Betsy and I myself, who all wrote columns, even if some of them were only about health and beauty. I don't know if Hilda could read, but she made startling hats. She went to a special school for making hats in New York and every day she wore a new hat to work, constructed by her own hands out of bits of straw or fur or ribbon or veiling in subtle, bizarre shades.

'That's amazing,' I said. 'Amazing.' I missed Doreen. She would have murmured some fine, scalding remark about Hilda's miraculous furpiece to cheer me up.

I felt very low. I had been unmasked only that morning by

Jay Cee herself, and I felt now that all the uncomfortable suspicions I had about myself were coming true, and I couldn't hide the truth much longer. After nineteen years of running after good marks and prizes and grants of one sort and another, I was letting up, slowing down, dropping clean out of the race.

'Why didn't you come along to the fur show with us?' Betsy asked. I had the impression she was repeating herself, and that she'd asked me the same question a minute ago, only I couldn't have been listening. 'Did you go off with Doreen?'

'No,' I said, 'I wanted to go to the fur show, but Jay Cee called up and made me come into the office.' That wasn't quite true about wanting to go to the show, but I tried to convince myself now that it was true, so I could be really wounded about what Jay Cee had done.

I told Betsy how I had been lying in bed that morning planning to go to the fur show. What I didn't tell her was that Doreen had come into my room earlier and said, 'What do you want to go to that assy show for, Lenny and I are going to Coney Island, so why don't you come along? Lenny can get you a nice fellow, the day's shot to hell anyhow with that luncheon and then the film première in the afternoon, so nobody'll miss us.'

For a minute I was tempted. The show certainly did seem stupid. I have never cared for furs. What I decided to do in the end was to lie in bed as long as I wanted to and then go to Central Park and spend the day lying in the grass, the longest grass I could find in that bald, duck-ponded wilderness.

I told Doreen I would not go to the show or the luncheon or the film première, but that I would not go to Coney Island either, I would stay in bed. After Doreen left, I wondered why I couldn't go the whole way doing what I should any more. This made me sad and tired. Then I wondered why I couldn't go the

27

whole way doing what I shouldn't, the way Doreen did, and this made me even sadder and more tired.

I didn't know what time it was, but I'd heard the girls bustling and calling in the hall and getting ready for the fur show, and then I'd heard the hall go still, and as I lay on my back in bed staring up at the blank, white ceiling the stillness seemed to grow bigger and bigger until I felt my eardrums would burst with it. Then the phone rang.

I stared at the phone for a minute. The receiver shook a bit in its bone-coloured cradle, so I could tell it was really ringing. I thought I might have given my phone number to somebody at a dance or a party and then forgotten clean about it. I lifted the receiver and spoke in a husky, receptive voice.

'Hello?'

'Jay Cee here,' Jay Cee rapped out with brutal promptitude. 'I wondered if you happened to be planning to come into the office today?'

I sank down into the sheets. I couldn't understand why Jay Cee thought I'd be coming into the office. We had these mimeographed schedule cards so we could keep track of all our activities, and we spent a lot of mornings and afternoons away from the office going to affairs in town. Of course, some of the affairs were optional.

There was quite a pause. Then I said meekly, 'I thought I was going to the fur show.' Of course I hadn't thought any such thing, but I couldn't figure out what else to say.

'I told her I thought I was going to the fur show,' I said to Betsy. 'But she told me to come into the office, she wanted to have a little talk with me, and there was some work to do.'

'Oh-oh!' Betsy said sympathetically. She must have seen the tears that plopped down into my dessert dish of meringue and brandy ice-cream, because she pushed over her own untouched dessert and I started absently on that when I'd finished my own. I felt a bit awkward about the tears, but they were real enough. Jay Cee had said some terrible things to me.

When I made my wan entrance into the office at about ten o'clock, Jay Cee stood up and came round her desk to shut the door, and I sat in the swivel chair in front of my typewriter table facing her, and she sat in the swivel chair behind her desk facing me, with the window full of potted plants, shelf after shelf of them, springing up at her back like a tropical garden.

'Doesn't your work interest you, Esther?'

'Oh, it does, it does,' I said. 'It interests me very much.' I felt like yelling the words, as if that might make them more convincing, but I controlled myself.

All my life I'd told myself studying and reading and writing and working like mad was what I wanted to do, and it actually seemed to be true, I did everything well enough and got all A's, and by the time I made it to college nobody could stop me.

I was college correspondent for the town *Gazette* and editor of the literary magazine and secretary of Honour Board, which deals with academic and social offences and punishments – a popular office, and I had a well-known woman poet and professor on the faculty championing me for graduate school at the biggest universities in the east, and promises of full scholarships all the way, and now I was apprenticed to the best editor on any intellectual fashion magazine, and what did I do but balk and balk like a dull cart horse?

'I'm very interested in everything.' The words fell with a hollow flatness on to Jay Cee's desk, like so many wooden nickels.

'I'm glad of that,' Jay Cee said a bit waspishly. 'You can learn a lot in this month on the magazine, you know, if you just roll up your shirt-cuffs. The girl who was here before you didn't bother with any of the fashion show stuff. She went straight from this office on to *Time*.'

'My!' I said, in the same sepulchral tone. 'That was quick!'

'Of course, you have another year at college yet,' Jay Cee went on a little more mildly. 'What do you have in mind after you graduate?'

What I always thought I had in mind was getting some big scholarship to graduate school or a grant to study all over Europe, and then I thought I'd be a professor and write books of poems or write books of poems and be an editor of some sort. Usually I had these plans on the tip of my tongue.

'I don't really know,' I heard myself say. I felt a deep shock, hearing myself say that, because the minute I said it, I knew it was true.

It sounded true, and I recognized it, the way you recognize some nondescript person that's been hanging around your door for ages and then suddenly comes up and introduces himself as your real father and looks exactly like you, so you know he really is your father, and the person you thought all your life was your father is a sham.

'I don't really know.'

'You'll never get anywhere like that.' Jay Cee paused. 'What languages do you have?'

'Oh, I can read a bit of French, I guess, and I've always wanted to learn German.' I'd been telling people I'd always wanted to learn German for about five years.

My mother spoke German during her childhood in America and was stoned for it during the First World War by the children at school. My German-speaking father, dead since I was nine, came from some manic-depressive hamlet in the black heart of Prussia. My younger brother was at that moment on the Experiment in International Living in Berlin and speaking German like a native.

What I didn't say was that each time I picked up a German dictionary or a German book, the very sight of those dense, black, barbed-wire letters made my mind shut like a clam.

'I've always thought I'd like to go into publishing.' I tried to recover a thread that might lead me back to my old, bright salesmanship. 'I guess what I'll do is apply at some publishing house.'

'You ought to read French and German,' Jay Cee said mercilessly, 'and probably several other languages as well, Spanish and Italian – better still, Russian. Hundreds of girls flood into New York every June thinking they'll be editors. You need to offer something more than the run-of-the-mill person. You better learn some languages.'

I hadn't the heart to tell Jay Cee there wasn't one scrap of space on my senior year schedule to learn languages in. I was taking one of those honours programmes that teaches you to think independently, and except for a course in Tolstoy and Dostoevsky and a seminar in advanced poetry-composition, I would spend my whole time writing on some obscure theme in the works of James Joyce. I hadn't picked out my theme yet, because I hadn't got round to reading *Finnegans Wake*, but my professor was very excited about my thesis and had promised to give me some leads on images about twins.

'I'll see what I can do,' I told Jay Cee. 'I probably might just fit in one of those double-barrelled, accelerated courses in elementary German they've rigged up.' I thought at the time I might actually do this. I had a way of persuading my Class Dean to let me do irregular things. She regarded me as a sort of interesting experiment.

At college I had to take a required course in physics and chemistry. I had already taken a course in botany and done very well. I never answered one test question wrong the whole year, and for a while I toyed with the idea of being a botanist and studying the wild grasses in Africa or the South American rain forests, because you can win big grants to study off-beat things like that in queer areas much more easily than winning grants to study art in Italy or English in England, there's not so much competition.

Botany was fine, because I loved cutting up leaves and putting them under the microscope and drawing diagrams of bread mould and the odd, heart-shaped leaf in the sex cycle of the fern, it seemed so real to me.

The day I went into physics class it was death.

A short dark man with a high, lisping voice, named Mr Manzi, stood in front of the class in a tight blue suit holding a little wooden ball. He put the ball on a steep grooved slide and let it run down to the bottom. Then he started talking about let a equal acceleration and let t equal time and suddenly he was scribbling letters and numbers and equals signs all over the blackboard and my mind went dead.

I took the physics book back to my dormitory. It was a huge book on porous mimeographed paper – four hundred pages long with no drawings or photographs, only diagrams and formulas – between brick-red cardboard covers. This book was written by Mr Manzi to explain physics to college girls, and if it worked on us he would try to have it published.

Well, I studied those formulas, I went to class and watched balls roll down slides and listened to bells ring and by the end of the semester most of the other girls had failed and I had a straight A. I heard Mr Manzi saying to a bunch of the girls who were complaining that the course was too hard, 'No, it can't be too hard, because one girl got a straight A.' 'Who is it? Tell us,' they said, but he shook his head and didn't say anything and gave me a sweet little conspiring smile.

That's what gave me the idea of escaping the next semester of chemistry. I may have made a straight A in physics, but I was panic-struck. Physics made me sick the whole time I learned it. What I couldn't stand was this shrinking everything into letters and numbers. Instead of leaf shapes and enlarged diagrams of the holes the leaves breathe through and fascinating words like carotene and xanthophyll on the blackboard, there were these hideous, cramped, scorpion-lettered formulas in Mr Manzi's special red chalk.

I knew chemistry would be worse, because I'd seen a big chart of the ninety-odd elements hung up in the chemistry lab, and all the perfectly good words like gold and silver and cobalt and aluminium were shortened to ugly abbreviations with different decimal numbers after them. If I had to strain my brain with any more of that stuff I would go mad. I would fail outright. It was only by a horrible effort of will that I had dragged myself through the first half of the year.

So I went to my Class Dean with a clever plan.

My plan was that I needed the time to take a course in Shakespeare, since I was, after all, an English major. She knew and I knew perfectly well I would get a straight A again in the chemistry course, so what was the point of my taking the exams, why couldn't I just go to the classes and look on and take it all in and forget about marks or credits? It was a case of honour among honourable people, and the content meant more than the form, and marks were really a bit silly anyway, weren't they, when you knew you'd always get an A? My plan was strengthened by the fact that the college had just dropped the second year of required science for the classes after me anyway, so my class was the last to suffer under the old ruling.

Mr Manzi was in perfect agreement with my plan. I think it flattered him that I enjoyed his classes so much I would take them for no materialistic reason like credit and an A, but for the sheer beauty of chemistry itself. I thought it was quite ingenious of me to suggest sitting in on the chemistry course even after I'd changed over to Shakespeare. It was quite an unnecessary gesture and made it seem I simply couldn't bear to give chemistry up.

Of course, I would never have succeeded with this scheme if I hadn't made that A in the first place. And if my Class Dean had known how scared and depressed I was, and how I seriously contemplated desperate remedies such as getting a doctor's certificate that I was unfit to study chemistry, the formulas made me dizzy and so on, I'm sure she wouldn't have listened to me for a minute, but would have made me take the course regardless.

As it happened, the Faculty Board passed my petition, and my Class Dean told me later that several of the professors were touched by it. They took it as a real step in intellectual maturity.

I had to laugh when I thought about the rest of that year. I went to the chemistry class five times a week and didn't miss a single one. Mr Manzi stood at the bottom of the big, rickety old amphitheatre, making blue flames and red flares and clouds of yellow stuff by pouring the contents of one test-tube into another, and I shut his voice out of my ears by pretending it was only a mosquito in the distance and sat back enjoying the bright lights and the coloured fires and wrote page after page of villanelles and sonnets.

Mr Manzi would glance at me now and then and see me writing, and send up a sweet little appreciative smile. I guess he thought I was writing down all those formulas not for exam time, like the other girls, but because his presentation fascinated me so much I couldn't help it.

Chapter Four

I don't know just why my successful evasion of chemistry should have floated into my mind there in Jay Cee's office.

All the time she talked to me, I saw Mr Manzi standing on thin air in back of Jay Cee's head, like something conjured up out of a hat, holding his little wooden ball and the test-tube that billowed a great cloud of yellow smoke the day before Easter vacation and smelt of rotten eggs and made all the girls and Mr Manzi laugh.

I felt sorry for Mr Manzi. I felt like going down to him on my hands and knees and apologizing for being such an awful liar.

Jay Cee handed me a pile of story manuscripts and spoke to me much more kindly. I spent the rest of the morning reading the stories and typing out what I thought of them on the pink Interoffice Memo sheets and sending them into the office of Betsy's editor to be read by Betsy the next day. Jay Cee interrupted me now and then to tell me something practical or a bit of gossip.

Jay Cee was going to lunch that noon with two famous writers, a man and a lady. The man had just sold six short stories to the *New Yorker* and six to Jay Cee. This surprised me, as I didn't know magazines bought stories in lots of six, and I was staggered by the thought of the amount of money six stories would probably bring in. Jay Cee said she had to be very careful at this lunch, because the lady writer wrote stories too, but she had never had any in the *New Yorker* and Jay Cee had only taken one from her in five years. Jay Cee had to flatter the more famous man at the same time as she was careful not to hurt the less famous lady.

When the cherubs in Jay Cee's French wall-clock waved their wings up and down and put the little gilt trumpets to their lips and pinged out twelve notes one after the other, Jay Cee told me I'd done enough work for the day, and to go off to the *Ladies' Day* tour and banquet and to the film première, and she would see me bright and early tomorrow.

Then she slipped a suit jacket over her lilac blouse, pinned a hat of imitation lilacs on the top of her head, powdered her nose briefly and adjusted her thick spectacles. She looked terrible, but very wise. As she left the office, she patted my shoulder with one lilac-gloved hand.

'Don't let the wicked city get you down.'

I sat quietly in my swivel chair for a few minutes and thought about Jay Cee. I tried to imagine what it would be like if I were Ee Gee, the famous editor, in an office full of potted rubber plants and African violets my secretary had to water each morning. I wished I had a mother like Jay Cee. Then I'd know what to do.

My own mother wasn't much help. My mother had taught shorthand and typing to support us ever since my father died, and secretly she hated it and hated him for dying and leaving no money because he didn't trust life insurance salesmen. She was always on to me to learn shorthand after college, so I'd have a practical skill as well as a college degree. 'Even the apostles were tent-makers,' she'd say. 'They had to live, just the way we do.'

*

I dabbled my fingers in the bowl of warm water a *Ladies' Day* waitress set down in place of my two empty ice-cream dishes. Then I wiped each finger carefully with my linen napkin which was still quite clean. Then I folded the linen napkin and laid it between my lips and brought my lips down on it precisely. When I put the napkin back on the table a fuzzy pink lip-shape bloomed right in the middle of it like a tiny heart.

I thought what a long way I had come.

The first time I saw a finger-bowl was at the home of my benefactress. It was the custom at my college, the little freckled lady in the Scholarships Office told me, to write to the person whose scholarship you had, if they were still alive, and thank them for it.

I had the scholarship of Philomena Guinea, a wealthy novelist who went to my college in the early nineteen-hundreds and had her first novel made into a silent film with Bette Davis as well as a radio serial that was still running, and it turned out she was alive and lived in a large mansion not far from my grandfather's country club.

So I wrote Philomena Guinea a long letter in coal-black ink on grey paper with the name of the college embossed on it in red. I wrote what the leaves looked like in autumn when I bicycled out into the hills, and how wonderful it was to live on a campus instead of commuting by bus to a city college and having to live at home, and how all knowledge was opening up before me and perhaps one day I would be able to write great books the way she did.

I had read one of Mrs Guinea's books in the town library – the college library didn't stock them for some reason – and it was crammed from beginning to end with long, suspenseful questions: 'Would Evelyn discern that Gladys knew Roger in her past? wondered Hector feverishly' and 'How could Donald marry her when he learned of the child Elsie, hidden

37

away with Mrs Rollmop on the secluded country farm? Griselda demanded of her bleak, moonlit pillow.' These books earned Philomena Guinea, who later told me she had been very stupid at college, millions and millions of dollars.

Mrs Guinea answered my letter and invited me to lunch at her home. That was where I saw my first finger-bowl.

The water had a few cherry blossoms floating in it, and I thought it must be some clear sort of Japanese after-dinner soup and ate every bit of it, including the crisp little blossoms. Mrs Guinea never said anything, and it was only much later, when I told a débutante I knew at college about the dinner, that I learned what I had done.

When we came out of the sunnily lit interior of the *Ladies' Day* offices, the streets were grey and fuming with rain. It wasn't the nice kind of rain that rinses you clean, but the sort of rain I imagine they must have in Brazil. It flew straight down from the sky in drops the size of coffee saucers and hit the hot sidewalks with a hiss that sent clouds of steam writhing up from the gleaming, dark concrete.

My secret hope of spending the afternoon alone in Central Park died in the glass egg-beater of *Ladies' Day*'s revolving doors. I found myself spewed out through the warm rain and into the dim, throbbing cave of a cab, together with Betsy and Hilda and Emily Ann Offenbach, a prim little girl with a bun of red hair and a husband and three children in Teaneck, New Jersey.

The movie was very poor. It starred a nice blonde girl who looked like June Allyson but was really somebody else, and a sexy black-haired girl who looked like Elizabeth Taylor but was also somebody else, and two big, broad-shouldered bone-heads with names like Rick and Gil.

It was a football romance and it was in technicolour.

I hate technicolour. Everybody in a technicolour movie seems to feel obliged to wear a lurid new costume in each new scene and to stand around like a clothes-horse with a lot of very green trees or very yellow wheat or very blue ocean rolling away for miles and miles in every direction.

Most of the action in this picture took place in the football stands, with the two girls waving and cheering in smart suits with orange chrysanthemums the size of cabbages on their lapels, or in a ballroom, where the girls swooped across the floor with their dates, in dresses like something out of *Gone With the Wind*, and then sneaked off into the powder-room to say nasty intense things to each other.

Finally I could see the nice girl was going to end up with the nice football hero and the sexy girl was going to end up with nobody, because the man named Gil had only wanted a mistress and not a wife all along and was now packing off to Europe on a single ticket.

At about this point I began to feel peculiar. I looked round me at all the rows of rapt little heads with the same silver glow on them at the front and the same black shadow on them at the back, and they looked like nothing more or less than a lot of stupid moon-brains.

I felt in terrible danger of puking. I didn't know whether it was the awful movie giving me a stomach-ache or all that caviar I had eaten.

'I'm going back to the hotel,' I whispered to Betsy through the half-dark.

Betsy was staring at the screen with deadly concentration. 'Don't you feel good?' she whispered, barely moving her lips.

'No,' I said. 'I feel like hell.'

'So do I, I'll come back with you.'

We slipped out of our seats and said Excuse me Excuse me Excuse me down the length of our row, while the people grumbled and hissed and shifted their rain boots and umbrellas to let us pass, and I stepped on as many feet as I could because it took my mind off this enormous desire to puke that was ballooning up in front of me so fast I couldn't see round it.

The remains of a tepid rain were still sifting down when we stepped out into the street.

Betsy looked a fright. The bloom was gone from her cheeks and her drained face floated in front of me, green and sweating. We fell into one of those yellow checkered cabs that are always waiting at the kerb when you are trying to decide whether or not you want a taxi, and by the time we reached the hotel I had puked once and Betsy had puked twice.

The cab driver took the corners with such momentum that we were thrown together first on one side of the back seat and then on the other. Each time one of us felt sick, she would lean over quietly as if she had dropped something and was picking it up off the floor, and the other one would hum a little and pretend to be looking out the window.

The cab driver seemed to know what we were doing, even so.

'Hey,' he protested, driving through a light that had just turned red, 'you can't do that in my cab, you better get out and do it in the street.'

But we didn't say anything, and I guess he figured we were almost at the hotel so he didn't make us get out until we pulled up in front of the main entrance.

We didn't dare wait to add up the fare. We stuffed a pile of silver into the cabby's hand and dropped a couple of kleenexes to cover the mess on the floor, and ran in through the lobby and on to the empty elevator. Luckily for us, it was a quiet time of day. Betsy was sick again in the elevator and I held her head, and then I was sick and she held mine.

Usually after a good puke you feel better right away. We hugged each other and then said good-bye and went off to opposite ends of the hall to lie down in our own rooms. There is nothing like puking with somebody to make you into old friends.

But the minute I'd shut the door behind me and undressed and dragged myself on to the bed, I felt worse than ever. I felt I just had to go to the toilet. I struggled into my white bathrobe with the blue cornflowers on it and staggered down to the bathroom.

Betsy was already there. I could hear her groaning behind the door, so I hurried on around the corner to the bathroom in the next wing. I thought I would die, it was so far.

I sat on the toilet and leaned my head over the edge of the washbowl and I thought I was losing my guts and my dinner both. The sickness rolled through me in great waves. After each wave it would fade away and leave me limp as a wet leaf and shivering all over and then I would feel it rising up in me again, and the glittering white torture-chamber tiles under my feet and over my head and on all four sides closed in and squeezed me to pieces.

I don't know how long I kept at it. I let the cold water in the bowl go on running loudly with the stopper out, so anybody who came by would think I was washing my clothes, and then when I felt reasonably safe I stretched out on the floor and lay quite still.

It didn't seem to be summer any more. I could feel the winter shaking my bones and banging my teeth together, and the big white hotel towel I had dragged down with me lay under my head numb as a snowdrift.

I thought it very bad manners for anybody to pound on a bathroom door the way some person was pounding. They could just go around the corner and find another bathroom the way I had done and leave me in peace. But the person kept banging and pleading with me to let them in and I thought I dimly recognized the voice. It sounded a bit like Emily Ann Offenbach.

'Just a minute,' I said then. My words bungled out thick as molasses.

I pulled myself together and slowly rose and flushed the toilet for the tenth time and slopped the bowl clean and rolled up the towel so the vomit stains didn't show very clearly and unlocked the door and stepped out into the hall.

I knew it would be fatal if I looked at Emily Ann or anybody else so I fixed my eyes glassily on a window that swam at the end of the hall and put one foot in front of the other.

The next thing I had a view of was somebody's shoe.

It was a stout shoe of cracked black leather and quite old, with tiny air holes in a scalloped pattern over the toe and a dull polish, and it was pointed at me. It seemed to be placed on a hard green surface that was hurting my right cheekbone.

I kept very still, waiting for a clue that would give me some notion of what to do. A little to the left of the shoe I saw a vague heap of blue cornflowers on a white ground and this made me want to cry. It was the sleeve of my own bathrobe I was looking at, and my left hand lay pale as a cod at the end of it.

'She's all right now.'

The voice came from a cool, rational region far above my head. For a minute I didn't think there was anything strange about it, and then I thought it was strange. It was a man's voice, and no men were allowed to be in our hotel at any time of the night or day.

'How many others are there?' the voice went on.

42

I listened with interest. The floor seemed wonderfully solid. It was comforting to know I had fallen and could fall no farther.

'Eleven, I think,' a woman's voice answered. I figured she must belong to the black shoe. 'I think there's eleven more of 'um, but one's missin' so there's oney ten.'

'Well, you get this one to bed and I'll take care of the rest.'

I heard a hollow boomp boomp in my right ear that grew fainter and fainter. Then a door opened in the distance, and there were voices and groans, and the door shut again.

Two hands slid under my armpits and the woman's voice said, 'Come, come, lovey, we'll make it yet,' and I felt myself being half lifted, and slowly the doors began to move by, one by one, until we came to an open door and went in.

The sheet on my bed was folded back, and the woman helped me lie down and covered me up to the chin and rested for a minute in the bedside armchair, fanning herself with one plump, pink hand. She wore gilt-rimmed spectacles and a white nurse's cap.

'Who are you?' I asked in a faint voice.

'I'm the hotel nurse.'

'What's the matter with me?'

'Poisoned,' she said briefly. 'Poisoned, the whole lot of you. I never seen anythin' like it. Sick here, sick there, whatever have you young ladies been stuffin' yourselves with?'

'Is everybody else sick too?' I asked with some hope.

'The whole of your lot,' she affirmed with relish. 'Sick as dogs and cryin' for ma.'

The room hovered around me with great gentleness, as if the chairs and the tables and the walls were withholding their weight out of sympathy for my sudden frailty.

'The doctor's given you an injection,' the nurse said from the doorway. 'You'll sleep now.'

And the door took her place like a sheet of blank paper, and then a larger sheet of paper took the place of the door, and I drifted toward it and smiled myself to sleep.

Somebody was standing by my pillow with a white cup.

'Drink this,' they said.

I shook my head. The pillow crackled like a wad of straw.

'Drink this and you'll feel better.'

A thick white china cup was lowered under my nose. In the wan light that might have been evening and might have been dawn I contemplated the clear amber liquid. Pads of butter floated on the surface and a faint chickeny aroma fumed up to my nostrils.

My eyes moved tentatively to the skirt behind the cup. 'Betsy,' I said.

'Betsy nothing, it's me.'

I raised my eyes then, and saw Doreen's head silhouetted against the paling window, her blonde hair lit at the tips from behind like a halo of gold. Her face was in shadow, so I couldn't make out her expression, but I felt a sort of expert tenderness flowing from the ends of her fingers. She might have been Betsy or my mother or a fern-scented nurse.

I bent my head and took a sip of the broth. I thought my mouth must be made of sand. I took another sip and then another and another until the cup was empty.

I felt purged and holy and ready for a new life.

Doreen set the cup on the window-sill and lowered herself into the armchair. I noticed that she made no move to take out a cigarette, and as she was a chain-smoker this surprised me.

'Well, you almost died,' she said finally.

'I guess it was all that caviar.'

'Caviar nothing! It was the crabmeat. They did tests on it and it was chock-full of ptomaine.'

I had a vision of the celestially white kitchens on *Ladies' Day* stretching into infinity. I saw avocado pear after avocado pear being stuffed with crabmeat and mayonnaise and photographed under brilliant lights. I saw the delicate, pink-mottled claw-meat poking seductively through its blanket of mayonnaise and the bland yellow pear cup with its rim of alligator-green cradling the whole mess.

Poison.

'Who did tests?' I thought the doctor might have pumped somebody's stomach and then analyzed what he found in his hotel laboratory.

'Those dodos on *Ladies' Day*. As soon as you all started keeling over like ninepins somebody called into the office and the office called across to *Ladies' Day* and they did tests on everything left over from the big lunch. Ha!'

'Ha!' I echoed hollowly. It was good to have Doreen back.

'They sent presents,' she added. 'They're in a big carton out in the hall.'

'How did they get here so fast?'

'Special express delivery, what do you think? They can't afford to have the lot of you running around saying you got poisoned at *Ladies' Day*. You could sue them for every penny they own if you just knew some smart law man.'

'What are the presents?' I began to feel if it was a good enough present I wouldn't mind about what happened, because I felt so pure as a result.

'Nobody's opened the box yet, they're all out flat. I'm supposed to be carting soup into everybody, seeing as I'm the only one on my feet, but I brought you yours first.'

'See what the present is,' I begged. Then I remembered and said, 'I've a present for you as well.'

Doreen went out into the hall. I could hear her rustling around for a minute and then the sound of paper tearing.

45

Finally she came back carrying a thick book with a glossy cover and people's names printed all over it.

'*The Thirty Best Short Stories of the Year.*' She dropped the book in my lap. 'There's eleven more of them out there in that box. I suppose they thought it'd give you something to read while you were sick.' She paused. 'Where's mine?'

I fished in my pocket-book and handed Doreen the mirror with her name and the daisies on it. Doreen looked at me and I looked at her and we both burst out laughing.

'You can have my soup if you want,' she said. 'They put twelve soups on the tray by mistake and Lenny and I stuffed down so many hotdogs while we were waiting for the rain to stop I couldn't eat another mouthful.'

'Bring it in,' I said. 'I'm starving.'

Chapter Five

At seven the next morning the telephone rang.

Slowly I swam up from the bottom of a black sleep. I already had a telegram from Jay Cee stuck in my mirror, telling me not to bother to come into work but to rest for a day and get completely well, and how sorry she was about the bad crabmeat, so I couldn't imagine who would be calling.

I reached out and hitched the receiver on to my pillow so the mouthpiece rested on my collarbone and the earpiece lay on my shoulder.

'Hello?'

A man's voice said, 'Is that Miss Esther Greenwood?' I thought I detected a slight foreign accent.

'It certainly is,' I said.

'This is Constantin Something-or-Other.'

I couldn't make out the last name, but it was full of S's and K's. I didn't know any Constantin, but I hadn't the heart to say so.

Then I remembered Mrs Willard and her simultaneous interpreter.

'Of course, of course!' I cried, sitting up and clutching the phone to me with both hands.

I'd never have given Mrs Willard credit for introducing me to a man named Constantin.

I collected men with interesting names. I already knew a Socrates. He was tall and ugly and intellectual and the son of some big Greek movie producer in Hollywood, but also a Catholic, which ruined it for both of us. In addition to Socrates I knew a White Russian named Attila at the Boston School of Business Administration.

Gradually I realized that Constantin was trying to arrange a meeting for us later in the day.

'Would you like to see the UN this afternoon?'

'I can already see the UN,' I told him, with a little hysterical giggle.

He seemed nonplussed.

'I can see it from my window.' I thought perhaps my English was a touch too fast for him.

There was a silence.

Then he said, 'Maybe you would like a bite to eat afterwards.'

I detected the vocabulary of Mrs Willard and my heart sank. Mrs Willard always invited you for a bite to eat. I remembered that this man had been a guest at Mrs Willard's house when he first came to America – Mrs Willard had one of these arrangements where you open your house to foreigners and then when you go abroad they open their houses to you.

I now saw quite clearly that Mrs Willard had simply traded her open house in Russia for my bite to eat in New York.

'Yes, I would like a bite to eat,' I said stiffly. 'What time will you come?'

'I'll call for you in my car about two. It's the Amazon, isn't it?'

'Yes.'

'Ah, I know where that is.'

For a moment I thought his tone was laden with special meaning, and then I figured that probably some of the girls at

48

the Amazon were secretaries at the UN and maybe he had taken one of them out at one time. I let him hang up first, and then I hung up and lay back in the pillows, feeling grim.

There I went again, building up a glamorous picture of a man who would love me passionately the minute he met me, and all out of a few prosy nothings. A duty tour of the UN and a post-UN sandwich!

I tried to jack up my morale.

Probably Mrs Willard's simultaneous interpreter would be short and ugly and I would come to look down on him in the end the way I looked down on Buddy Willard. This thought gave me a certain satisfaction. Because I did look down on Buddy Willard, and although everybody still thought I would marry him when he came out of the TB place, I knew I would never marry him if he were the last man on earth.

Buddy Willard was a hypocrite.

Of course, I didn't know he was a hypocrite at first. I thought he was the most wonderful boy I'd ever seen. I'd adored him from a distance for five years before he even looked at me, and then there was a beautiful time when I still adored him and he started looking at me, and then just as he was looking at me more and more I discovered quite by accident what an awful hypocrite he was, and now he wanted me to marry him and I hated his guts.

The worst part of it was I couldn't come straight out and tell him what I thought of him, because he caught TB before I could do that, and now I had to humour him along till he got well again and could take the unvarnished truth.

I decided not to go down to the cafeteria for breakfast. It would only mean getting dressed, and what was the point of getting dressed if you were staying in bed for the morning? I could have called down and asked for a breakfast tray in my room, I guess, but then I would have to tip the person who brought it up and I never knew how much to tip. I'd had some very unsettling experiences trying to tip people in New York.

When I first arrived at the Amazon a dwarfish, bald man in a bellhop's uniform carried my suitcase up in the elevator and unlocked my room for me. Of course I rushed immediately to the window and looked out to see what the view was. After a while I was aware of this bellhop turning on the hot and cold taps in my washbowl and saying 'This is the hot and this is the cold' and switching on the radio and telling me the names of all the New York stations and I began to get uneasy, so I kept my back to him and said firmly, 'Thank you for bringing up my suitcase.'

'Thank you thank you thank you. Ha!' he said in a very nasty insinuating tone, and before I could wheel round to see what had come over him he was gone, shutting the door behind him with a rude slam.

Later, when I told Doreen about his curious behaviour, she said, 'You ninny, he wanted his tip.'

I asked how much I should have given and she said a quarter at least and thirty-five cents if the suitcase was too heavy. Now I could have carried that suitcase to my room perfectly well by myself, only the bellhop seemed so eager to do it that I let him. I thought that sort of service came along with what you paid for your hotel room.

I hate handing over money to people for doing what I could just as easily do myself, it makes me nervous.

Doreen said ten per cent was what you should tip a person, but I somehow never had the right change and I'd have felt awfully silly giving somebody half a dollar and saying, 'Fifteen cents of this is a tip for you, please give me thirty-five cents back.'

The first time I took a taxi in New York I tipped the driver ten cents. The fare was a dollar, so I thought ten cents was exactly right and gave the driver my dime with a little flourish and a smile. But he only held it in the palm of his hand and stared and stared at it, and when I stepped out of the cab, hoping I had not handed him a Canadian dime by mistake, he started yelling, 'Lady I gotta live like you and everybody else,' in a loud voice which scared me so much I broke into a run. Luckily he was stopped at a traffic light or I think he would have driven along beside me yelling in that embarrassing way.

When I asked Doreen about this she said the tipping percentage might well have risen from ten to fifteen per cent since she was last in New York. Either that, or that particular cab-driver was an out and out louse.

I reached for the book the people from *Ladies' Day* had sent.

When I opened it a card fell out. The front of the card showed a poodle in a flowered bedjacket sitting in a poodle basket with a sad face, and the inside of the card showed the poodle lying down in the basket with a little smile, sound asleep under an embroidered sampler that said, 'You'll get well best with lots and lots of rest'. At the bottom of the card somebody had written, 'Get well quick! from all of your good friends at *Ladies' Day*' in lavender ink.

I flipped through one story after another until finally I came to a story about a fig-tree.

This fig-tree grew on a green lawn between the house of a Jewish man and a convent, and the Jewish man and a beautiful dark nun kept meeting at the tree to pick the ripe figs, until one day they saw an egg hatching in a bird's nest on a branch of the tree, and as they watched the little bird peck its way out of the egg, they touched the backs of their hands together, and then the nun didn't come out to pick figs with the Jewish man any more but a mean-faced Catholic kitchen-maid came to pick them instead and counted up the figs the man picked after they were both through to be sure he hadn't picked any more than she had, and the man was furious.

I thought it was a lovely story, especially the part about the fig-tree in winter under the snow and then the fig-tree in spring with all the green fruit. I felt sorry when I came to the last page. I wanted to crawl in between those black lines of print the way you crawl through a fence, and go to sleep under that beautiful big green fig-tree.

It seemed to me Buddy Willard and I were like that Jewish man and that nun, although of course we weren't Jewish or Catholic but Unitarian. We had met together under our own imaginary fig-tree, and what we had seen wasn't a bird coming out of an egg but a baby coming out of a woman, and then something awful happened and we went our separate ways.

As I lay there in my white hotel bed feeling lonely and weak, I thought of Buddy Willard lying even lonelier and weaker than I was up in that sanatorium in the Adirondacks, and I felt like a heel of the worst sort. In his letters Buddy kept telling me how he was reading poems by a poet who was also a doctor and how he'd found out about some famous dead Russian short story writer who had been a doctor too, so maybe doctors and writers could get along fine after all.

Now this was a very different tune from what Buddy Willard had been singing all the two years we were getting to know each other. I remember the day he smiled at me and said, 'Do you know what a poem is, Esther?'

'No, what?' I said.

'A piece of dust.' And he looked so proud of having thought of this that I just stared at his blond hair and his blue eyes and his white teeth – he had very long, strong white teeth – and said 'I guess so.'

It was only in the middle of New York a whole year later that I finally thought of an answer to that remark.

I spent a lot of time having imaginary conversations with Buddy Willard. He was a couple of years older than I was and very scientific, so he could always prove things. When I was with him I had to work to keep my head above water.

These conversations I had in my mind usually repeated the beginnings of conversations I'd really had with Buddy, only they finished with me answering him back quite sharply, instead of just sitting around and saying 'I guess so'.

Now, lying on my back in bed, I imagined Buddy saying, 'Do you know what a poem is, Esther?'

'No, what?' I would say.

'A piece of dust.'

Then just as he was smiling and starting to look proud, I would say, 'So are the cadavers you cut up. So are the people you think you're curing. They're dust as dust as dust. I reckon a good poem lasts a whole lot longer than a hundred of those people put together.'

And of course Buddy wouldn't have any answer to that, because what I said was true. People were made of nothing so much as dust, and I couldn't see that doctoring all that dust was a bit better than writing poems people would remember and repeat to themselves when they were unhappy or sick and couldn't sleep.

My trouble was I took everything Buddy Willard told me as the honest-to-God truth. I remember the first night he kissed me. It was after the Yale Junior Prom.

It was strange, the way Buddy had invited me to that Prom.

He popped into my house out of the blue one Christmas vacation, wearing a thick white turtleneck sweater and looking so handsome I could hardly stop staring and said, 'I might drop over to see you at college some day, all right?'

I was flabbergasted. I only saw Buddy at church on Sundays when we were both home from college, and then at a distance, and I couldn't figure what had put it into his head to run over and see me – he had run the two miles between our houses for cross-country practice, he said.

Of course, our mothers were good friends. They had gone to school together and then both married their professors and settled down in the same town, but Buddy was always off on a scholarship at prep school in the fall or earning money by fighting blister rust in Montana in the summer, so our mothers being old school chums really didn't matter a bit.

After this sudden visit I didn't hear a word from Buddy until one fine Saturday morning in early March. I was up in my room at college, studying about Peter the Hermit and Walter the Penniless for my history exam on the crusades the coming Monday when the hall phone rang.

Usually people are supposed to take turns answering the hall phone, but as I was the only freshman on a floor with all seniors they made me answer it most of the time. I waited a minute to see if anybody would beat me to it. Then I figured everybody was probably out playing squash or away on weekends, so I answered it myself.

'Is that you, Esther?' the girl on watch downstairs said, and when I said Yes, she said, 'There's a man to see you.'

I was surprised to hear this, because of all the blind dates I'd had that year not one called me up again for a second date. I just didn't have any luck. I hated coming downstairs sweaty-handed and curious every Saturday night and having some senior introduce me to her aunt's best friend's son and finding some pale, mushroomy fellow with protruding ears or buck teeth or a bad leg. I didn't think I deserved it. After all, I wasn't crippled in any way, I just studied too hard, I didn't know when to stop.

Well, I combed my hair and put on some more lipstick and took my history book – so I could say I was on my way to the library if it turned out to be somebody awful – and went down, and there was Buddy Willard leaning against the mail table in a khaki zipper jacket and blue dungarees and frayed grey sneakers and grinning up at me.

'I just came over to say hello,' he said.

I thought it odd he should come all the way up from Yale even hitch-hiking, as he did, to save money, just to say hello.

'Hello,' I said. 'Let's go out and sit on the porch.'

I wanted to go out on the porch because the girl on watch was a nosey senior and eyeing me curiously. She obviously thought Buddy had made a big mistake.

We sat side by side in two wicker rocking-chairs. The sunlight was clean and windless and almost hot.

'I can't stay more than a few minutes,' Buddy said.

'Oh, come on, stay for lunch,' I said.

'Oh, I can't do that. I'm up here for the Sophomore Prom with Joan.'

I felt like a prize idiot.

'How *is* Joan?' I asked coldly.

Joan Gilling came from our home town and went to our church and was a year ahead of me at college. She was a big wheel – president of her class and a physics major and the college hockey champion. She always made me feel squirmy with her starey pebble-coloured eyes and her gleaming tombstone teeth and her breathy voice. She was big as a horse, too. I began to think Buddy had pretty poor taste.

'Oh Joan,' he said. 'She asked me up to this dance two months ahead of time and her mother asked my mother if I would take her, so what could I do?'

'Well, why did you say you'd take her if you didn't want to?' I asked meanly.

'Oh, I like Joan. She never cares whether you spend any money on her or not and she enjoys doing things out-of-doors.

55

The last time she came down to Yale for house week-end we went on a bicycle trip to East Rock and she's the only girl I haven't had to push up hills. Joan's all right.'

I went cold with envy. I had never been to Yale, and Yale was the place all the seniors in my house liked to go best on week-ends. I decided to expect nothing from Buddy Willard. If you expect nothing from somebody you are never disappointed.

'You better go and find Joan then,' I said in a matter-of-fact voice. 'I've a date coming any minute and he won't like seeing me sitting around with you.'

'A date?' Buddy looked surprised. 'Who is it?'

'It's two,' I said, 'Peter the Hermit and Walter the Penniless.'

Buddy didn't say anything, so I said, 'Those are their nicknames.'

Then I added, 'They're from Dartmouth.'

I guess Buddy never read much history, because his mouth stiffened. He swung up from the wicker rocking-chair and gave it a sharp little unnecessary push. Then he dropped a pale blue envelope with a Yale crest into my lap.

'Here's a letter I meant to leave for you if you weren't in. There's a question in it you can answer by mail. I don't feel like asking you about it right now.'

After Buddy had gone I opened the letter. It was a letter inviting me to the Yale Junior Prom.

I was so surprised I let out a couple of yips and ran into the house shouting, 'I'm going I'm going I'm going.' After the bright white sun on the porch it looked pitch-dark in there, and I couldn't make out a thing. I found myself hugging the senior on watch. When she heard I was going to the Yale Junior Prom she treated me with amazement and respect.

Oddly enough, things changed in the house after that. The seniors on my floor started speaking to me and every now and then one of them would answer the phone quite spontaneously and nobody made any more nasty loud remarks outside my door about people wasting their golden college days with their noses stuck in a book.

Well all during the Junior Prom Buddy treated me like a friend or a cousin.

We danced about a mile apart the whole time, until during 'Auld Lang Syne' he suddenly rested his chin on the top of my head as if he were very tired. Then in the cold, black, three o'clock wind we walked very slowly the five miles back to the house where I was sleeping in the living-room on a couch that was too short because it only cost fifty cents a night instead of two dollars like most of the other places with proper beds.

I felt dull and flat and full of shattered visions.

I had imagined Buddy would fall in love with me that weekend and that I wouldn't have to worry about what I was doing on any more Saturday nights the rest of the year. Just as we approached the house where I was staying Buddy said, 'Let's go up to the chemistry lab.'

I was aghast. 'The *chemistry* lab?'

'Yes.' Buddy reached for my hand. 'There's a beautiful view up there behind the chemistry lab.'

And sure enough, there was a sort of hilly place behind the chemistry lab from which you could see the lights of a couple of the houses in New Haven.

I stood pretending to admire them while Buddy got a good footing on the rough soil. While he kissed me I kept my eyes open and tried to memorize the spacing of the house lights so I would never forget them.

Finally Buddy stepped back. 'Wow!' he said.

'Wow what?' I said, surprised. It had been a dry, uninspiring little kiss, and I remember thinking it was too bad both our

57

mouths were so chapped from walking five miles in that cold wind.

'Wow, it makes me feel terrific to kiss you.'

I modestly didn't say anything.

'I guess you go out with a lot of boys,' Buddy said then.

'Well, I guess I do.' I thought I must have gone out with a different boy for every week in the year.

'Well, I have to study a lot.'

'So do I,' I put in hastily. 'I have to keep my scholarship after all.'

'Still, I think I could manage to see you every third week-end.'

'That's nice.' I was almost fainting and dying to get back to college and tell everybody.

Buddy kissed me again in front of the house steps, and the next fall, when his scholarship to Medical School came through, I went there to see him instead of to Yale and it was there I found out how he had fooled me all those years and what a hypocrite he was.

I found out on the day we saw the baby born.

Chapter Six

I had kept begging Buddy to show me some really interesting hospital sights, so one Friday I cut all my classes and came down for a long week-end and he gave me the works.

I started out by dressing in a white coat and sitting on a tall stool in a room with four cadavers, while Buddy and his friends cut them up. These cadavers were so unhuman-looking they didn't bother me a bit. They had stiff, leathery, purple-black skin and they smelt like old pickle jars.

After that, Buddy took me out into a hall where they had some big glass bottles full of babies that had died before they were born. The baby in the first bottle had a large white head bent over a tiny curled-up body the size of a frog. The baby in the next bottle was bigger and the baby next to that one was bigger still and the baby in the last bottle was the size of a normal baby and he seemed to be looking at me and smiling a little piggy smile.

I was quite proud of the calm way I stared at all these gruesome things. The only time I jumped was when I leaned my elbow on Buddy's cadaver's stomach to watch him dissect a lung. After a minute or two I felt this burning sensation in my elbow and it occurred to me the cadaver might just be half alive since it was still warm, so I leapt off my stool with a small exclamation. Then Buddy explained the burning was only from the pickling fluid, and I sat back in my old position.

In the hour before lunch Buddy took me to a lecture on sickle-cell anaemia and some other depressing diseases, where they wheeled sick people out on to the platform and asked them questions and then wheeled them off and showed coloured slides.

One slide I remember showed a beautiful laughing girl with a black mole on her cheek. 'Twenty days after that mole appeared the girl was dead,' the doctor said, and everybody went very quiet for a minute and then the bell rang, so I never really found out what the mole was or why the girl died.

In the afternoon we went to see a baby born.

First we found a linen closet in the hospital corridor where Buddy took out a white mask for me to wear and some gauze.

A tall fat medical student, big as Sidney Greenstreet, lounged nearby, watching Buddy wind the gauze round and round my head until my hair was completely covered and only my eyes peered out over the white mask.

The medical student gave an unpleasant little snicker. 'At least your mother loves you,' he said.

I was so busy thinking how very fat he was and how unfortunate it must be for a man and especially a young man to be fat, because what woman could stand leaning over that big stomach to kiss him, that I didn't immediately realize what this student had said to me was an insult. By the time I figured he must consider himself quite a fine fellow and had thought up a cutting remark about how only a mother loves a fat man, he was gone.

Buddy was examining a queer wooden plaque on the wall with a row of holes in it, starting from a hole about the size of a silver dollar and ending with one the size of a dinner-plate.

'Fine, fine,' he said to me. 'There's somebody about to have a baby this minute.'

At the door of the delivery room stood a thin, stoop-shouldered medical student Buddy knew.

'Hello, Will,' Buddy said. 'Who's on the job?'

'I am,' Will said gloomily, and I noticed little drops of sweat beading his high pale forehead. 'I am, and it's my first.'

Buddy told me Will was a third-year man and had to deliver eight babies before he could graduate.

Then he noticed a bustle at the far end of the hall and some men in lime-green coats and skull-caps and a few nurses came moving towards us in a ragged procession wheeling a trolley with a big white lump on it.

'You oughtn't to see this,' Will muttered in my ear. 'You'll never want to have a baby if you do. They oughtn't to let women watch. It'll be the end of the human race.'

Buddy and I laughed, and then Buddy shook Will's hand and we all went into the room.

I was so struck by the sight of the table where they were lifting the woman I didn't say a word. It looked like some awful torture table, with these metal stirrups sticking up in mid-air at one end and all sorts of instruments and wires and tubes I couldn't make out properly at the other.

Buddy and I stood together by the window, a few feet away from the woman, where we had a perfect view.

The woman's stomach stuck up so high I couldn't see her face or the upper part of her body at all. She seemed to have nothing but an enormous spider-fat stomach and two little ugly spindly legs propped in the high stirrups, and all the time the baby was being born she never stopped making this unhuman whooing noise.

Later Buddy told me the woman was on a drug that would make her forget she'd had any pain and that when she swore and groaned she really didn't know what she was doing because she was in a kind of twilight sleep.

I thought it sounded just like the sort of drug a man would invent. Here was a woman in terrible pain, obviously feeling every bit of it or she wouldn't groan like that, and she would go straight home and start another baby, because the drug would make her forget how bad the pain had been, when all the time, in some secret part of her, that long, blind, doorless and windowless corridor of pain was waiting to open up and shut her in again.

The head doctor, who was supervising Will, kept saying to the woman, 'Push down, Mrs Tomolillo, push down, that's a good girl, push down,' and finally through the split, shaven place between her legs, lurid with disinfectant, I saw a dark fuzzy thing appear.

'The baby's head,' Buddy whispered under cover of the woman's groans.

But the baby's head stuck for some reason, and the doctor told Will he'd have to make a cut. I heard the scissors close on the woman's skin like cloth and the blood began to run down – a fierce, bright red. Then all at once the baby seemed to pop out into Will's hands, the colour of a blue plum and floured with white stuff and streaked with blood, and Will kept saying, 'I'm going to drop it, I'm going to drop it, I'm going to drop it,' in a terrified voice.

'No, you're not,' the doctor said, and took the baby out of Will's hands and started massaging it, and the blue colour went away and the baby started to cry in a lorn, croaky voice and I could see it was a boy.

The first thing that baby did was pee in the doctor's face. I told Buddy later I didn't see how that was possible, but he said it was quite possible, though unusual, to see something like that happen.

As soon as the baby was born the people in the room divided up into two groups, the nurses tying a metal dog-tag on the baby's wrist and swabbing its eyes with cotton on the end of a stick and wrapping it up and putting it in a canvas-sided cot, while the doctor and Will started sewing up the woman's cut with a needle and a long thread.

I think somebody said, 'It's a boy, Mrs Tomolillo,' but the woman didn't answer or raise her head.

'Well, how was it?' Buddy asked with a satisfied expression as we walked across the green quadrangle to his room.

'Wonderful,' I said. 'I could see something like that every day.'

I didn't feel up to asking him if there were any other ways to have babies. For some reason the most important thing to me was actually seeing the baby come out of you yourself and making sure it was yours. I thought if you had to have all that pain anyway you might just as well stay awake.

I had always imagined myself hitching up on to my elbows on the delivery table after it was all over – dead white, of course, with no make-up and from the awful ordeal, but smiling and radiant, with my hair down to my waist, and reaching out for my first little squirmy child and saying its name, whatever it was.

'Why was it all covered with flour?' I asked then, to keep the conversation going, and Buddy told me about the waxy stuff that guarded the baby's skin.

When we were back in Buddy's room, which reminded me of nothing so much as a monk's cell, with its bare walls and bare bed and bare floor and the desk loaded with Gray's *Anatomy* and other thick gruesome books, Buddy lit a candle and un-corked a bottle of Dubonnet. Then we lay down side by side on the bed and Buddy sipped his wine while I read aloud 'somewhere I have never travelled' and other poems from a book I'd brought.

Buddy said he figured there must be something in poetry if a girl like me spent all her days over it, so each time we met I read him some poetry and explained to him what I found in it. It was Buddy's idea. He always arranged our week-ends so we'd never regret wasting our time in any way. Buddy's father was a teacher, and I think Buddy could have been a teacher as well, he was always trying to explain things to me and introduce me to new knowledge.

Suddenly, after I finished a poem, he said, 'Esther, have you ever seen a man?'

The way he said it I knew he didn't mean a regular man or a man in general, I knew he meant a man naked.

'No,' I said. 'Only statues.'

'Well, don't you think you would like to see me?'

I didn't know what to say. My mother and my grandmother had started hinting around to me a lot lately about what a fine, clean boy Buddy Willard was, coming from such a fine, clean family, and how everybody at church thought he was a model person, so kind to his parents and to older people, as well as so athletic and so handsome and so intelligent.

All I'd heard about, really, was how fine and clean Buddy was and how he was the kind of person a girl should stay fine and clean for. So I didn't really see the harm in anything Buddy would think up to do.

'Well, all right, I guess so,' I said.

I stared at Buddy while he unzipped his chino pants and took them off and laid them on a chair and then took off his underpants that were made of something like nylon fishnet.

'They're cool,' he explained, 'and my mother says they wash easily.'

Then he just stood there in front of me and I kept on staring at him. The only thing I could think of was turkey neck and turkey gizzards and I felt very depressed.

64

Buddy seemed hurt I didn't say anything. 'I think you ought to get used to me like this,' he said. 'Now let me see you.'

But undressing in front of Buddy suddenly appealed to me about as much as having my Posture Picture taken at college, where you have to stand naked in front of a camera, knowing all the time that a picture of you stark naked, both full view and side view, is going into the college gym files to be marked A B C or D depending on how straight you are.

'Oh, some other time,' I said.

'All right.' Buddy got dressed again.

Then we kissed and hugged a while and I felt a little better. I drank the rest of the Dubonnet and sat cross-legged at the end of Buddy's bed and asked for a comb. I began to comb my hair down over my face so Buddy couldn't see it. Suddenly I said, 'Have you ever had an affair with anyone, Buddy?'

I don't know what made me say it, the words just popped out of my mouth. I never thought for one minute that Buddy Willard would have an affair with anyone. I expected him to say, 'No, I have been saving myself for when I get married to somebody pure and a virgin like you.'

But Buddy didn't say anything, he just turned pink.

'Well, have you?'

'What do you mean, an affair?' Buddy asked then in a hollow voice.

'You know, have you ever gone to bed with anyone?' I kept rhythmically combing the hair down over the side of my face nearest to Buddy, and I could feel the little electric filaments clinging to my hot cheeks and I wanted to shout, 'Stop, stop, don't tell me, don't say anything.' But I didn't, I just kept still.

'Well, yes, I have,' Buddy said finally.

I almost fell over. From the first night Buddy Willard kissed me and said I must go out with a lot of boys, he made me feel I was much more sexy and experienced than he was and that everything he did like hugging and kissing and petting was simply what I made him feel like doing out of the blue, he couldn't help it and didn't know how it came about.

Now I saw he had only been pretending all this time to be so innocent.

'Tell me about it.' I combed my hair slowly over and over, feeling the teeth of the comb dig into my cheek at every stroke. 'Who was it?'

Buddy seemed relieved I wasn't angry. He even seemed relieved to have somebody to tell about how he was seduced.

Of course, somebody had seduced Buddy, Buddy hadn't started it and it wasn't really his fault. It was this waitress at the hotel he worked at as a busboy the last summer on Cape Cod. Buddy had noticed her staring at him queerly and shoving her breasts up against him in the confusion of the kitchen, so finally one day he asked her what the trouble was and she looked him straight in the eye and said, 'I want you.'

'Served up with parsley?' Buddy had laughed innocently.

'No,' she had said. 'Some night.'

And that's how Buddy had lost his pureness and his virginity.

At first I thought he must have slept with the waitress only the once, but when I asked how many times, just to make sure, he said he couldn't remember but a couple of times a week for the rest of the summer. I multiplied three by ten and got thirty, which seemed beyond all reason.

After that something in me just froze up.

Back at college I started asking a senior here and a senior there what they would do if a boy they knew suddenly told them he'd slept thirty times with some slutty waitress one summer, smack in the middle of knowing them. But these seniors said most boys were like that and you couldn't honestly accuse them of anything until you were at least pinned or engaged to be married.

66

Actually, it wasn't the idea of Buddy sleeping with some-body that bothered me. I mean I'd read about all sorts of people sleeping with each other, and if it had been any other boy I would merely have asked him the most interesting details, and maybe gone out and slept with somebody myself just to even things up, and then thought no more about it.

What I couldn't stand was Buddy's pretending I was so sexy and he was so pure, when all the time he'd been having an affair with that tarty waitress and must have felt like laughing in my face.

'What does your mother think about this waitress?' I asked Buddy that week-end.

Buddy was amazingly close to his mother. He was always quoting what she said about the relationship between a man and a woman, and I knew Mrs Willard was a real fanatic about virginity for men and women both. When I first went to her house for supper she gave me a queer, shrewd, searching look, and I knew she was trying to tell whether I was a virgin or not.

Just as I thought, Buddy was embarrassed. 'Mother asked me about Gladys,' he admitted.

'Well, what did you say?'

'I said Gladys was free, white and twenty-one.'

Now I knew Buddy would never talk to his mother as rudely as that for my sake. He was always saying how his mother said, 'What a man wants is a mate and what a woman wants is infinite security,' and, 'What a man is is an arrow into the future and what a woman is is the place the arrow shoots off from,' until it made me tired.

Every time I tried to argue, Buddy would say his mother still got pleasure out of his father and wasn't that wonderful for people their age, it must mean she really knew what was what.

Well, I had just decided to ditch Buddy Willard for once and for all, not because he'd slept with that waitress but because he didn't have the honest guts to admit it straight off to everybody and face up to it as part of his character, when the phone in the hall rang and somebody said in a little knowing singsong, 'It's for you, Esther, it's from Boston.'

I could tell right away something must be wrong, because Buddy was the only person I knew in Boston, and he never called me long distance because it was so much more expensive than letters. Once, when he had a message he wanted me to get almost immediately, he went all round his entry at medical school asking if anybody was driving up to my college that week-end, and sure enough, somebody was, so he gave them a note for me and I got it the same day. He didn't even have to pay for a stamp.

It was Buddy all right. He told me that the annual fall chest X-ray showed he had caught TB and he was going off on a scholarship for medical students who caught TB to a TB place in the Adirondacks. Then he said I hadn't written since that last week-end and he hoped nothing was the matter between us, and would I please try to write him at least once a week and come to visit him at this TB place in my Christmas vacation?

I had never heard Buddy so upset. He was very proud of his perfect health and was always telling me it was psychosomatic when my sinuses blocked up and I couldn't breathe. I thought this an odd attitude for a doctor to have and perhaps he should study to be a psychiatrist instead, but of course I never came right out and said so.

I told Buddy how sorry I was about the TB and promised to write, but when I hung up I didn't feel one bit sorry. I only felt a wonderful relief.

I thought the TB might just be a punishment for living the kind of double life Buddy lived and feeling so superior to people. And I thought how convenient it would be now I didn't have to announce to everybody at college I had broken off with Buddy and start the boring business of blind dates all over again.

I simply told everyone that Buddy had TB and we were practically engaged, and when I stayed in to study on Saturday nights they were extremely kind to me because they thought I was so brave, working the way I did just to hide a broken heart.

Chapter Seven

Of course, Constantin was much too short, but in his own way he was handsome, with light brown hair and dark blue eyes and a lively, challenging expression. He could almost have been an American, he was so tan and had such good teeth, but I could tell straight away that he wasn't. He had what no American man I've ever met has had, and that's intuition.

From the start Constantin guessed I wasn't any protégée of Mrs Willard's. I raised an eyebrow here and dropped a dry little laugh there, and pretty soon we were both openly raking Mrs Willard over the coals and I thought, 'This Constantin won't mind if I'm too tall and don't know enough languages and haven't been to Europe, he'll see through all that stuff to what I really am.'

Constantin drove me to the UN in his old green convertible with cracked, comfortable brown leather seats and the top down. He told me his tan came from playing tennis, and when we were sitting there side by side flying down the streets in the open sun he took my hand and squeezed it, and I felt happier than I had been since I was about nine and running along the hot white beaches with my father the summer before he died.

And while Constantin and I sat in one of those hushed plush auditoriums in the UN, next to a stern muscular Russian girl with no make-up who was a simultaneous interpreter like

Constantin, I thought how strange it had never occurred to me before that I was only purely happy until I was nine years old.

After that – in spite of the Girl Scouts and the piano lessons and the water-colour lessons and the dancing lessons and the sailing camp, all of which my mother scrimped to give me, and college, with crewing in the mist before breakfast and black-bottom pies and the little new firecrackers of ideas going off every day – I had never been really happy again.

I stared through the Russian girl in her double-breasted grey suit, rattling off idiom after idiom in her own unknowable tongue – which Constantin said was the most difficult part, because the Russians didn't have the same idioms as our idioms – and I wished with all my heart I could crawl into her and spend the rest of my life barking out one idiom after another. It mightn't make me any happier, but it would be one more little pebble of efficiency among all the other pebbles.

Then Constantin and the Russian girl interpreter and the whole bunch of black and white and yellow men arguing down there behind their labelled microphones seemed to move off at a distance. I saw their mouths going up and down without a sound, as if they were sitting on the deck of a departing ship, stranding me in the middle of a huge silence.

I started adding up all the things I couldn't do.

I began with cooking.

My grandmother and my mother were such good cooks that I left everything to them. They were always trying to teach me one dish or another, but I would just look on and say, 'Yes, yes, I see,' while the instructions slid through my head like water, and then I'd always spoil what I did so nobody would ask me to do it again.

I remember Jody, my best and only girl-friend at college in my freshman year, making me scrambled eggs at her house one morning. They tasted unusual, and when I asked her if she had put in anything extra, she said cheese and garlic salt. I asked who told her to do that, and she said nobody, she just thought it up. But then, she was practical and a sociology major.

I didn't know shorthand either.

This meant I couldn't get a good job after college. My mother kept telling me nobody wanted a plain English major. But an English major who knew shorthand was something else again. Everybody would want her. She would be in demand among all the up-and-coming young men and she would transcribe letter after thrilling letter.

The trouble was, I hated the idea of serving men in any way. I wanted to dictate my own thrilling letters. Besides, those little shorthand symbols in the book my mother showed me seemed just as bad as let t equal time and let s equal the total distance.

My list grew longer.

I was a terrible dancer. I couldn't carry a tune. I had no sense of balance, and when we had to walk down a narrow board with our hands out and a book on our heads in gym class I always fell over. I couldn't ride a horse or ski, the two things I wanted to do most, because they cost too much money. I couldn't speak German or read Hebrew or write Chinese. I didn't even know where most of the odd out-of-the-way countries the UN men in front of me represented fitted in on the map.

For the first time in my life, sitting there in the sound-proof heart of the UN building between Constantin who could play tennis as well as simultaneously interpret and the Russian girl who knew so many idioms, I felt dreadfully inadequate. The trouble was, I had been inadequate all along, I simply hadn't thought about it.

The one thing I was good at was winning scholarships and prizes, and that era was coming to an end.

I felt like a racehorse in a world without race-tracks or a

champion college footballer suddenly confronted by Wall Street and a business suit, his days of glory shrunk to a little gold cup on his mantel with a date engraved on it like the date on a tombstone.

I saw my life branching out before me like the green fig-tree in the story.

From the tip of every branch, like a fat purple fig, a wonderful future beckoned and winked. One fig was a husband and a happy home and children, and another fig was a famous poet and another fig was a brilliant professor, and another fig was Ee Gee, the amazing editor, and another fig was Europe and Africa and South America, and another fig was Constantin and Socrates and Attila and a pack of other lovers with queer names and off-beat professions, and another fig was an Olympic lady crew champion, and beyond and above these figs were many more figs I couldn't quite make out.

I saw myself sitting in the crotch of this fig-tree, starving to death, just because I couldn't make up my mind which of the figs I would choose. I wanted each and every one of them, but choosing one meant losing all the rest, and, as I sat there, unable to decide, the figs began to wrinkle and go black, and, one by one, they plopped to the ground at my feet.

Constantin's restaurant smelt of herbs and spices and sour cream. All the time I had been in New York I had never found such a restaurant. I only found those Heavenly Hamburger places, where they serve giant hamburgers and soup-of-the-day and four kinds of fancy cake at a very clean counter facing a long glarey mirror.

To reach this restaurant we had to climb down seven dimly-lit steps into a sort of cellar.

Travel posters plastered the smoke-dark walls, like so many picture windows overlooking Swiss lakes and Japanese mountains and African velds, and thick, dusty bottle-candles that seemed for centuries to have wept their coloured waxes red over blue over green in a fine, three-dimensional lace, cast a circle of light round each table where the faces floated, flushed and flamelike themselves.

I don't know what I ate, but I felt immensely better after the first mouthful. It occurred to me that my vision of the fig-tree and all the fat figs that withered and fell to earth might well have arisen from the profound void of an empty stomach.

Constantin kept refilling our glasses with a sweet Greek wine that tasted of pine bark, and I found myself telling him how I was going to learn German and go to Europe and be a war correspondent like Maggie Higgins.

I felt so fine by the time we came to the yoghurt and strawberry jam that I decided I would let Constantin seduce me.

Ever since Buddy Willard had told me about that waitress I had been thinking I ought to go out and sleep with somebody myself. Sleeping with Buddy wouldn't count, though, because he would still be one person ahead of me, it would have to be with somebody else.

The only boy I ever actually discussed going to bed with was a bitter, hawk-nosed Southerner from Yale, who came up to college one week-end only to find his date had eloped with a taxi-driver the day before. As the girl had lived in my house and as I was the only one home that particular night, it was my job to cheer him up.

At the local coffee-shop, hunched in one of the secretive, high-backed booths with hundreds of people's names gouged into the wood, we drank cup after cup of black coffee and talked frankly about sex.

This boy – his name was Eric – said he thought it disgusting the way all the girls at my college stood around on the porches under the porch lights and in the bushes in plain view, necking madly before the one o'clock curfew, so everybody passing by could see them. A million years of evolution, Eric said bitterly, and what are we? Animals.

Then Eric told me how he had slept with his first woman.

He went to a Southern prep school that specialized in building all-round gentlemen, and by the time you graduated it was an unwritten rule that you had to have known a woman. Known in the Biblical sense, Eric said.

So one Saturday Eric and a few of his classmates took a bus into the nearest city and visited a notorious whorehouse. Eric's whore hadn't even taken off her dress. She was a fat, middle-aged woman with dyed red hair and suspiciously thick lips and rat-coloured skin and she wouldn't turn off the light, so he had had her under a fly-spotted twenty-five watt bulb, and it was nothing like it was cracked up to be. It was boring as going to the toilet.

I said maybe if you loved a woman it wouldn't seem so boring, but Eric said it would be spoiled by thinking this woman too was just an animal like the rest, so if he loved anybody he would never go to bed with her. He'd go to a whore if he had to and keep the woman he loved free of all that dirty business.

It had crossed my mind at the time that Eric might be a good person to go to bed with, since he had already done it and, unlike the usual run of boys, didn't seem dirty-minded or silly when he talked about it. But then Eric wrote me a letter saying he thought he might really be able to love me, I was so intelligent and cynical and yet had such a kind face, surprisingly like his older sister's; so I knew it was no use, I was the type he would never go to bed with, and wrote him I was unfortunately about to marry a childhood sweetheart.

75

The more I thought about it the better I liked the idea of being seduced by a simultaneous interpreter in New York City. Constantin seemed mature and considerate in every way. There were no people I knew he would want to brag to about it, the way college boys bragged about sleeping with girls in the backs of cars to their room-mates or their friends on the basketball team. And there would be a pleasant irony in sleeping with a man Mrs Willard had introduced me to, as if she were, in a roundabout way, to blame for it.

When Constantin asked if I would like to come up to his apartment to hear some balalaika records I smiled to myself. My mother had always told me never under any circumstances to go with a man to a man's rooms after an evening out, it could mean only the one thing.

'I'm very fond of balalaika music,' I said.

Constantin's room had a balcony, and the balcony overlooked the river, and we could hear the hooing of the tugs down in the darkness. I felt moved and tender and perfectly certain about what I was going to do.

I knew I might have a baby, but that thought hung far and dim in the distance and didn't trouble me at all. There was no one hundred per cent sure way not to have a baby, it said in an article my mother cut out of the *Reader's Digest* and mailed to me at college. This article was written by a married woman lawyer with children and called 'In Defence of Chastity'.

It gave all the reasons a girl shouldn't sleep with anybody but her husband and then only after they were married.

The main point of the article was that a man's world is different from a woman's world and a man's emotions are different from a woman's emotions and only marriage can bring the two worlds and the two different sets of emotions together properly. My mother said this was something a girl didn't know about till it was too late, so she had to take the

76

advice of people who were already experts, like a married woman.

This woman lawyer said the best men wanted to be pure for their wives, and even if they weren't pure, they wanted to be the ones to teach their wives about sex. Of course they would try to persuade a girl to have sex and say they would marry her later, but as soon as she gave in, they would lose all respect for her and start saying that if she did that with them she would do that with other men and they would end up making her life miserable.

The woman finished her article by saying better be safe than sorry and besides, there was no sure way of not getting stuck with a baby and then you'd really be in a pickle.

Now the one thing this article didn't seem to me to consider was how a girl felt.

It might be nice to be pure and then to marry a pure man, but what if he suddenly confessed he wasn't pure after we were married, the way Buddy Willard had? I couldn't stand the idea of a woman having to have a single pure life and a man being able to have a double life, one pure and one not.

Finally I decided that if it was so difficult to find a red-blooded intelligent man who was still pure by the time he was twenty-one I might as well forget about staying pure myself and marry somebody who wasn't pure either. Then when he started to make my life miserable I could make his miserable as well.

When I was nineteen, pureness was the great issue.

Instead of the world being divided up into Catholics and Protestants or Republicans and Democrats or white men and black men or even men and women, I saw the world divided into people who had slept with somebody and people who hadn't, and this seemed the only really significant difference between one person and another.

I thought a spectacular change would come over me the day I crossed the boundary line.

I thought it would be the way I'd feel if I ever visited Europe. I'd come home, and if I looked closely into the mirror I'd be able to make out a little white Alp at the back of my eye. Now I thought that if I looked into the mirror tomorrow I'd see a doll-size Constantin sitting in my eye and smiling out at me.

Well for about an hour we lounged on Constantin's balcony in two separate sling-back chairs with the victrola playing and the balalaika records stacked between us. A faint milky light diffused from the street lights or the half-moon or the cars or the stars, I couldn't tell what, but apart from holding my hand Constantin showed no desire to seduce me whatsoever.

I asked if he was engaged or had any special girl friend, thinking maybe that's what was the matter, but he said no, he made a point of keeping clear of such attachments.

At last I felt a powerful drowsiness drifting through my veins from all the pine-bark wine I had drunk.

'I think I'll go in and lie down,' I said.

I strolled casually into the bedroom and stooped over to nudge off my shoes. The clean bed bobbed before me like a safe boat. I stretched full-length and shut my eyes. Then I heard Constantin sigh and come in from the balcony. One by one his shoes clonked on to the floor, and he lay down by my side.

I looked at him secretly from under a fall of hair.

He was lying on his back, his hands under his head, staring at the ceiling. The starched white sleeves of his shirt, rolled up to the elbows, glimmered eerily in the half-dark and his tan skin seemed almost black. I thought he must be the most beautiful man I'd ever seen.

I thought if only I had a keen, shapely bone-structure to my face or could discuss politics shrewdly or was a famous writer Constantin might find me interesting enough to sleep with.

And then I wondered if as soon as he came to like me he would sink into ordinariness, and if as soon as he came to love me I would find fault after fault, the way I did with Buddy Willard and the boys before him.

The same thing happened over and over:

I would catch sight of some flawless man off in the distance, but as soon as he moved closer I immediately saw he wouldn't do at all.

That's one of the reasons I never wanted to get married. The last thing I wanted was infinite security and to be the place an arrow shoots off from. I wanted change and excitement and to shoot off in all directions myself, like the coloured arrows from a Fourth of July rocket.

I woke to the sound of rain.

It was pitch dark. After a while I deciphered the faint outlines of an unfamiliar window. Every so often a beam of light appeared out of thin air, traversed the wall like a ghostly, exploratory finger, and slid off into nothing again.

Then I heard the sound of somebody breathing.

At first I thought it was only myself, and that I was lying in the dark in my hotel room after being poisoned. I held my breath, but the breathing kept on.

A green eye glowed on the bed before me. It was divided into quarters like a compass. I reached out slowly and closed my hand on it. I lifted it up. With it came an arm, heavy as a dead man's, but warm with sleep.

Constantin's watch said three o'clock.

He was lying in his shirt and trousers and stocking feet just as I had left him when I dropped asleep, and as my eyes grew used to the darkness I made out his pale eyelids and his straight nose and his tolerant, shapely mouth, but they seemed insubstantial, as if drawn on fog. For a few minutes I leaned over, studying him. I had never fallen asleep beside a man before.

I tried to imagine what it would be like if Constantin were my husband.

It would mean getting up at seven and cooking him eggs and bacon and toast and coffee and dawdling about in my night-gown and curlers after he'd left for work to wash up the dirty plates and make the bed, and then when he came home after a lively, fascinating day he'd expect a big dinner, and I'd spend the evening washing up even more dirty plates till I fell into bed, utterly exhausted.

This seemed a dreary and wasted life for a girl with fifteen years of straight A's, but I knew that's what marriage was like, because cook and clean and wash was just what Buddy Willard's mother did from morning till night, and she was the wife of a university professor and had been a private school teacher herself.

Once when I visited Buddy I found Mrs Willard braiding a rug out of strips of wool from Mr Willard's old suits. She'd spent weeks on that rug, and I had admired the tweedy browns and greens and blues patterning the braid, but after Mrs Willard was through, instead of hanging the rug on the wall the way I would have done, she put it down in place of her kitchen mat, and in a few days it was soiled and dull and indistinguishable from any mat you could buy for under a dollar in the Five and Ten.

And I knew that in spite of all the roses and kisses and restaurant dinners a man showered on a woman before he married her, what he secretly wanted when the wedding service ended was for her to flatten out underneath his feet like Mrs Willard's kitchen mat.

Hadn't my own mother told me that as soon as she and my father left Reno on their honeymoon – my father had been married before, so he needed a divorce – my father said to her, 'Whew, that's a relief, now we can stop pretending and be ourselves'? – and from that day on my mother never had a minute's peace.

I also remembered Buddy Willard saying in a sinister, knowing way that after I had children I would feel differently, I wouldn't want to write poems any more. So I began to think maybe it was true that when you were married and had children it was like being brainwashed, and afterwards you went about numb as a slave in some private, totalitarian state.

As I stared down at Constantin the way you stare down at a bright, unattainable pebble at the bottom of a deep well, his eyelids lifted and he looked through me, and his eyes were full of love. I watched dumbly as a little shutter of recognition clicked across the blur of tenderness and the wide pupils went glossy and depthless as patent leather.

Constantin sat up, yawning. 'What time is it?'

'Three,' I said in a flat voice. 'I better go home. I have to be at work first thing in the morning.'

'I'll drive you.'

As we sat back to back on our separate sides of the bed fumbling with our shoes in the horrid cheerful white light of the bed lamp, I sensed Constantin turn round. 'Is your hair always like that?'

'Like what?'

He didn't answer but reached over and put his hand at the root of my hair and ran his fingers out slowly to the tip ends like a comb. A little electric shock flared through me, and I sat quite still. Ever since I was small I loved feeling somebody comb my hair. It made me go all sleepy and peaceful.

'Ah, I know what it is,' Constantin said. 'You've just washed it.'

And he bent to lace up his tennis shoes.

An hour later I lay in my hotel bed, listening to the rain. It didn't even sound like rain, it sounded like a tap running. The ache in the middle of my left shin bone came to life, and I abandoned any hope of sleep before seven, when my radio-alarm clock would rouse me with its hearty renderings of Sousa.

Every time it rained the old leg-break seemed to remember itself, and what it remembered was a dull hurt.

Then I thought, 'Buddy Willard made me break that leg.'

Then I thought, 'No, I broke it myself. I broke it on purpose to pay myself back for being such a heel.'

Chapter Eight

Mr Willard drove me up to the Adirondacks.

It was the day after Christmas and a grey sky bellied over us, fat with snow. I felt overstuffed and dull and disappointed, the way I always do the day after Christmas, as if whatever it was the pine boughs and the candles and the silver and gilt-ribboned presents and the birch-log fires and the Christmas turkey and the carols at the piano promised never came to pass.

At Christmas I almost wished I was a Catholic.

First Mr Willard drove and then I drove. I don't know what we talked about, but as the countryside, already deep under old falls of snow, turned us a bleaker shoulder, and as the fir trees crowded down from the grey hills to the road edge, so darkly green they looked black, I grew gloomier and gloomier.

I was tempted to tell Mr Willard to go ahead alone, I would hitch-hike home.

But one glance at Mr Willard's face – the silver hair in its boyish crewcut, the clear eyes, the pink cheeks, all frosted like a sweet wedding cake with the innocent, trusting expression – and I knew I couldn't do it. I'd have to see the visit through to the end.

At midday the greyness paled a bit, and we parked in an icy turn-off and shared out the tunafish sandwiches and the oatmeal cookies and the apples and the thermos of black coffee Mrs Willard had packed for our lunch.

Mr Willard eyed me kindly. Then he cleared his throat and brushed a few last crumbs from his lap. I could tell he was going to say something serious, because he was very shy, and I'd heard him clear his throat in that same way before giving an important economics lecture.

'Nelly and I have always wanted a daughter.'

For one crazy minute I thought Mr Willard was going to announce that Mrs Willard was pregnant and expecting a baby girl. Then he said, 'But I don't see how any daughter could be nicer than you.'

Mr Willard must have thought I was crying because I was so glad he wanted to be a father to me. 'There, there,' he patted my shoulder and cleared his throat once or twice. 'I think we understand each other.'

Then he opened the car door on his side and strolled round to my side, his breath shaping tortuous smoke signals in the grey air. I moved over to the seat he had left and he started the car and we drove on.

I'm not sure what I expected of Buddy's sanatorium.

I think I expected a kind of wooden chalet perched up on top of a small mountain, with rosy-cheeked young men and women, all very attractive but with hectic glittering eyes, lying covered with thick blankets on outdoor balconies.

'TB is like living with a bomb in your lung,' Buddy had written to me at college. 'You just lie around very quietly hoping it won't go off.'

I found it hard to imagine Buddy lying quietly. His whole philosophy of life was to be up and doing every second. Even when we went to the beach in the summer he never lay down to drowse in the sun the way I did. He ran back and forth or played ball or did a little series of rapid push-ups to use the time.

Mr Willard and I waited in the reception room for the end of the afternoon rest cure.

The colour scheme of the whole sanatorium seemed to be based on liver. Dark, glowering woodwork, burnt-brown leather chairs, walls that might once have been white but had succumbed under a spreading malady of mould or damp. A mottled brown linoleum sealed off the floor.

On a low coffee-table, with circular and semi-circular stains bitten into the dark veneer, lay a few wilted numbers of *Time* and *Life*. I flipped to the middle of the nearest magazine. The face of Eisenhower beamed up at me, bald and blank as the face of a foetus in a bottle.

After a while I became aware of a sly, leaking noise. For a minute I thought the walls had begun to discharge the moisture that must saturate them, but then I saw the noise came from a small fountain in one corner of the room.

The fountain spurted a few inches into the air from a rough length of pipe, threw up its hands, collapsed and drowned its ragged dribble in a stone basin of yellowing water. The basin was paved with the white hexagonal tiles one finds in public lavatories.

A buzzer sounded. Doors opened and shut in the distance. Then Buddy came in.

'Hello, Dad.'

Buddy hugged his father, and promptly, with a dreadful brightness, came over to me and held out his hand. I shook it. It felt moist and fat.

Mr Willard and I sat together on a leather couch. Buddy perched opposite us on the edge of a slippery armchair. He kept smiling, as if the corners of his mouth were strung up on invisible wire.

The last thing I expected was for Buddy to be fat. All the time I thought of him at the sanatorium I saw shadows carving themselves under his cheekbones and his eyes burning out of almost fleshless sockets.

But everything concave about Buddy had suddenly turned convex. A pot belly swelled under the tight white nylon shirt and his cheeks were round and ruddy as marzipan fruit. Even his laugh sounded plump.

Buddy's eyes met mine. 'It's the eating,' he said. 'They stuff us day after day and then just make us lie around. But I'm allowed out on walk-hours now, so don't worry, I'll thin down in a couple of weeks.' He jumped up, smiling like a glad host. 'Would you like to see my room?'

I followed Buddy, and Mr Willard followed me, through a pair of swinging doors set with panes of frosted glass down a dim, liver-coloured corridor smelling of floor wax and lysol and another vaguer odour, like bruised gardenias.

Buddy threw open a brown door, and we filed into the narrow room.

A lumpy bed, shrouded by a thin white spread, pencil-striped with blue, took up most of the space. Next to it stood a bed table with a pitcher and a water glass and the silver twig of a thermometer poking up from a jar of pink disinfectant. A second table, covered with books and papers and off-kilter clay pots – baked and painted, but not glazed – squeezed itself between the bed foot and the closet door.

'Well,' Mr Willard breathed, 'it looks comfortable enough.'

Buddy laughed.

'What are these?' I picked up a clay ashtray in the shape of a lilypad, with the veinings carefully drawn in yellow on a murky green ground. Buddy didn't smoke.

'That's an ashtray,' Buddy said. 'It's for you.'

I put the tray down. 'I don't smoke.'

'I know,' Buddy said. 'I thought you might like it, though.'

'Well,' Mr Willard rubbed one papery lip against another. 'I guess I'll be getting on. I guess I'll be leaving you two young people . . .'

'Fine, Dad. You be getting on.'

I was surprised. I had thought Mr Willard was going to stay the night before driving me back the next day.

'Shall I come too?'

'No, no.' Mr Willard peeled a few bills from his wallet and handed them to Buddy. 'See that Esther gets a comfortable seat on the train. She'll stay a day or so, maybe.'

Buddy escorted his father to the door.

I felt Mr Willard had deserted me. I thought he must have planned it all along, but Buddy said No, his father simply couldn't stand the sight of sickness and especially his own son's sickness, because he thought all sickness was sickness of the will. Mr Willard had never been sick a day in his life.

I sat down on Buddy's bed. There simply wasn't anywhere else to sit.

Buddy rummaged among his papers in a businesslike way. Then he handed me a thin, grey magazine. 'Turn to page eleven.'

The magazine was printed somewhere in Maine and full of stencilled poems and descriptive paragraphs separated from each other by asterisks. On page eleven I found a poem titled 'Florida Dawn'. I skipped down through image after image about water-melon lights and turtle-green palms and shells fluted like bits of Greek architecture.

'Not bad.' I thought it was dreadful.

'Who wrote it?' Buddy asked with an odd, pigeony smile.

My eye dropped to the name on the lower right-hand corner of the page. B. S. Willard.

'I don't know.' Then I said, 'Of course I know, Buddy. You wrote it.'

Buddy edged over to me.

I edged back. I had very little knowledge about TB, but it seemed to me an extremely sinister disease, the way it went on so invisibly. I thought Buddy might well be sitting in his own little murderous aura of TB germs.

'Don't worry,' Buddy laughed. 'I'm not positive.'

'Positive?'

'You won't catch anything.'

Buddy stopped for a breath, the way you do in the middle of climbing something very steep.

'I want to ask you a question.' He had a disquieting new habit of boring into my eyes with his look as if actually bent on piercing my head, the better to analyse what went on inside it.

'I'd thought of asking it by letter.'

I had a fleeting vision of a pale blue envelope with a Yale crest on the back flap.

'But then I decided it would be better if I waited until you came up, so I could ask you in person.' He paused. 'Well, don't you want to know what it is?'

'What?' I said in a small, unpromising voice.

Buddy sat down beside me. He put his arm around my waist and brushed the hair from my ear. I didn't move. Then I heard him whisper, 'How would you like to be Mrs Buddy Willard?'

I had an awful impulse to laugh.

I thought how that question would have bowled me over at any time in my five- or six-year period of adoring Buddy Willard from a distance.

Buddy saw me hesitate.

'Oh, I'm in no shape now, I know,' he said quickly. 'I'm still on P.A.S. and I may yet lose a rib or two, but I'll be back at med school by next fall. A year from this spring at the latest . . .'

'I think I should tell you something, Buddy.'

'I know,' Buddy said stiffly. 'You've met someone.'

'No, it's not that.'

'What is it, then?'

'I'm never going to get married.'

'You're crazy.' Buddy brightened. 'You'll change your mind.'

'No. My mind's made up.'

But Buddy just went on looking cheerful.

'Remember,' I said, 'that time you hitch-hiked back to college with me after Skit Night?'

'I remember.'

'Remember how you asked me where would I like to live best, the country or the city?'

'And you said . . .'

'And I said I wanted to live in the country and in the city both?'

Buddy nodded.

'And you,' I continued with sudden force, 'laughed and said I had the perfect set-up of a true neurotic and that that question came from some questionnaire you'd had in psychology class that week?'

Buddy's smile dimmed.

'Well, you were right. I *am* neurotic. I could never settle down in either the country *or* the city.'

'You could live between them,' Buddy suggested helpfully. 'Then you could go to the city sometimes and to the country sometimes.'

'Well, what's so neurotic about that?'

Buddy didn't answer.

'Well?' I rapped out, thinking, 'You can't coddle these sick people, it's the worst thing for them, it'll spoil them to bits.'

'Nothing,' Buddy said in a pale, still voice.

'Neurotic, ha!' I let out a scornful laugh. 'If neurotic is

wanting two mutually exclusive things at one and the same time, then I'm neurotic as hell. I'll be flying back and forth between one mutually exclusive thing and another for the rest of my days.'

Buddy put his hand on mine.

'Let me fly with you.'

I stood at the top of the ski slope on Mount Pisgah, looking down. I had no business to be up there. I had never skied before in my life. Still, I thought I would enjoy the view while I had the chance.

At my left, the rope tow deposited skier after skier on the snowy summit which, packed by much crossing and re-crossing and slightly melted in the noon sun, had hardened to the consistency and polish of glass. The cold air punished my lungs and sinuses to a visionary clearness.

On every side of me the red and blue and white jacketed skiers tore away down the blinding slope like fugitive bits of an American flag. From the foot of the ski run, the imitation log cabin lodge piped its popular songs into the overhang of silence.

Gazing down on the Jungfrau
From our chalet for two . . .

The lilt and boom threaded by me like an invisible rivulet in a desert of snow. One careless, superb gesture, and I would be hurled into motion down the slope towards the small khaki spot in the sidelines, among the spectators, which was Buddy Willard.

All morning Buddy had been teaching me how to ski.

First, Buddy borrowed skis and ski poles from a friend of his in the village, and ski boots from a doctor's wife whose feet were only one size larger than my own, and a red ski jacket from a student nurse. His persistence in the face of mulishness was astounding.

Then I remembered that at medical school Buddy had won a prize for persuading the most relatives of dead people to have their dead ones cut up whether they needed it or not, in the interests of science. I forget what the prize was, but I could just see Buddy in his white coat with his stethoscope sticking out of a side pocket like part of his anatomy, smiling and bowing and talking those numb, dumb relatives into signing the post-mortem papers.

Next, Buddy borrowed a car from his own doctor, who'd had TB himself and was very understanding, and we drove off as the buzzer for walk-hour rasped along the sunless sanatorium corridors.

Buddy had never skied before either, but he said that the elementary principles were quite simple, and as he'd often watched the ski instructors and their pupils he could teach me all I'd need to know.

For the first half-hour I obediently herring-boned up a small slope, pushed off with my poles and coasted straight down. Buddy seemed pleased with my progress.

'That's fine, Esther,' he observed, as I negotiated my slope for the twentieth time. 'Now let's try you on the rope tow.'

I stopped in my tracks, flushed and panting.

'But Buddy, I don't know how to zigzag yet. All those people coming down from the top know how to zigzag.'

'Oh, you need only go half-way. Then you won't gain very much momentum.'

And Buddy accompanied me to the rope tow and showed me how to let the rope run through my hands, and then told me to close my fingers round it and go up.

It never occurred to me to say no.

I wrapped my fingers around the rough, bruising snake of a

rope that slithered through them, and went up.

But the rope dragged me, wobbling and balancing, so rapidly I couldn't hope to dissociate myself from it half-way. There was a skier in front of me and a skier behind me, and I'd have been knocked over and stuck full of skis and poles the minute I let go, and I didn't want to make trouble, so I hung quietly on.

At the top, though, I had second thoughts.

Buddy singled me out, hesitating there in the red jacket. His arms chopped the air like khaki windmills. Then I saw he was signalling me to come down a path that had opened in the middle of the weaving skiers. But as I poised, uneasy, with a dry throat, the smooth white path from my feet to his feet grew blurred.

A skier crossed it from the left, another crossed it from the right, and Buddy's arms went on waving feebly as antennae from the other side of a field swarming with tiny moving animalcules like germs, or bent, bright exclamation marks.

I looked up from that churning amphitheatre to the view beyond it.

The great, grey eye of the sky looked back at me, its mist-shrouded sun focusing all the white and silent distances that poured from every point of the compass, hill after pale hill, to stall at my feet.

The interior voice nagging me not to be a fool – to save my skin and take off my skis and walk down, camouflaged by the scrub pines bordering the slope – fled like a disconsolate mosquito. The thought that I might kill myself formed in my mind coolly as a tree or a flower.

I measured the distance to Buddy with my eye.

His arms were folded, now, and he seemed of a piece with the split-rail fence behind him – numb, brown and inconsequential.

Edging to the rim of the hilltop, I dug the spikes of my poles into the snow and pushed myself into a flight I knew I couldn't stop by skill or any belated access of will.

I aimed straight down.

A keen wind that had been hiding itself struck me full in the mouth and raked the hair back horizontal on my head. I was descending, but the white sun rose no higher. It hung over the suspended waves of the hills, an insentient pivot without which the world would not exist.

A small, answering point in my own body flew towards it. I felt my lungs inflate with the inrush of scenery – air, mountains, trees, people. I thought, 'This is what it is to be happy.'

I plummeted down past the zigzaggers, the students, the experts, through year after year of doubleness and smiles and compromise, into my own past.

People and trees receded on either hand like the dark sides of a tunnel as I hurtled on to the still, bright point at the end of it, the pebble at the bottom of the well, the white sweet baby cradled in its mother's belly.

My teeth crunched a gravelly mouthful. Ice water seeped down my throat.

Buddy's face hung over me, near and huge, like a distracted planet. Other faces showed themselves up in back of his. Behind them, black dots swarmed on a plane of whiteness. Piece by piece, as at the strokes of a dull godmother's wand, the old world sprang back into position.

'You were doing fine,' a familiar voice informed my ear, 'until that man stepped into your path.'

People were unfastening my bindings and collecting my ski poles from where they poked skyward, askew, in their separate snowbanks. The lodge fence propped itself at my back.

93

Buddy bent to pull off my boots and the several pairs of white wool socks that padded them. His plump hand shut on my left foot, then inched up my ankle, closing and probing, as if feeling for a concealed weapon.

A dispassionate white sun shone at the summit of the sky. I wanted to hone myself on it till I grew saintly and thin and essential as the blade of a knife.

'I'm going up,' I said. 'I'm going to do it again.'

'No, you're not.'

A queer, satisfied expression came over Buddy's face.

'No, you're not,' he repeated with a final smile. 'Your leg's broken in two places. You'll be stuck in a cast for months.'

Chapter Nine

'I'm so glad they're going to die.'

Hilda arched her cat-limbs in a yawn, buried her head in her arms on the conference table and went back to sleep. A wisp of bilious green straw perched on her brow like a tropical bird.

Bile green. They were promoting it for fall, only Hilda, as usual, was half a year ahead of time. Bile green with black, bile green with white, bile green with nile green, its kissing cousin.

Fashion blurbs, silver and full of nothing, sent up their fishy bubbles in my brain. They surfaced with a hollow pop.

I'm so glad they're going to die.

I cursed the luck that had timed my arrival in the hotel cafeteria to coincide with Hilda's. After a late night I felt too dull to think up the excuse that would take me back to my room for the glove, the handkerchief, the umbrella, the notebook I forgot. My penalty was the long, dead walk from the frosted glass doors of the Amazon to the strawberry-marble slab of our entry on Madison Avenue.

Hilda moved like a mannequin the whole way.

'That's a lovely hat, did you make it?'

I half-expected Hilda to turn on me and say, 'You sound sick', but she only extended and then retracted her swanny neck.

'Yes.'

The night before I'd seen a play where the heroine was

possessed by a dybbuk, and when the dybbuk spoke from her mouth its voice sounded so cavernous and deep you couldn't tell whether it was a man or a woman. Well Hilda's voice sounded just like the voice of that dybbuk.

She stared at her reflection in the glossed shop windows as if to make sure, moment by moment, that she continued to exist. The silence between us was so profound I thought part of it must be my fault.

So I said, 'Isn't it awful about the Rosenbergs?'

The Rosenbergs were to be electrocuted late that night.

'Yes!' Hilda said, and at last I felt I had touched a human string in the cat's cradle of her heart. It was only as the two of us waited for the others in the tomb-like morning gloom of the conference room that Hilda amplified that Yes of hers.

'It's awful such people should be alive.'

She yawned then, and her pale orange mouth opened on a large darkness. Fascinated, I stared at the blind cave behind her face until the two lips met and moved and the dybbuk spoke out of its hiding place, 'I'm so glad they're going to die.'

'Come on, give us a smile.'

I sat on the pink velvet love-seat in Jay Cee's office, holding a paper rose and facing the magazine photographer. I was the last of the twelve to have my picture taken. I had tried concealing myself in the powder-room, but it didn't work. Betsy had spied my feet under the doors.

I didn't want my picture taken because I was going to cry. I didn't know why I was going to cry, but I knew that if anybody spoke to me or looked at me too closely the tears would fly out of my eyes and the sobs would fly out of my throat and I'd cry for a week. I could feel the tears brimming and sloshing in me like water in a glass that is unsteady and too full.

This was the last round of photographs before the magazine went to press and we returned to Tulsa or Biloxi or Teaneck or Coos Bay or wherever we'd come from, and we were supposed to be photographed with props to show what we wanted to be.

Betsy held an ear of corn to show she wanted to be a farmer's wife, and Hilda held the bald, faceless head of a hatmaker's dummy to show she wanted to design hats, and Doreen held a gold-embroidered sari to show she wanted to be a social worker in India (she didn't really, she told me, she only wanted to get her hands on a sari).

When they asked me what I wanted to be I said I didn't know.

'Oh, sure you know,' the photographer said.

'She wants,' said Jay Cee wittily, 'to be everything.'

I said I wanted to be a poet.

Then they scouted about for something for me to hold.

Jay Cee suggested a book of poems, but the photographer said no, that was too obvious. It should be something that showed what inspired the poems. Finally Jay Cee unclipped the single, long-stemmed paper rose from her latest hat.

The photographer fiddled with his hot white lights. 'Show us how happy it makes you to write a poem.'

I stared through the frieze of rubber plant leaves in Jay Cee's window to the blue sky beyond. A few stagey cloud puffs were travelling from right to left. I fixed my eyes on the largest cloud, as if, when it passed out of sight, I might have the good luck to pass with it.

I felt it was very important to keep the line of my mouth level.

'Give us a smile.'

At last, obediently, like the mouth of a ventriloquist's dummy, my own mouth started to quirk up.

97

'Hey,' the photographer protested, with sudden foreboding, 'you look like you're going to cry.'

I couldn't stop.

I buried my face in the pink velvet façade of Jay Cee's love-seat and with immense relief the salt tears and miserable noises that had been prowling around in me all morning burst out into the room.

When I lifted my head, the photographer had vanished. Jay Cee had vanished as well. I felt limp and betrayed, like the skin shed by a terrible animal. It was a relief to be free of the animal, but it seemed to have taken my spirit with it, and everything else it could lay its paws on.

I fumbled in my pocketbook for the gilt compact with the mascara and the mascara brush and the eyeshadow and the three lipsticks and the side mirror. The face that peered back at me seemed to be peering from the grating of a prison cell after a prolonged beating. It looked bruised and puffy and all the wrong colours. It was a face that needed soap and water and Christian tolerance.

I started to paint it with small heart.

Jay Cee breezed back after a decent interval with an armful of manuscripts.

'These'll amuse you,' she said. 'Have a good read.'

Every morning a snowy avalanche of manuscripts swelled the dust-grey piles in the office of the Fiction Editor. Secretly, in studies and attics and schoolrooms all over America, people must be writing. Say someone or other finished a manuscript every minute; in five minutes that would be five manuscripts stacked on the Fiction Editor's desk. Within the hour there would be sixty, crowding each other on to the floor. And in a year . . .

I smiled, seeing a pristine, imaginary manuscript floating in mid-air, with Esther Greenwood typed in the upper-right hand corner. After my month on the magazine I'd applied for a summer school course with a famous writer where you sent in the manuscript of a story and he read it and said whether you were good enough to be admitted into his class.

Of course, it was a very small class, and I had sent in my story a long time ago and hadn't heard from the writer yet, but I was sure I'd find the letter of acceptance waiting on the mail table at home.

I decided I'd surprise Jay Cee and send in a couple of the stories I wrote in this class under a pseudonym. Then one day the Fiction Editor would come in to Jay Cee personally and plop the stories down on her desk and say, 'Here's something a cut above the usual,' and Jay Cee would agree and accept them and ask the author to lunch and it would be me.

'Honestly,' Doreen said, 'this one'll be different.'

'Tell me about him,' I said stonily.

'He's from Peru.'

'They're squat,' I said. 'They're ugly as Aztecs.'

'No, no, no, sweetie, I've already met him.'

We were sitting on my bed in a mess of dirty cotton dresses and laddered nylons and grey underwear, and for ten minutes Doreen had been trying to persuade me to go to a country club dance with a friend of somebody Lenny knew which, she insisted, was a very different thing from a friend of Lenny's, but as I was catching the eight o'clock train home the next morning I felt I should make some attempt to pack.

I also had a dim idea that if I walked the streets of New York by myself all night something of the city's mystery and magnificence might rub off on to me at last.

But I gave it up.

It was becoming more and more difficult for me to decide to

do anything in those last days. And when I eventually *did* decide to do something, such as packing a suitcase, I only dragged all my grubby, expensive clothes out of the bureau and the closet and spread them on the chairs and the bed and the floor and then sat and stared at them, utterly perplexed. They seemed to have a separate, mulish identity of their own that refused to be washed and folded and stowed.

'It's these clothes,' I told Doreen. 'I just can't face these clothes when I come back.'

'That's easy.'

And in her beautiful, one-track way, Doreen started to snatch up slips and stockings and the elaborate strapless bra, full of steel springs – a free gift from the Primrose Corset Company, which I'd never had the courage to wear – and finally, one by one, the sad array of queerly-cut forty dollar dresses . . .

'Hey, leave that one out. I'm wearing it.'

Doreen extricated a black scrap from her bundle and dropped it in my lap. Then, snowballing the rest of the clothes into one soft, conglomerate mass, she stuffed them out of sight under the bed.

Doreen knocked on the green door with the gold knob.

Scuffling and a man's laugh, cut short, sounded from inside. Then a tall boy in shirtsleeves and a blond crewcut inched the door open and peered out.

'Baby!' he roared.

Doreen disappeared in his arms. I thought it must be the person Lenny knew.

I stood quietly in the doorway in my black sheath and my black stole with the fringe, yellower than ever, but expecting less. 'I am an observer,' I told myself, as I watched Doreen being handed into the room by the blond boy to another man, who was also tall, but dark, with slightly longer hair. This man was wearing an immaculate white suit, a pale blue shirt and a yellow satin tie with a bright stickpin.

I couldn't take my eyes off that stickpin.

A great white light seemed to shoot out of it, illuminating the room. Then the light withdrew into itself, leaving a dewdrop on a field of gold.

I put one foot in front of the other.

'That's a diamond,' somebody said, and a lot of people burst out laughing.

My nail tapped a glassy facet.

'Her first diamond.'

'Give it to her, Marco.'

Marco bowed and deposited the stickpin in my palm.

It dazzled and danced with light like a heavenly ice-cube. I slipped it quickly into my imitation jet bead evening bag and looked round. The faces were empty as plates, and nobody seemed to be breathing.

'Fortunately,' a dry, hard hand encircled my upper arm, 'I am escorting the lady for the rest of the evening. Perhaps,' the spark in Marco's eyes extinguished, and they went black, 'I shall perform some small service . . .'

Somebody laughed.

'. . . worthy of a diamond.'

The hand round my arm tightened. 'Ouch!'

Marco removed his hand. I looked down at my arm. A thumb-print purpled into view. Marco watched me. Then he pointed to the underside of my arm. 'Look there.'

I looked, and saw four, faint matching prints.

'You see, I am quite serious.'

Marco's small, flickering smile reminded me of a snake I'd teased in the Bronx Zoo. When I tapped my finger on the stout cage glass the snake had opened its clockwork jaws and seemed to smile. Then it struck and struck and struck at the invisible pane till I moved off.

I had never met a woman-hater before.

I could tell Marco was a woman-hater, because in spite of all the models and TV starlets in the room that night he paid attention to nobody but me. Not out of kindness or even curiosity, but because I'd happened to be dealt to him, like a playing card in a pack of identical cards.

A man in the country club band stepped up to the mike and started shaking those seedpod rattles that mean South American music.

Marco reached for my hand, but I hung on to my fourth daiquiri and stayed put. I'd never had a daiquiri before. The reason I had a daiquiri was because Marco ordered it for me, and I felt so grateful he hadn't asked what sort of drink I wanted that I didn't say a word, I just drank one daiquiri after another.

Marco looked at me.

'No,' I said.

'What do you mean, no?'

'I can't dance to that kind of music.'

'Don't be stupid.'

'I want to sit here and finish my drink.'

Marco bent towards me with a tight smile, and in one swoop my drink took wing and landed in a potted palm. Then Marco gripped my hand in such a way I had to choose between following him on to the floor or having my arm torn off.

'It's a tango.' Marco manoeuvred me out among the dancers. 'I love tangos.'

'I can't dance.'

'You don't have to dance. I'll do the dancing.'

Marco hooked an arm around my waist and jerked me up

against his dazzling white suit. Then he said, 'Pretend you are drowning.'

I shut my eyes, and the music broke over me like a rainstorm. Marco's leg slid forward against mine and my leg slid back and I seemed to be riveted to him, limb for limb, moving as he moved, without any will or knowledge of my own, and after a while I thought, 'It doesn't take two to dance, it only takes one,' and I let myself blow and bend like a tree in the wind.

'What did I tell you?' Marco's breath scorched my ear. 'You're a perfectly respectable dancer.'

I began to see why woman-haters could make such fools of women. Woman-haters were like gods: invulnerable and chock-full of power. They descended, and then they disappeared. You could never catch one.

After the South American music there was an interval.

Marco led me through the French doors into the garden. Lights and voices spilled from the ballroom window, but a few yards beyond the darkness drew up its barricade and sealed them off. In the infinitesimal glow of the stars, the trees and flowers were strewing their cool odours. There was no moon.

The box hedges shut behind us. A deserted golf course stretched away towards a few hilly clumps of trees, and I felt the whole desolate familiarity of the scene – the country club and the dance and the lawn with its single cricket.

I didn't know where I was, but it was somewhere in the wealthy suburbs of New York.

Marco produced a slim cigar and a silver lighter in the shape of a bullet. He set the cigar between his lips and bent over the small flare. His face, with its exaggerated shadows and planes of light, looked alien and pained, like a refugee's.

I watched him.

'Who are you in love with?' I said then.

For a minute Marco didn't say anything, he simply opened his mouth and breathed out a blue, vaporous ring.

'Perfect!' he laughed.

The ring widened and blurred, ghost-pale on the dark air.

Then he said, 'I am in love with my cousin.'

I felt no surprise.

'Why don't you marry her?'

'Impossible.'

'Why?'

Marco shrugged. 'She's my first cousin. She's going to be a nun.'

'Is she beautiful?'

'There's no one to touch her.'

'Does she know you love her?'

'Of course.'

I paused. The obstacle seemed unreal to me.

'If you love her,' I said, 'you'll love somebody else someday.'

Marco dashed his cigar underfoot.

The ground soared and struck me with a soft shock. Mud squirmed through my fingers. Marco waited until I half rose. Then he put both hands on my shoulders and flung me back.

'My dress . . .'

'Your dress!' The mud oozed and adjusted itself to my shoulder blades. 'Your dress!' Marco's face lowered cloudily over mine. A few drops of spit struck my lips. 'Your dress is black and the dirt is black as well.'

Then he threw himself face down as if he would grind his body through me and into the mud.

'It's happening,' I thought. 'It's happening. If I just lie here and do nothing it will happen.'

Marco set his teeth to the strap at my shoulder and tore my sheath to the waist. I saw the glimmer of bare skin, like a pale veil separating two bloody-minded adversaries.

'Slut!'

The word hissed by my ear.

'Slut!'

The dust cleared, and I had a full view of the battle.

I began to writhe and bite.

Marco weighed me to the earth.

'Slut!'

I gouged at his leg with the sharp heel of my shoe. He turned, fumbling for the hurt.

Then I fisted my fingers together and smashed them at his nose. It was like hitting the steel plate of a battleship. Marco sat up. I began to cry.

Marco pulled out a white handkerchief and dabbed his nose. Blackness, like ink, spread over the pale cloth.

I sucked at my salty knuckles.

'I want Doreen.'

Marco stared off across the golf links.

'I want Doreen. I want to go home.'

'Sluts, all sluts.' Marco seemed to be talking to himself. 'Yes or no, it is all the same.'

I poked Marco's shoulder.

'Where's Doreen?'

Marco snorted. 'Go to the parking lot. Look in the backs of all the cars.'

Then he spun round.

'My diamond.'

I got up and retrieved my stole from the darkness. I started to walk off. Marco sprang to his feet and blocked my path. Then, deliberately, he wiped his finger under his bloody nose and with two strokes stained my cheeks. 'I have earned my diamond with this blood. Give it to me.'

'I don't know where it is.'

Now I knew perfectly well that the diamond was in my

evening bag and that when Marco knocked me down my evening bag had soared, like a night bird, into the enveloping darkness. I began to think I would lead him away and then return on my own and hunt for it.

I had no idea what a diamond that size would buy, but whatever it was, I knew it would be a lot.

Marco took my shoulders in both hands.

'Tell me,' he said, giving each word equal emphasis. 'Tell me, or I'll break your neck.'

Suddenly I didn't care.

'It's in my imitation jet bead evening bag,' I said. 'Somewhere in the muck.'

I left Marco on his hands and knees, scrabbling in the darkness for another, smaller darkness that hid the light of his diamond from his furious eyes.

Doreen was not in the ballroom nor in the parking lot.

I kept to the fringe of the shadows so nobody would notice the grass plastered to my dress and shoes, and with my black stole I covered my shoulders and bare breasts.

Luckily for me, the dance was nearly over, and groups of people were leaving and coming out to the parked cars. I asked at one car after another until finally I found a car that had room and would drop me in the middle of Manhattan.

At that vague hour between dark and dawn, the sunroof of the Amazon was deserted.

Quiet as a burglar in my cornflower-sprigged bathrobe, I crept to the edge of the parapet. The parapet reached almost to my shoulders, so I dragged a folding chair from the stack against the wall, opened it, and climbed on to the precarious seat.

A stiff breeze lifted the hair from my head. At my feet, the city doused its lights in sleep, its buildings blackened, as if for a funeral.

It was my last night.

I grasped the bundle I carried and pulled at a pale tail. A strapless elasticized slip which, in the course of wear, had lost its elasticity, slumped into my hand. I waved it, like a flag of truce, once, twice . . . The breeze caught it, and I let go.

A white flake floated out into the night, and began its slow descent. I wondered on what street or rooftop it would come to rest.

I tugged at the bundle again.

The wind made an effort, but failed, and a batlike shadow sank towards the roof garden of the penthouse opposite.

Piece by piece, I fed my wardrobe to the night wind, and flutteringly, like a loved one's ashes, the grey scraps were ferried off, to settle here, there, exactly where I would never know, in the dark heart of New York.

Chapter Ten

The face in the mirror looked like a sick Indian.

I dropped the compact into my pocket-book and stared out of the train window. Like a colossal junkyard, the swamps and back lots of Connecticut flashed past, one broken-down fragment bearing no relation to another.

What a hotch-potch the world was!

I glanced down at my unfamiliar skirt and blouse.

The skirt was a green dirndl with tiny black, white and electric blue shapes swarming across it, and it stuck out like a lampshade. Instead of sleeves, the white eyelet blouse had frills at the shoulder, floppy as the wings of a new angel.

I'd forgotten to save any day clothes from the ones I let fly over New York, so Betsy had traded me a blouse and skirt for my bathrobe with the cornflowers on it.

A wan reflection of myself, white wings, brown ponytail and all, ghosted over the landscape.

'Pollyanna Cowgirl,' I said out loud.

A woman in the seat opposite looked up from her magazine.

I hadn't, at the last moment, felt like washing off the two diagonal lines of dried blood that marked my cheeks. They seemed touching, and rather spectacular, and I thought I would carry them around with me, like the relic of a dead lover, till they wore off of their own accord.

Of course, if I smiled or moved my face much, the blood would flake away in no time, so I kept my face immobile, and when I had to speak I spoke through my teeth, without disturbing my lips.

I didn't really see why people should look at me.

Plenty of people looked queerer than I did.

My grey suitcase rode on the rack over my head, empty except for *The Thirty Best Short Stories of the Year*, a white plastic sunglasses case and two dozen avocado pears, a parting present from Doreen.

The pears were unripe, so they would keep well, and whenever I lifted my suitcase up or down or simply carried it along, they cannoned from one end to the other with a special little thunder of their own.

'Root Wan Twenny Ate!' the conductor bawled.

The domesticated wilderness of pine, maple and oak rolled to a halt and stuck in the frame of the train window like a bad picture. My suitcase grumbled and bumped as I negotiated the long aisle.

I stepped from the air-conditioned compartment on to the station platform, and the motherly breath of the suburbs enfolded me. It smelt of lawn sprinklers and station-wagons and tennis rackets and dogs and babies.

A summer calm laid its soothing hand over everything, like death.

My mother was waiting by the glove-grey Chevrolet.

'Why lovey, what's happened to your face?'

'Cut myself,' I said briefly, and crawled into the back seat after my suitcase. I didn't want her staring at me the whole way home.

The upholstery felt slippery and clean.

My mother climbed behind the wheel and tossed a few letters into my lap, then turned her back.

The car purred into life.

'I think I should tell you right away,' she said, and I could see bad news in the set of her neck, 'you didn't make that writing course.'

The air punched out of my stomach.

All through June the writing course had stretched before me like a bright, safe bridge over the dull gulf of the summer. Now I saw it totter and dissolve, and a body in a white blouse and green skirt plummet into the gap.

Then my mouth shaped itself sourly.

I had expected it.

I slunk down on the middle of my spine, my nose level with the rim of the window, and watched the houses of outer Boston glide by. As the houses grew more familiar, I slunk still lower.

I felt it was very important not to be recognized.

The grey, padded car roof closed over my head like the roof of a prison van, and the white, shining, identical clapboard houses with their interstices of well-groomed green proceeded past, one bar after another in a large but escape-proof cage.

I had never spent a summer in the suburbs before.

The soprano screak of carriage wheels punished my ear. Sun, seeping through the blinds, filled the bedroom with a sulphurous light. I didn't know how long I had slept, but I felt one big twitch of exhaustion.

The twin bed next to mine was empty and unmade.

At seven I had heard my mother get up, slip into her clothes and tiptoe out of the room. Then the buzz of the orange squeezer sounded from downstairs, and the smell of coffee and bacon filtered under my door. Then the sink water ran from the tap and dishes clinked as my mother dried them and put them back in the cupboard.

Then the front door opened and shut. Then the car door opened and shut, and the motor went broom-broom and, edging off with a crunch of gravel, faded into the distance.

My mother was teaching shorthand and typing to a lot of city college girls and wouldn't be home till the middle of the afternoon.

The carriage wheels screaked past again. Somebody seemed to be wheeling a baby back and forth under my window.

I slipped out of bed and on to the rug, and quietly, on my hands and knees, crawled over to see who it was.

Ours was a small, white clapboard house set in the middle of a small green lawn on the corner of two peaceful suburban streets, but in spite of the little maple trees planted at intervals around our property, anybody passing along the sidewalk could glance up at the second storey windows and see just what was going on.

This was brought home to me by our next-door neighbour, a spiteful woman named Mrs Ockenden.

Mrs Ockenden was a retired nurse who had just married her third husband – the other two died in curious circumstances – and she spent an inordinate amount of time peering from behind the starched white curtains of her windows.

She had called my mother up twice about me – once to report that I had been sitting in front of the house for an hour under the streetlight and kissing somebody in a blue Plymouth, and once to say that I had better pull the blinds down in my room, because she had seen me half-naked getting ready for bed one night when she happened to be out walking her Scotch terrier.

With great care, I raised my eyes to the level of the window-sill.

A woman not five feet tall, with a grotesque, protruding stomach, was wheeling an old black baby carriage down the street. Two or three small children of various sizes, all pale, with smudgy faces and bare smudgy knees, wobbled along in the shadow of her skirts.

A serene, almost religious smile lit up the woman's face. Her head tilted happily back, like a sparrow egg perched on a duck egg, she smiled into the sun.

I knew the woman well.

It was Dodo Conway.

Dodo Conway was a Catholic who had gone to Barnard and then married an architect who had gone to Columbia and was also a Catholic. They had a big, rambling house up the street from us, set behind a morbid façade of pine trees, and surrounded by scooters, tricycles, doll carriages, toy fire trucks, baseball bats, badminton nets, croquet wickets, hamster cages and cocker spaniel puppies – the whole sprawling paraphernalia of suburban childhood.

Dodo interested me in spite of myself.

Her house was unlike all the others in our neighbourhood in its size (it was much bigger) and its colour (the second storey was constructed of dark brown clapboard and the first of grey stucco, studded with grey and purple golf-ball-shaped stones), and the pine trees completely screened it from view, which was considered unsociable in our community of adjoining lawns and friendly, waist-high hedges.

Dodo raised her six children – and would no doubt raise her seventh – on rice crispies, peanut-butter-and-marshmallow sandwiches, vanilla ice-cream and gallon upon gallon of Hoods milk. She got a special discount from the local milkman.

Everybody loved Dodo, although the swelling size of her family was the talk of the neighbourhood. The older people around, like my mother, had two children, and the younger, more prosperous ones had four, but nobody but Dodo was on the verge of a seventh. Even six was considered excessive, but then, everybody said, of course Dodo was a Catholic.

I watched Dodo wheel the youngest Conway up and down. She seemed to be doing it for my benefit.

Children made me sick.

A floorboard creaked, and I ducked down again, just as Dodo Conway's face, by instinct, or some gift of supernatural hearing, turned on the little pivot of its neck.

I felt her gaze pierce through the white clapboard and the pink, wallpaper roses and uncover me, crouching there behind the silver pickets of the radiator.

I crawled back into bed and pulled the sheet over my head. But even that didn't shut out the light, so I buried my head under the darkness of the pillow and pretended it was night. I couldn't see the point of getting up.

I had nothing to look forward to.

After a while I heard the telephone ringing in the downstairs hall. I stuffed the pillow into my ears and gave myself five minutes. Then I lifted my head from its bolt hole. The ringing had stopped.

Almost at once it started up again.

Cursing whatever friend, relative or stranger had sniffed out my homecoming, I padded barefoot downstairs. The black instrument on the hall table trilled its hysterical note over and over, like a nervous bird.

I picked up the receiver.

'Hullo,' I said, in a low, disguised voice.

'Hullo Esther, what's the matter, have you got laryngitis?'

It was my old friend Jody, calling from Cambridge.

Jody was working at the Co-op that summer and taking a lunchtime course in sociology. She and two other girls from my college had rented a big apartment from four Harvard law students, and I'd been planning to move in with them when my writing course began.

Jody wanted to know when they could expect me.

'I'm not coming,' I said. 'I didn't make the course.'

There was a small pause.

'He's an ass,' Jody said then. 'He doesn't know a good thing when he sees it.'

'My sentiments exactly.' My voice sounded strange and hollow in my ears.

'Come anyway. Take some other course.'

The notion of studying German or abnormal psychology flitted through my head. After all, I'd saved nearly the whole of my New York salary, so I could just about afford it.

But the hollow voice said, 'You better count me out.'

'Well,' Jody began, 'there's this other girl who wanted to come in with us if anybody dropped out . . .'

'Fine. Ask her.'

The minute I hung up I knew I should have said I would come. One more morning listening to Dodo Conway's baby carriage would drive me crazy. And I made a point of never living in the same house with my mother for more than a week.

I reached for the receiver.

My hand advanced a few inches, then retreated and fell limp. I forced it towards the receiver again, but again it stopped short, as if it had collided with a pane of glass.

I wandered into the dining-room.

Propped on the table I found a long, business-like letter from the summer school and a thin blue letter on left-over Yale stationery, addressed to me in Buddy Willard's lucid hand.

I slit open the summer school letter with a knife.

Since I wasn't accepted for the writing course, it said, I could choose some other course instead, but I should call in to the Admissions Office that same morning, or it would be too late to register, the courses were almost full.

I dialled the Admissions Office and listened to the zombie voice leave a message that Miss Esther Greenwood was cancelling all arrangements to come to summer school.

Then I opened Buddy Willard's letter.

Buddy wrote that he was probably falling in love with a nurse who also had TB, but his mother had rented a cottage in the Adirondacks for the month of July, and if I came along with her, he might well find his feeling for the nurse was a mere infatuation.

I snatched up a pencil and crossed out Buddy's message. Then I turned the letter paper over and on the opposite side wrote that I was engaged to a simultaneous interpreter and never wanted to see Buddy again as I did not want to give my children a hypocrite for a father.

I stuck the letter back in the envelope, scotch-taped it together, and readdressed it to Buddy, without putting on a new stamp. I thought the message was worth a good three cents.

Then I decided I would spend the summer writing a novel.

That would fix a lot of people.

I strolled into the kitchen, dropped a raw egg into a teacup of raw hamburger, mixed it up and ate it. Then I set up the card-table on the screened breezeway between the house and the garage.

A great wallowing bush of mock orange shut off the view of the street in front, the house wall and the garage wall took care of either side, and a clump of birches and a box hedge protected me from Mrs Ockenden at the back.

I counted out three hundred and fifty sheets of corrasable bond from my mother's stock in the hall closet, secreted away under a pile of old felt hats and clothes brushes and woollen scarves.

Back on the breezeway, I fed the first, virgin sheet into my old portable and rolled it up.

From another, distanced mind, I saw myself sitting on the breezeway, surrounded by two white clapboard walls, a mock orange bush and a clump of birches and a box hedge, small as a doll in a doll's house.

A feeling of tenderness filled my heart. My heroine would be myself, only in disguise. She would be called Elaine. Elaine. I counted the letters on my fingers. There were six letters in Esther, too. It seemed a lucky thing.

Elaine sat on the breezeway in an old yellow nightgown of her mother's waiting for something to happen. It was a sweltering morning in July, and drops of sweat crawled down her back, one by one, like slow insects.

I leaned back and read what I had written.

It seemed lively enough, and I was quite proud of the bit about the drops of sweat like insects, only I had the dim impression I'd probably read it somewhere else a long time ago.

I sat like that for about an hour, trying to think what would come next, and in my mind, the barefoot doll in her mother's old yellow nightgown sat and stared into space as well.

'Why honey, don't you want to get dressed?'

My mother took care never to tell me to do anything. She would only reason with me sweetly, like one intelligent, mature person with another.

'It's almost three in the afternoon.'

'I'm writing a novel,' I said. 'I haven't got time to change out of this and change into that.'

I lay on the couch on the breezeway and shut my eyes. I could hear my mother clearing the typewriter and the papers from the card-table and laying out the silver for supper, but I didn't move.

Inertia oozed like molasses through Elaine's limbs. That's what it must feel like to have malaria, she thought.

At that rate, I'd be lucky if I wrote a page a day.

Then I knew what the trouble was.

I needed experience.

How could I write about life when I'd never had a love affair or a baby or seen anybody die? A girl I knew had just won a prize for a short story about her adventures among the pygmies in Africa. How could I compete with that sort of thing?

By the end of supper my mother had convinced me I should study shorthand in the evenings. Then I would be killing two birds with one stone, writing a novel and learning something practical as well. I would also be saving a whole lot of money.

That same evening, my mother unearthed an old blackboard from the cellar and set it up on the breezeway. Then she stood at the blackboard and scribbled little curlicues in white chalk while I sat in a chair and watched.

At first I felt hopeful.

I thought I might learn shorthand in no time, and when the freckled lady in the Scholarships Office asked me why I hadn't worked to earn money in July and August, the way you were supposed to if you were a scholarship girl, I could tell her I had taken a free shorthand course instead, so I could support myself right after college.

The only thing was, when I tried to picture myself in some job, briskly jotting down line after line of shorthand, my mind went blank. There wasn't one job I felt like doing where you used shorthand. And, as I sat there and watched, the white chalk curlicues blurred into senselessness.

I told my mother I had a terrible headache, and went to bed.

An hour later the door inched open, and she crept into the

room. I heard the whisper of her clothes as she undressed. She climbed into bed. Then her breathing grew slow and regular.

In the dim light of the streetlamp that filtered through the drawn blinds, I could see the pin curls on her head glittering like a row of little bayonets.

I decided I would put off the novel until I had gone to Europe and had a lover, and that I would never learn a word of shorthand. If I never learned shorthand I would never have to use it.

I thought I would spend the summer reading *Finnegans Wake* and writing my thesis.

Then I would be way ahead when college started at the end of September, and able to enjoy my last year instead of swotting away with no make-up and stringy hair, on a diet of coffee and benzedrine, the way most of the seniors taking honours did, until they finished their thesis.

Then I thought I might put off college for a year and apprentice myself to a pottery maker.

Or work my way to Germany and be a waitress, until I was bilingual.

Then plan after plan started leaping through my head, like a family of scatty rabbits.

I saw the years of my life spaced along a road in the form of telephone poles, threaded together by wires. I counted one, two, three . . . nineteen telephone poles, and then the wires dangled into space, and try as I would, I couldn't see a single pole beyond the nineteenth.

The room blued into view, and I wondered where the night had gone. My mother turned from a foggy log into a slumbering, middle-aged woman, her mouth slightly open and a snore ravelling from her throat. The piggish noise irritated me, and for a while it seemed to me that the only way to stop it would be to take the column of skin and sinew from which it rose and twist it to silence between my hands.

I feigned sleep until my mother left for school, but even my eyelids didn't shut out the light. They hung the raw, red screen of their tiny vessels in front of me like a wound. I crawled between the mattress and the padded bedstead and let the mattress fall across me like a tombstone. It felt dark and safe under there, but the mattress was not heavy enough.

It needed about a ton more weight to make me sleep.

riverrun, past Eve and Adam's, from swerve of shore to bend of bay, brings us by a commodius vicus of recirculation back to Howth Castle and Environs . . .

The thick book made an unpleasant dent in my stomach.

riverrun, past Eve and Adam's . . .

I thought the small letter at the start might mean that nothing ever really began all new, with a capital, but that it just flowed on from what came before. Eve and Adam's was Adam and Eve, of course, but it probably signified something else as well.

Maybe it was a pub in Dublin.

My eyes sank through an alphabet soup of letters to the long word in the middle of the page.

bababadalgharaghtakamminarronnkonnbronntonnerronn-ruonnthunntrovarrhounawnskawntoohoohoordenenthurnuk!

I counted the letters. There were exactly a hundred of them. I thought this must be important.

Why should there be a hundred letters?

Haltingly, I tried the word aloud.

It sounded like a heavy wooden object falling downstairs, boomp boomp boomp, step after step. Lifting the pages of the book, I let them fan slowly by my eyes. Words, dimly familiar, but twisted all awry, like faces in a funhouse mirror, fled past, leaving no impression on the glassy surface of my brain.

I squinted at the page.

The letters grew barbs and rams' horns. I watched them separate, each from the other, and jiggle up and down in a silly way. Then they associated themselves in fantastic, untranslatable shapes, like Arabic or Chinese.

I decided to junk my thesis.

I decided to junk the whole honours programme and become an ordinary English major. I went to look up the requirements of an ordinary English major at my college.

There were lots of requirements, and I didn't have half of them. One of the requirements was a course in the eighteenth century. I hated the very idea of the eighteenth century, with all those smug men writing tight little couplets and being so dead keen on reason. So I'd skipped it. They let you do that in honours, you were much freer. I had been so free I'd spent most of my time on Dylan Thomas.

A friend of mine, also in honours, had managed never to read a word of Shakespeare; but she was a real expert on the *Four Quartets*.

I saw how impossible and embarrassing it would be for me to try to switch from my free programme into the stricter one. So I looked up the requirements for English majors at the city college where my mother taught.

They were even worse.

You had to know Old English and the History of the English Language and a representative selection of all that had been written from Beowulf to the present day.

This surprised me. I had always looked down on my mother's college, as it was co-ed, and filled with people who couldn't get scholarships to the big eastern colleges.

Now I saw that the stupidest person at my mother's college

knew more than I did. I saw they wouldn't even let me in through the door, let alone give me a large scholarship like the one I had at my own college.

I thought I'd better go to work for a year and think things over. Maybe I could study the eighteenth century in secret.

But I didn't know shorthand, so what could I do?

I could be a waitress or a typist.

But I couldn't stand the idea of being either one.

'You say you want more sleeping pills?'

'Yes.'

'But the ones I gave you last week are very strong.'

'They don't work any more.'

Teresa's large, dark eyes regarded me thoughtfully. I could hear the voices of her three children in the garden under the consulting-room window. My Aunt Libby had married an Italian, and Teresa was my aunt's sister-in-law and our family doctor.

I liked Teresa. She had a gentle, intuitive touch.

I thought it must be because she was Italian.

There was a little pause.

'What seems to be the matter?' Teresa said then.

'I can't sleep. I can't read.' I tried to speak in a cool, calm way, but the zombie rose up in my throat and choked me off. I turned my hands palm up.

'I think,' Teresa tore off a white slip from her prescription pad and wrote down a name and address, 'you'd better see another doctor I know. He'll be able to help you more than I can.'

I peered at the writing, but I couldn't read it.

'Doctor Gordon,' Teresa said. 'He's a psychiatrist.'

Chapter Eleven

Doctor Gordon's waiting-room was hushed and beige.

The walls were beige, and the carpets were beige, and the upholstered chairs and sofas were beige. There were no mirrors or pictures, only certificates from different medical schools, with Doctor Gordon's name in Latin, hung about the walls. Pale green loopy ferns and spiked leaves of a much darker green filled the ceramic pots on the end-table and the coffee-table and the magazine-table.

At first I wondered why the room felt so safe. Then I realized it was because there were no windows.

The air-conditioning made me shiver.

I was still wearing Betsy's white blouse and dirndl skirt. They drooped a bit now, as I hadn't washed them in my three weeks at home. The sweaty cotton gave off a sour but friendly smell.

I hadn't washed my hair for three weeks, either.

I hadn't slept for seven nights.

My mother told me I must have slept, it was impossible not to sleep in all that time, but if I slept, it was with my eyes wide open, for I had followed the green, luminous course of the second hand and the minute hand and the hour hand of the bedside clock through their circles and semi-circles, every night for seven nights, without missing a second, or a minute, or an hour.

The reason I hadn't washed my clothes or my hair was because it seemed so silly.

I saw the days of the year stretching ahead like a series of bright, white boxes, and separating one box from another was sleep, like a black shade. Only for me, the long perspective of shades that set off one box from the next had suddenly snapped up, and I could see day after day after day glaring ahead of me like a white, broad, infinitely desolate avenue.

It seemed silly to wash one day when I would only have to wash again the next.

It made me tired just to think of it.

I wanted to do everything once and for all and be through with it.

Doctor Gordon twiddled a silver pencil.

'Your mother tells me you are upset.'

I curled in the cavernous leather chair and faced Doctor Gordon across an acre of highly polished desk.

Doctor Gordon waited. He tapped his pencil – tap, tap, tap – across the neat green field of his blotter.

His eyelashes were so long and thick they looked artificial. Black plastic reeds fringing two green, glacial pools.

Doctor Gordon's features were so perfect he was almost pretty.

I hated him the minute I walked in through the door.

I had imagined a kind, ugly, intuitive man looking up and saying 'Ah!' in an encouraging way, as if he could see something I couldn't, and then I would find words to tell him how I was so scared, as if I were being stuffed farther and farther into a black, airless sack with no way out.

Then he would lean back in his chair and match the tips of his fingers together in a little steeple and tell me why I couldn't sleep and why I couldn't read and why I couldn't eat and why everything people did seemed so silly, because they only died in the end.

And then, I thought, he would help me, step by step, to be myself again.

But Doctor Gordon wasn't like that at all. He was young and good-looking, and I could see right away he was conceited.

Doctor Gordon had a photograph on his desk, in a silver frame, that half faced him and half faced my leather chair. It was a family photograph, and it showed a beautiful dark-haired woman, who could have been Doctor Gordon's sister, smiling out over the heads of two blond children.

I think one child was a boy and one was a girl, but it may have been that both children were boys or that both were girls, it is hard to tell when children are so small. I think there was also a dog in the picture, towards the bottom – a kind of aire-dale or a golden retriever – but it may have only been the pattern in the woman's skirt.

For some reason the photograph made me furious.

I didn't see why it should be turned half towards me unless Doctor Gordon was trying to show me right away that he was married to some glamorous woman and I'd better not get any funny ideas.

Then I thought, how could this Doctor Gordon help me anyway, with a beautiful wife and beautiful children and a beautiful dog haloing him like the angels on a Christmas card?

'Suppose you try and tell me what you think is wrong.'

I turned the words over suspiciously, like round, sea-polished pebbles that might suddenly put out a claw and change into something else.

What did I *think* was wrong?

That made it sound as if nothing was *really* wrong, I only *thought* it was wrong.

In a dull, flat voice – to show I was not beguiled by his good looks or his family photograph – I told Doctor Gordon about not sleeping and not eating and not reading. I didn't tell him about the handwriting, which bothered me most of all.

That morning I had tried to write a letter to Doreen, down in West Virginia, asking whether I could come and live with her and maybe get a job at her college waiting on table or something.

But when I took up my pen, my hand made big, jerky letters like those of a child, and the lines sloped down the page from left to right almost diagonally, as if they were loops of string lying on the paper, and someone had come along and blown them askew.

I knew I couldn't send a letter like that, so I tore it up in little pieces and put them in my pocket-book, next to my all-purpose compact, in case the psychiatrist asked to see them.

But of course Doctor Gordon didn't ask to see them, as I hadn't mentioned them, and I began to feel pleased at my cleverness. I thought I only need tell him what I wanted to, and that I could control the picture he had of me by hiding this and revealing that, all the while he thought he was so smart.

The whole time I was talking, Doctor Gordon bent his head as if he were praying, and the only noise apart from the dull, flat voice was the tap, tap, tap of Doctor Gordon's pencil at the same point on the green blotter, like a stalled walking-stick.

When I had finished, Doctor Gordon lifted his head.

'Where did you say you went to college?'

Baffled, I told him. I didn't see where college fitted in.

'Ah!' Doctor Gordon leaned back in his chair, staring into the air over my shoulder with a reminiscent smile.

I thought he was going to tell me his diagnosis, and that perhaps I had judged him too hastily and too unkindly. But he only said, 'I remember your college well. I was up there, during the war. They had a WAC station, didn't they? Or was it WAVES?'

I said I didn't know.

'Yes, a WAC station, I remember now. I was doctor for the lot, before I was sent overseas. My, they were a pretty bunch of girls.'

Doctor Gordon laughed.

Then, in one smooth move, he rose to his feet and strolled towards me round the corner of his desk. I wasn't sure what he meant to do, so I stood up as well.

Doctor Gordon reached for the hand that hung at my right side and shook it.

'See you next week, then.'

The full, bosomy elms made a tunnel of shade over the yellow and red brick fronts along Commonwealth Avenue, and a trolley-car was threading itself towards Boston down its slim, silver track. I waited for the trolley to pass, then crossed to the grey Chevrolet at the opposite curb.

I could see my mother's face, anxious and sallow as a slice of lemon, peering up at me through the windshield.

'Well, what did he say?'

I pulled the car door shut. It didn't catch. I pushed it out and drew it in again with a dull slam.

'He said he'll see me next week.'

My mother sighed.

Doctor Gordon cost twenty-five dollars an hour.

'Hi there, what's your name?'

'Elly Higginbottom.'

The sailor fell into step beside me, and I smiled.

I thought there must be as many sailors on the Common as there were pigeons. They seemed to come out of a dun-coloured recruiting house on the far side, with blue and white

'Join the Navy' posters stuck up on billboards round it and all over the inner walls.

'Where do you come from, Elly?'

'Chicago.'

I had never been to Chicago, but I knew one or two boys who went to Chicago University, and it seemed the sort of place where unconventional, mixed-up people would come from.

'You sure are a long way from home.'

The sailor put his arm around my waist, and for a long time we walked around the Common like that, the sailor stroking my hip through the green dirndl skirt, and me smiling mysteriously and trying not to say anything that would show I was from Boston and might at any moment meet Mrs Willard, or one of my mother's other friends, crossing the Common after tea on Beacon Hill or shopping in Filene's Basement.

I thought if I ever did get to Chicago, I might change my name to Elly Higginbottom for good. Then nobody would know I had thrown up a scholarship at a big eastern women's college and mucked up a month in New York and refused a perfectly solid medical student for a husband who would one day be a member of the A.M.A. and earn pots of money.

In Chicago, people would take me for what I was.

I would be simple Elly Higginbottom, the orphan. People would love me for my sweet, quiet nature. They wouldn't be after me to read books and write long papers on the twins in James Joyce. And one day I might just marry a virile, but tender, garage mechanic and have a big cowy family, like Dodo Conway.

If I happened to feel like it.

'What do you want to do when you get out of the Navy?' I asked the sailor suddenly.

It was the longest sentence I had said, and he seemed taken aback. He pushed his white cup-cake cap to one side and scratched his head.

'Well, I dunno, Elly,' he said. 'I might just go to college on the G.I. Bill.'

I paused. Then I said suggestively, 'You ever thought of opening a garage?'

'Nope,' said the sailor. 'Never have.'

I peered at him from the corner of my eye. He didn't look a day over sixteen.

'Do you know how old I am?' I said accusingly.

The sailor grinned at me. 'Nope, and I don't care either.'

It occurred to me that this sailor was really remarkably handsome. He looked Nordic and virginal. Now I was simple-minded it seemed I attracted clean, handsome people.

'Well, I'm thirty,' I said, and waited.

'Gee, Elly, you don't look it.' The sailor squeezed my hip.

Then he glanced quickly from left to right. 'Listen, Elly, if we go round to those steps over there, under the monument, I can kiss you.'

At that moment I noticed a brown figure in sensible flat brown shoes striding across the Common in my direction. From the distance, I couldn't make out any features on the dime-sized face, but I knew it was Mrs Willard.

'Could you please tell me the way to the subway?' I said to the sailor in a loud voice.

'Huh?'

'The subway that goes out to the Deer Island Prison?'

When Mrs Willard came up I would have to pretend I was only asking the sailor directions, and didn't really know him at all.

'Take your hands off me,' I said between my teeth.

'Say Elly, what's up?'

The woman approached and passed by without a look or a nod, and of course it wasn't Mrs Willard. Mrs Willard was at her cottage in the Adirondacks.

I fixed the woman's receding back with a vengeful stare.

'Say, Elly . . .'

'I thought it was somebody I knew,' I said. 'Some blasted lady from this orphan home in Chicago.'

The sailor put his arm around me again.

'You mean you got no mom and dad, Elly?'

'No.' I let out a tear that seemed ready. It made a little hot track down my cheek.

'Say Elly, don't cry. This lady, was she mean to you?'

'She was . . . she was *aw*ful!'

The tears came in a rush, then, and while the sailor was holding me and patting them dry with a big, clean, white, linen handkerchief in the shelter of an American elm, I thought what an awful woman that lady in the brown suit had been, and how she, whether she knew it or not, was responsible for my taking the wrong turn here and the wrong path there and for everything bad that happened after that.

'Well, Esther, how do you feel this week?'

Doctor Gordon cradled his pencil like a slim, silver bullet.

'The same.'

'The same?' He quirked an eyebrow, as if he didn't believe it.

So I told him again, in the same dull, flat voice, only it was angrier this time, because he seemed so slow to understand, how I hadn't slept for fourteen nights and how I couldn't read or write or swallow very well.

Doctor Gordon seemed unimpressed.

I dug into my pocket-book and found the scraps of my letter to Doreen. I took them out and let them flutter on to Doctor

Gordon's immaculate green blotter. They lay there, dumb as daisy petals in a summer meadow.

'What,' I said, 'do you think of that?'

I thought Doctor Gordon must immediately see how bad the handwriting was, but he only said, 'I think I would like to speak to your mother. Do you mind?'

'No.' But I didn't like the idea of Doctor Gordon talking to my mother one bit. I thought he might tell her I should be locked up. I picked up every scrap of my letter to Doreen, so Doctor Gordon couldn't piece them together and see I was planning to run away, and walked out of his office without another word.

I watched my mother grow smaller and smaller until she disappeared into the door of Doctor Gordon's office building. Then I watched her grow larger and larger as she came back to the car.

'Well?' I could tell she had been crying.

My mother didn't look at me. She started the car.

Then she said, as we glided under the cool, deep-sea shade of the elms, 'Doctor Gordon doesn't think you've improved at all. He thinks you should have some shock treatments at his private hospital in Walton.'

I felt a sharp stab of curiosity, as if I had just read a terrible newspaper headline about somebody else.

'Does he mean *live* there?'

'No,' my mother said, and her chin quivered.

I thought she must be lying.

'You tell me the truth,' I said, 'or I'll never speak to you again.'

'Don't I *al*ways tell you the truth?' my mother said, and burst into tears.

After two hours on a narrow ledge seven storeys above a concrete parking lot and gathered crowds, Mr George Pollucci let himself be helped to safety through a nearby window by Sgt Will Kilmartin of the Charles Street police force.

I cracked open a peanut from the ten cent bag I had bought to feed the pigeons, and ate it. It tasted dead, like a bit of old tree bark.

I brought the newspaper close up to my eyes to get a better view of George Pollucci's face, spotlighted like a three-quarter moon against a vague background of brick and black sky. I felt he had something important to tell me, and that whatever it was might just be written on his face.

But the smudgy crags of George Pollucci's features melted away as I peered at them, and resolved themselves into a regular pattern of dark and light and medium grey dots.

The inky black newspaper paragraph didn't tell why Mr Pollucci was on the ledge, or what Sgt Kilmartin did to him when he finally got him in through the window.

The trouble about jumping was that if you didn't pick the right number of storeys, you might still be alive when you hit bottom. I thought seven storeys must be a safe distance.

I folded the paper and wedged it between the slats of the park bench. It was what my mother called a scandal sheet, full of the local murders and suicides and beatings and robbings, and just about every page had a half-naked lady on it with her breasts surging over the edge of her dress and her legs arranged so you could see to her stocking tops.

I didn't know why I had never bought any of these papers before. They were the only things I could read. The little paragraphs between the pictures ended before the letters had a chance to get cocky and wiggle about. At home, all I ever saw was the *Christian Science Monitor*, which appeared on the door-step at five o'clock every day but Sunday and treated suicides and sex crimes and aeroplane crashes as if they didn't happen.

A big white swan full of little children approached my bench, then turned round a bosky islet covered with ducks and paddled back under the dark arch of the bridge. Everything I looked at seemed bright and extremely tiny.

I saw, as if through the keyhole of a door I couldn't open, myself and my younger brother, knee-high and holding rabbit-eared balloons, climb aboard a swanboat and fight for a seat at the edge, over the peanut-shell-paved water. My mouth tasted of cleanness and peppermint. If we were good at the dentist's, my mother always bought us a swanboat ride.

I circled the Public Garden – over the bridge and under the blue-green monuments, past the American flag flower-bed and the entrance where you could have your picture taken in an orange-and-white striped canvas booth for twenty-five cents – reading the names of the trees.

My favourite tree was the Weeping Scholar Tree. I thought it must come from Japan. They understood things of the spirit in Japan.

They disembowelled themselves when anything went wrong.

I tried to imagine how they would go about it. They must have an extremely sharp knife. No, probably two extremely sharp knives. Then they would sit down, cross-legged, a knife in either hand. Then they would cross their hands and point a knife at each side of their stomach. They would have to be naked, or the knife would get stuck in their clothes.

Then in one quick flash, before they had time to think twice, they would jab the knives in and zip them round, one on the upper crescent and one on the lower crescent, making a full circle. Then their stomach skin would come loose, like a plate, and their insides would fall out, and they would die.

It must take a lot of courage to die like that.

My trouble was I hated the sight of blood.

I thought I might stay in the park all night.

The next morning Dodo Conway was driving my mother and me to Walton, and if I was to run away before it was too late, now was the time. I looked in my pocket-book and counted out a dollar bill and seventy-nine cents in dimes and nickels and pennies.

I had no idea how much it would cost to get to Chicago, and I didn't dare go to the bank and draw out all my money, because I thought Doctor Gordon might well have warned the bank clerk to intercept me if I made any obvious move.

Hitch-hiking occurred to me, but I had no idea which of all the routes out of Boston led to Chicago. It's easy enough to find directions on a map, but I had very little knowledge of directions when I was smack in the middle of somewhere. Every time I wanted to figure what was east or what was west it seemed to be noon, or cloudy, which was no help at all, or night-time, and except for the Big Dipper and Cassiopeia's Chair, I was hopeless at stars, a failing which always disheartened Buddy Willard.

I decided to walk to the bus terminal and inquire about the fares to Chicago. Then I might go to the bank and withdraw precisely that amount, which would not cause so much suspicion.

I had just strolled in through the glass doors of the terminal and was browsing over the rack of coloured tour leaflets and schedules, when I realized that the bank in my home town would be closed, as it was already mid-afternoon, and I couldn't get any money out till the next day.

My appointment at Walton was for ten o'clock.

At that moment, the loudspeaker crackled into life and started announcing the stops of a bus getting ready to leave in the parking lot outside. The voice on the loudspeaker went bockle bockle bockle, the way they do, so you can't understand a word, and then, in the middle of all the static, I heard a familiar name clear as A on the piano in the middle of all the tuning instruments of an orchestra.

It was a stop two blocks from my house.

I hurried out into the hot, dusty, end-of-July afternoon, sweating and sandy-mouthed, as if late for a difficult interview, and boarded the red bus, whose motor was already running.

I handed my fare to the driver, and silently, on gloved hinges, the door folded shut at my back.

Chapter Twelve

Doctor Gordon's private hospital crowned a grassy rise at the end of a long, secluded drive that had been whitened with broken quahog shells. The yellow clapboard walls of the large house, with its encircling veranda, gleamed in the sun, but no people strolled on the green dome of the lawn.

As my mother and I approached the summer heat bore down on us, and a cicada started up, like an aerial lawnmower, in the heart of a copper beech tree at the back. The sound of the cicada only served to underline the enormous silence.

A nurse met us at the door.

'Will you wait in the living-room, please. Doctor Gordon will be with you presently.'

What bothered me was that everything about the house seemed normal, although I knew it must be chock-full of crazy people. There were no bars on the windows that I could see, and no wild or disquieting noises. Sunlight measured itself out in regular oblongs on the shabby, but soft red carpets, and a whiff of fresh-cut grass sweetened the air.

I paused in the doorway of the living-room.

For a minute I thought it was the replica of a lounge in a guest house I visited once on an island off the coast of Maine. The French doors let in a dazzle of white light, a grand piano filled the far corner of the room, and people in summer clothes were sitting about at card tables and in the lopsided wicker armchairs one so often finds at down-at-heel seaside resorts.

Then I realized that none of the people were moving.

I focused more closely, trying to pry some clue from their stiff postures. I made out men and women, and boys and girls who must be as young as I, but there was a uniformity to their faces, as if they had lain for a long time on a shelf, out of the sunlight, under siftings of pale, fine dust.

Then I saw that some of the people were indeed moving, but with such small, birdlike gestures I had not at first discerned them.

A grey-faced man was counting out a deck of cards, one, two, three, four . . . I thought he must be seeing if it was a full pack, but when he had finished counting, he started over again. Next to him, a fat lady played with a string of wooden beads. She drew all the beads up to one end of the string. Then click, click, click, she let them fall back on each other.

At the piano, a young girl leafed through a few sheets of music, but when she saw me looking at her, she ducked her head crossly and tore the sheets in half.

My mother touched my arm, and I followed her into the room.

We sat, without speaking, on a lumpy sofa that creaked each time one stirred.

Then my gaze slid over the people to the blaze of green beyond the diaphanous curtains, and I felt as if I were sitting in the window of an enormous department store. The figures around me weren't people, but shop dummies, painted to resemble people and propped up in attitudes counterfeiting life.

I climbed after Doctor Gordon's dark-jacketed back.

Downstairs, in the hall, I had tried to ask him what the shock treatment would be like, but when I opened my mouth no words came out, my eyes only widened and stared at the smiling, familiar face that floated before me like a plate full of assurances.

At the top of the stairs, the garnet-coloured carpet stopped. A plain, brown linoleum, tacked to the floor, took its place, and extended down a corridor lined with shut white doors. As I followed Doctor Gordon, a door opened somewhere in the distance, and I heard a woman shouting.

All at once a nurse popped around the corner of the corridor ahead of us leading a woman in a blue bathrobe with shaggy, waist-length hair. Doctor Gordon stepped back, and I flattened against the wall.

As the woman was dragged by, waving her arms and struggling in the grip of the nurse, she was saying, 'I'm going to jump out of the window, I'm going to jump out of the window, I'm going to jump out of the window.'

Dumpy and muscular in her smudge-fronted uniform, the wall-eyed nurse wore such thick spectacles that four eyes peered out at me from behind the round, twin panes of glass. I was trying to tell which eyes were the real eyes and which the false eyes, and which of the real eyes was the wall-eye and which the straight eye, when she brought her face up to mine with a large, conspiratorial grin and hissed, as if to reassure me, 'She thinks she's going to jump out the window but she can't jump out the window because they're all barred!'

And as Doctor Gordon led me into a bare room at the back of the house, I saw that the windows in that part were indeed barred, and that the room door and the closet door and the drawers of the bureau and everything that opened and shut was fitted with a keyhole so it could be locked up.

I lay down on the bed.

The wall-eyed nurse came back. She unclasped my watch

and dropped it in her pocket. Then she started tweaking the hairpins from my hair.

Doctor Gordon was unlocking the closet. He dragged out a table on wheels with a machine on it and rolled it behind the head of the bed. The nurse started swabbing my temples with a smelly grease.

As she leaned over to reach the side of my head nearest the wall, her fat breast muffled my face like a cloud or a pillow. A vague, medicinal stench emanated from her flesh.

'Don't worry,' the nurse grinned down at me. 'Their first time everybody's scared to death.'

I tried to smile, but my skin had gone stiff, like parchment.

Doctor Gordon was fitting two metal plates on either side of my head. He buckled them into place with a strap that dented my forehead, and gave me a wire to bite.

I shut my eyes.

There was a brief silence, like an indrawn breath.

Then something bent down and took hold of me and shook me like the end of the world. Whee-ee-ee-ee-ee, it shrilled, through an air crackling with blue light, and with each flash a great jolt drubbed me till I thought my bones would break and the sap fly out of me like a split plant.

I wondered what terrible thing it was that I had done.

I was sitting in a wicker chair, holding a small cocktail glass of tomato juice. The watch had been replaced on my wrist, but it looked odd. Then I realized it had been fastened upside down. I sensed the unfamiliar positioning of the hairpins in my hair.

'How do you feel?'

An old metal floor lamp surfaced in my mind. One of the few relics of my father's study, it was surmounted by a copper bell which held the light bulb, and from which a frayed, tiger-coloured cord ran down the length of the metal stand to a socket in the wall.

One day I'd decided to move this lamp from the side of my mother's bed to my desk at the other end of the room. The cord would be long enough, so I didn't unplug it. I closed both hands around the lamp and the fuzzy cord and gripped them tight.

Then something leapt out of the lamp in a blue flash and shook me till my teeth rattled, and I tried to pull my hands off, but they were stuck, and I screamed, or a scream was torn from my throat, for I didn't recognize it, but heard it soar and quaver in the air like a violently disembodied spirit.

Then my hands jerked free, and I fell back on to my mother's bed. A small hole, blackened as if with pencil lead, pitted the centre of my right palm.

'How do you feel?'

'All right.'

But I didn't. I felt terrible.

'Which college did you say you went to?'

I said what college it was.

'Ah!' Doctor Gordon's face lighted with a slow, almost tropical smile. 'They had a WAC station up there, didn't they, during the war?'

My mother's knuckles were bone-white, as if the skin had worn off them in the hour of waiting. She looked past me to Doctor Gordon, and he must have nodded, or smiled, because her face relaxed.

'A few more shock treatments, Mrs Greenwood,' I heard Doctor Gordon say, 'and I think you'll notice a wonderful improvement.'

The girl was still sitting on the piano stool, the torn sheet of music splayed at her feet like a dead bird. She stared at me, and I stared back. Her eyes narrowed. She stuck out her tongue.

My mother was following Doctor Gordon to the door. I lingered behind, and when their backs were turned, I rounded on the girl and thumbed both ears at her. She pulled her tongue in, and her face went stony.

I walked out into the sun.

Panther-like in a dapple of tree shadow, Dodo Conway's black station wagon lay in wait.

The station wagon had been ordered originally by a wealthy society lady, black, without a speck of chrome, and with black leather upholstery, but when it came, it depressed her. It was the dead spit of a hearse, she said, and everybody else thought so too, and nobody would buy it, so the Conways drove it home, cut-price, and saved themselves a couple of hundred dollars.

Sitting in the front seat, between Dodo and my mother, I felt dumb and subdued. Every time I tried to concentrate, my mind glided off, like a skater, into a large empty space, and pirouetted there, absently.

'I'm through with that Doctor Gordon,' I said, after we had left Dodo and her black wagon behind the pines. 'You can call him up and tell him I'm not coming next week.'

My mother smiled. 'I knew my baby wasn't like that.'

I looked at her. 'Like what?'

'Like those awful people. Those awful dead people at that hospital.' She paused. 'I knew you'd decide to be all right again.'

STARLET SUCCUMBS AFTER SIXTY-EIGHT HOUR COMA.

I felt in my pocket-book among the paper scraps and the compact and the peanut shells and the dimes and nickels and the blue jiffy box containing nineteen Gillette blades, till I unearthed the snapshot I'd had taken that afternoon in the orange-and-white striped booth.

I brought it up next to the smudgy photograph of the dead

140

girl. It matched, mouth for mouth, nose for nose. The only difference was the eyes. The eyes in the snapshot were open, and those in the newspaper photograph were closed. But I knew if the dead girl's eyes were to be thumbed wide, they would look out at me with the same dead, black, vacant expression as the eyes in the snapshot.

I stuffed the snapshot back in my pocket-book.

'I will just sit here in the sun on this park bench five minutes more by the clock on that building over there,' I told myself 'and then I will go somewhere and do it.'

I summoned my little chorus of voices.

Doesn't your work interest you, Esther?

You know, Esther, you've got the perfect set-up of a true neurotic.

You'll never get anywhere like that, you'll never get anywhere like that, you'll never get anywhere like that.

Once, on a hot summer night, I had spent an hour kissing a hairy, ape-shaped law student from Yale because I felt sorry for him, he was so ugly. When I had finished, he said, 'I have you taped, baby. You'll be a prude at forty.'

'Factitious!' my creative writing professor at college scrawled on a story of mine called 'The Big Weekend'.

I hadn't known what factitious meant, so I looked it up in the dictionary.

Factitious: artificial, sham.

You'll never get anywhere like that.

I hadn't slept for twenty-one nights.

I thought the most beautiful thing in the world must be shadow, the million moving shapes and cul-de-sacs of shadow. There was shadow in bureau drawers and closets and suitcases, and shadow under houses and trees and stones, and shadow at the back of people's eyes and smiles, and shadow, miles and miles and miles of it, on the night side of the earth.

I looked down at the two flesh-coloured band-aids forming a cross on the calf of my right leg.

That morning I had made a start.

I had locked myself in the bathroom, and run a tub full of warm water, and taken out a Gillette blade.

When they asked some old Roman philosopher or other how he wanted to die, he said he would open his veins in a warm bath. I thought it would be easy, lying in the tub and seeing the redness flower from my wrists, flush after flush through the clear water, till I sank to sleep under a surface gaudy as poppies.

But when it came right down to it, the skin of my wrist looked so white and defenceless that I couldn't do it. It was as if what I wanted to kill wasn't in that skin or the thin blue pulse that jumped under my thumb, but somewhere else, deeper, more secret, and a whole lot harder to get at.

It would take two motions. One wrist, then the other wrist. Three motions, if you counted changing the razor from hand to hand. Then I would step into the tub and lie down.

I moved in front of the medicine cabinet. If I looked in the mirror while I did it, it would be like watching somebody else, in a book or a play.

But the person in the mirror was paralysed and too stupid to do a thing.

Then I thought, maybe I ought to spill a little blood for practice, so I sat on the edge of the tub and crossed my right ankle over my left knee. Then I lifted my right hand with the razor and let it drop of its own weight, like a guillotine, on to the calf of my leg.

I felt nothing. Then I felt a small, deep thrill, and a bright seam of red welled up at the lip of the slash. The blood gathered darkly, like fruit, and rolled down my ankle into the cup of my black patent leather shoe.

I thought of getting into the tub then, but I realized my dallying had used up the better part of the morning, and that my mother would probably come home and find me before I was done.

So I bandaged the cut, packed up my Gillette blades and caught the eleven-thirty bus to Boston.

'Sorry, baby, there's no subway to the Deer Island Prison, it's on a niland.'

'No, it's not on an island, it used to be on an island, but they filled up the water with dirt and now it joins on to the mainland.'

'There's no subway.'

'I've got to get there.'

'Hey,' the fat man in the ticket booth peered at me through the grating, 'don't cry. Who you got there, honey, some relative?'

People shoved and bumped by me in the artificially lit dark, hurrying after the trains that rumbled in and out of intestinal tunnels under Scollay Square. I could feel the tears start to spurt from the screwed-up nozzles of my eyes.

'It's my *father*.'

The fat man consulted a diagram on the wall of his booth. 'Here's how you do,' he said, 'you take a car from the track over there and get off at Orient Heights and then hop a bus with The Point on it.' He beamed at me. 'It'll run you straight to the prison gate.'

'Hey you!' A young fellow in a blue uniform waved from the hut.

I waved back and kept on going.

'Hey you!'

I stopped, and walked slowly over to the hut that perched like a circular living-room on the waste of sands.

'Hey, you can't go any further. That's prison property, no trespassers allowed.'

'I thought you could go anyplace along the beach,' I said. 'So long as you stayed under the tideline.'

The fellow thought a minute.

Then he said, 'Not this beach.'

He had a pleasant, fresh face.

'You've a nice place here,' I said. 'It's like a little house.'

He glanced back into the room, with its braided rug and chintz curtains. He smiled.

'We even got a coffee pot.'

'I used to live near here.'

'No kidding. I was born and brought up in this town myself.'

I looked across the sands to the parking lot and the barred gate, and past the barred gate to the narrow road, lapped by the ocean on both sides, that led out to the one-time island.

The red brick buildings of the prison looked friendly, like the buildings of a seaside college. On a green hump of lawn to the left, I could see small white spots and slightly larger pink spots moving about. I asked the guard what they were, and he said, 'Them's pigs 'n' chickens.'

I was thinking that if I'd had the sense to go on living in that old town I might just have met this prison guard in school and married him and had a parcel of kids by now. It would be nice, living up by the sea with piles of little kids and pigs and chickens, wearing what my grandmother called wash dresses, and sitting about in some kitchen with bright linoleum and fat arms, drinking pots of coffee.

'How do you get into that prison?'

'You get a pass.'

'No, how do you get *locked* in?'

'Oh,' the guard laughed, 'you steal a car, you rob a store.'

'You got any murderers in there?'

'No. Murderers go to a big state place.'

'Who else is in there?'

'Well, the first day of winter we get these old bums out of Boston. They heave a brick through a window, and then they get picked up and spend the winter out of the cold, with TV and plenty to eat, and basketball games on the weekend.'

'That's nice.'

'Nice if you like it,' said the guard.

I said good-bye and started to move off, glancing back over my shoulder only once. The guard still stood in the door-way of his observation booth, and when I turned he lifted his arm in a salute.

The log I sat on was lead-heavy and smelled of tar. Under the stout, grey cylinder of the water tower on its commanding hill, the sandbar curved out into the sea. At high tide the bar completely submerged itself.

I remembered that sandbar well. It harboured, in the crook of its inner curve, a particular shell that could be found nowhere else on the beach.

The shell was thick, smooth, big as a thumb joint, and usually white, although sometimes pink or peach-coloured. It resembled a sort of modest conch.

'Mummy, that girl's *still* sitting there.'

I looked up, idly, and saw a small, sandy child being dragged up from the sea's edge by a skinny, bird-eyed woman in red shorts and a red-and-white polka-dotted halter.

I hadn't counted on the beach being overrun with summer people. In the ten years of my absence, fancy blue and pink and pale green shanties had sprung up on the flat sands of the Point like a crop of tasteless mushrooms, and the silver aeroplanes and cigar-shaped blimps had given way to jets that scoured the rooftops in their loud offrush from the airport across the bay.

I was the only girl on the beach in a skirt and high heels, and it occurred to me I must stand out. I had removed my patent leather shoes after a while, for they foundered badly in the sand. It pleased me to think they would be perched there on the silver log, pointing out to sea, like a sort of soul-compass, after I was dead.

I fingered the box of razors in my pocket-book.

Then I thought how stupid I was. I had the razors, but no warm bath.

I considered renting a room. There must be a boarding house among all those summer places. But I had no luggage. That would create suspicion. Besides, in a boarding house other people are always wanting to use the bathroom. I'd hardly have time to do it and step into the tub when somebody would be pounding at the door.

The gulls on their wooden stilts at the tip of the bar miaowed like cats. Then they flapped up, one by one, in their ash-coloured jackets, circling my head and crying.

'Say, lady, you better not sit out here, the tide's coming in.'

The small boy squatted a few feet away. He picked up a round purple stone and lobbed it into the water. The water swallowed it with a resonant plop. Then he scrabbled around, and I heard the dry stones clank together like money.

He skimmed a flat stone over the dull green surface, and it skipped seven times before it sliced out of sight.

'Why don't you go home?' I said.

The boy skipped another, heavier stone. It sank after the second bounce.

'Don't want to.'

'Your mother's looking for you.'

'She is not.' He sounded worried.

'If you go home, I'll give you some candy.'

The boy hitched closer. 'What kind?'

But I knew without looking into my pocket-book that all I had was peanut shells.

'I'll give you some money to buy some candy.'

'Ar-*thur*!'

A woman was indeed coming out on the sandbar, slipping and no doubt cursing to herself, for her lips went up and down between her clear, peremptory calls.

'Ar-*thur*!'

She shaded her eyes with one hand, as if this helped her discern us through the thickening sea dusk.

I could sense the boy's interest dwindle as the pull of his mother increased. He began to pretend he didn't know me. He kicked over a few stones, as if searching for something, and edged off.

I shivered.

The stones lay lumpish and cold under my bare feet. I thought longingly of the black shoes on the beach. A wave drew back, like a hand, then advanced and touched my foot.

The drench seemed to come off the sea floor itself, where blind white fish ferried themselves by their own light through the great polar cold. I saw sharks' teeth and whales' earbones littered about down there like gravestones.

I waited, as if the sea could make my decision for me.

A second wave collapsed over my feet, lipped with white froth, and the chill gripped my ankles with a mortal ache.

My flesh winced, in cowardice, from such a death.

I picked up my pocket-book and started back over the cold stones to where my shoes kept their vigil in the violet light.

Chapter Thirteen

'Of course his mother killed him.'

I looked at the mouth of the boy Jody had wanted me to meet. His lips were thick and pink and a baby face nestled under the silk of white-blond hair. His name was Cal, which I thought must be short for something, but I couldn't think what it would be short for, unless it was California.

'How can you be sure she killed him?' I said.

Cal was supposed to be very intelligent, and Jody had said over the phone that he was cute and I would like him. I wondered, if I'd been my old self, if I would have liked him.

It was impossible to tell.

'Well, first she says No no no, and then she says Yes.'

'But then she says No no again.'

Cal and I lay side by side on an orange and green striped towel on a mucky beach across the swamps from Lynn. Jody and Mark, the boy she was pinned to, were swimming. Cal hadn't wanted to swim, he had wanted to talk, and we were arguing about this play where a young man finds out he has a brain disease, on account of his father fooling around with unclean women, and in the end his brain, which has been softening all along, snaps completely, and his mother is debating whether to kill him or not.

I had a suspicion that my mother had called Jody and

begged her to ask me out, so I wouldn't sit around in my room all day with the shades drawn. I didn't want to go at first, because I thought Jody would notice the change in me, and that anybody with half an eye would see I didn't have a brain in my head.

But all during the drive north, and then east, Jody had joked and laughed and chattered and not seemed to mind that I only said, 'My' or 'Gosh' or 'You don't say'.

We browned hotdogs on the public grills at the beach, and by watching Jody and Mark and Cal very carefully I managed to cook my hotdog just the right amount of time and didn't burn it or drop it into the fire, the way I was afraid of doing. Then, when nobody was looking, I buried it in the sand.

After we ate, Jody and Mark ran down to the water hand-in-hand, and I lay back, staring into the sky, while Cal went on and on about this play.

The only reason I remembered this play was because it had a mad person in it, and everything I had ever read about mad people stuck in my mind, while everything else flew out.

'But it's the Yes that matters,' Cal said. 'It's the Yes she'll come back to in the end.'

I lifted my head and squinted out at the bright blue plate of the sea – a bright blue plate with a dirty rim. A big round grey rock, like the upper half of an egg, poked out of the water about a mile from the stony headland.

'What was she going to kill him with? I forget.'

I hadn't forgotten. I remembered perfectly well, but I wanted to hear what Cal would say.

'Morphia powders.'

'Do you suppose they have morphia powders in America?'

Cal considered a minute. Then he said, 'I wouldn't think so. They sound awfully old-fashioned.'

I rolled over on to my stomach and squinted at the view in

the other direction, towards Lynn. A glassy haze rippled up from the fires in the grills and the heat on the road, and through the haze, as through a curtain of clear water, I could make out a smudgy skyline of gas tanks and factory stacks and derricks and bridges.

It looked one hell of a mess.

I rolled on to my back again and made my voice casual. 'If you were going to kill yourself, how would you do it?'

Cal seemed pleased. 'I've often thought of that. I'd blow my brains out with a gun.'

I was disappointed. It was just like a man to do it with a gun. A fat chance I had of laying my hands on a gun. And even if I did, I wouldn't have a clue as to what part of me to shoot at.

I'd already read in the papers about people who'd tried to shoot themselves, only they ended up shooting an important nerve and getting paralysed, or blasting their face off, but being saved, by surgeons and a sort of miracle, from dying outright.

The risks of a gun seemed great.

'What kind of a gun?'

'My father's shotgun. He keeps it loaded. I'd just have to walk into his study one day and,' Cal pointed a finger to his temple and made a comical, screwed-up face, 'click!' He widened his pale grey eyes and looked at me.

'Does your father happen to live near Boston?' I asked idly.

'Nope. In Clacton-on-Sea. He's English.'

Jody and Mark ran up hand-in-hand, dripping and shaking off water drops like two loving puppies. I thought there would be too many people, so I stood up and pretended to yawn.

'I guess I'll go for a swim.'

Being with Jody and Mark and Cal was beginning to weigh on my nerves, like a dull wooden block on the strings of a piano. I was afraid that at any moment my control would snap, and I would start babbling about how I couldn't read and couldn't write and how I must be just about the only person who had stayed awake for a solid month without dropping dead of exhaustion.

A smoke seemed to be going up from my nerves like the smoke from the grills and the sun-saturated road. The whole landscape – beach and headland and sea and rock – quavered in front of my eyes like a stage backcloth.

I wondered at what point in space the silly, sham blue of the sky turned black.

'You swim too, Cal.'

Jody gave Cal a playful little push.

'Ohhh,' Cal hid his face in the towel. 'It's too cold.'

I started to walk towards the water.

Somehow, in the broad, shadowless light of noon, the water looked amiable and welcoming.

I thought drowning must be the kindest way to die, and burning the worst. Some of those babies in the jars that Buddy Willard showed me had gills, he said. They went through a stage where they were just like fish.

A little, rubbishy wavelet, full of candy wrappers and orange peel and seaweed, folded over my foot.

I heard the sand thud behind me, and Cal came up.

'Let's swim to that rock over there.' I pointed at it.

'Are you crazy? That's a mile out.'

'What are you?' I said. 'Chicken?'

Cal took me by the elbow and jostled me into the water. When we were waist high, he pushed me under. I surfaced, splashing, my eyes seared with salt. Underneath, the water was green and semi-opaque as a hunk of quartz.

I started to swim, a modified dogpaddle, keeping my face towards the rock. Cal did a slow crawl. After a while he put his head up and treaded water.

'Can't make it.' He was panting heavily.

'Okay. You go back.'

I thought I would swim out until I was too tired to swim back. As I paddled on, my heartbeat boomed like a dull motor in my ears.

I am I am I am.

That morning I had tried to hang myself.

I had taken the silk cord of my mother's yellow bathrobe as soon as she left for work, and, in the amber shade of the bedroom, fashioned it into a knot that slipped up and down on itself. It took me a long time to do this, because I was poor at knots and had no idea how to make a proper one.

Then I hunted around for a place to attach the rope.

The trouble was, our house had the wrong kind of ceilings. The ceilings were low, white and smoothly plastered, without a light fixture or a wood beam in sight. I thought with longing of the house my grandmother had before she sold it to come and live with us, and then with my Aunt Libby.

My grandmother's house was built in the fine, nineteenth-century style, with lofty rooms and sturdy chandelier brackets and high closets with stout rails across them, and an attic where nobody ever went, full of trunks and parrot cages and dressmaker's dummies and overhead beams thick as a ship's timbers.

But it was an old house, and she'd sold it, and I didn't know anybody else with a house like that.

After a discouraging time of walking about with the silk cord dangling from my neck like a yellow cat's tail and finding no place to fasten it, I sat on the edge of my mother's bed and tried pulling the cord tight.

But each time I would get the cord so tight I could feel a rushing in my ears and a flush of blood in my face my hands would weaken and let go, and I would be all right again.

Then I saw that my body had all sorts of little tricks, such as making my hands go limp at the crucial second, which would save it, time and again, whereas if I had the whole say, I would be dead in a flash.

I would simply have to ambush it with whatever sense I had left, or it would trap me in its stupid cage for fifty years without any sense at all. And when people found out my mind had gone, as they would have to, sooner or later, in spite of my mother's guarded tongue, they would persuade her to put me into an asylum where I could be cured.

Only my case was incurable.

I had bought a few paperbacks on abnormal psychology at the drug store and compared my symptoms with the symptoms in the books, and sure enough, my symptoms tallied with the most hopeless cases.

The only thing I could read, beside the scandal sheets, were these abnormal psychology books. It was as if some slim opening had been left, so I could learn all I needed to know about my case to end it in the proper way.

I wondered, after the hanging fiasco, if I shouldn't just give it up and turn myself over to the doctors, but then I remembered Doctor Gordon and his private shock machine. Once I was locked up they could use that on me all the time.

And I thought of how my mother and brother and friends would visit me, day after day, hoping I would be better. Then their visits would slacken off, and they would give up hope. They would grow old. They would forget me.

They would be poor, too.

They would want me to have the best of care at first, so they would sink all their money in a private hospital like Doctor Gordon's. Finally, when the money was used up, I would be moved to a state hospital, with hundreds of people like me, in a big cage in the basement.

The more hopeless you were, the further away they hid you.

Cal had turned around and was swimming in.

As I watched, he dragged himself slowly out of the neck-deep sea. Against the khaki-coloured sand and the green shore wavelets, his body was bisected for a moment, like a white worm. Then it crawled completely out of the green and on to the khaki and lost itself among dozens and dozens of other worms that were wriggling or just lolling about between the sea and the sky.

I paddled my hands in the water and kicked my feet. The egg-shaped rock didn't seem to be any nearer than it had been when Cal and I had looked at it from the shore.

Then I saw it would be pointless to swim as far as the rock, because my body would take that excuse to climb out and lie in the sun, gathering strength to swim back.

The only thing to do was to drown myself then and there.

So I stopped.

I brought my hands to my breast, ducked my head, and dived, using my hands to push the water aside. The water pressed in on my eardrums and on my heart. I fanned myself down, but before I knew where I was, the water had spat me up into the sun, and the world was sparkling all about me like blue and green and yellow semi-precious stones.

I dashed the water from my eyes.

I was panting, as after a strenuous exertion, but floating, without effort.

I dived, and dived again, and each time popped up like a cork.

The grey rock mocked me, bobbing on the water easy as a lifebuoy.

I knew when I was beaten.

I turned back.

The flowers nodded like bright, knowledgeable children as I trundled them down the hall.

I felt silly in my sage-green volunteer's uniform, and superfluous, unlike the white-uniformed doctors and nurses, or even the brown-uniformed scrubwomen with their mops and their buckets of grimy water, who passed me without a word.

If I had been getting paid, no matter how little, I could at least count this a proper job, but all I got for a morning of pushing round magazines and candy and flowers was a free lunch.

My mother said the cure for thinking too much about yourself was helping somebody who was worse off than you, so Teresa had arranged for me to sign on as a volunteer at our local hospital. It was difficult to be a volunteer at this hospital, because that's what all the Junior League women wanted to do, but luckily for me, a lot of them were away on vacation.

I had hoped they would send me to a ward with some really gruesome cases, who would see through my numb, dumb face to how I meant well, and be grateful. But the head of the volunteers, a society lady at our church, took one look at me and said, 'You're on maternity.'

So I rode the elevator up three flights to the maternity ward and reported to the head nurse. She gave me the trolley of flowers. I was supposed to put the right vases at the right beds in the right rooms.

But before I came to the door of the first room I noticed that a lot of the flowers were droopy and brown at the edges. I thought it would be discouraging for a woman who'd just had a baby to see somebody plonk down a big bouquet of dead flowers in front of her, so I steered the trolley to a wash-basin in an alcove in the hall and began to pick out all the flowers that were dead.

Then I picked out all those that were dying.

There was no waste-basket in sight, so I crumpled the flowers up and laid them in the deep white basin. The basin felt cold as a tomb. I smiled. This must be how they laid the bodies away in the hospital morgue. My gesture, in its small way, echoed the larger gesture of the doctors and nurses.

I swung the door of the first room open and walked in, dragging my trolley. A couple of nurses jumped up, and I had a confused impression of shelves and medicine cabinets.

'What do you want?' one of the nurses demanded sternly. I couldn't tell one from the other, they all looked just alike.

'I'm taking the flowers round.'

The nurse who had spoken put a hand on my shoulder and led me out of the room, manoeuvring the trolley with her free, expert hand. She flung open the swinging doors of the room next to that one and bowed me in. Then she disappeared.

I could hear giggles in the distance till a door shut and cut them off.

There were six beds in the room, and each had a woman in it. The women were all sitting up and knitting or riffling through magazines or putting their hair in pincurls and chattering like parrots in a parrot house.

I had thought they would be sleeping, or lying quiet and pale, so I could tiptoe round without any trouble and match the bed numbers to the numbers inked on adhesive tape on the vases, but before I had a chance to get my bearings, a bright, jazzy blonde with a sharp, triangular face beckoned to me.

I approached her, leaving the trolley in the middle of the floor, but then she made an impatient gesture, and I saw she wanted me to bring the trolley too.

I wheeled the trolley over to her bedside with a helpful smile.

'Hey, where's my larkspur?' A large, flabby lady from across the ward raked me with an eagle eye.

The sharp-faced blonde bent over the trolley. 'Here are my yellow roses,' she said, 'but they're all mixed up with some lousy iris.'

Other voices joined the voices of the first two women. They sounded cross and loud and full of complaint.

I was opening my mouth to explain that I had thrown a bunch of dead larkspur in the sink, and that some of the vases I had weeded out looked skimpy, there were so few flowers left, so I had joined a few of the bouquets together to fill them out, when the swinging door flew open and a nurse stalked in to see what the commotion was.

'Listen, nurse, I had this big bunch of larkspur Larry brought last night.'

'She's loused up my yellow roses.'

Unbuttoning the green uniform as I ran, I stuffed it, in passing, into the washbasin with the rubbish of dead flowers. Then I took the deserted side steps down to the street two at a time, without meeting another soul.

'Which way is the graveyard?'

The Italian in the black leather jacket stopped and pointed down an alley behind the white Methodist church. I remembered the Methodist church. I had been a Methodist for the first nine years of my life, before my father died and we moved and turned Unitarian.

My mother had been a Catholic before she was a Methodist. My grandmother and my grandfather and my Aunt Libby were all still Catholics. My Aunt Libby had broken away from the Catholic Church at the same time my mother did, but then she'd fallen in love with an Italian Catholic, so she'd gone back again.

Lately I had considered going into the Catholic Church myself. I knew that Catholics thought killing yourself was an awful sin. But perhaps, if this was so, they might have a good way to persuade me out of it.

Of course, I didn't believe in life after death or the virgin birth or the Inquisition or the infallibility of that little monkey-faced Pope or anything, but I didn't have to let the priest see this, I could just concentrate on my sin, and he would help me repent.

The only trouble was, Church, even the Catholic Church, didn't take up the whole of your life. No matter how much you knelt and prayed, you still had to eat three meals a day and have a job and live in the world.

I thought I might see how long you had to be a Catholic before you became a nun, so I asked my mother, thinking she'd know the best way to go about it.

My mother had laughed at me. 'Do you think they'll take somebody like you, right off the bat? Why you've got to know all these catechisms and credos and believe in them, lock, stock and barrel. A girl with your sense!'

Still, I imagined myself going to some Boston priest – it would have to be Boston, because I didn't want any priest in my home town to know I'd thought of killing myself. Priests were terrible gossips.

I would be in black, with my dead white face, and I would throw myself at this priest's feet and say, 'O Father, help me.'

But that was before people had begun to look at me in a funny way, like those nurses in the hospital.

I was pretty sure the Catholics wouldn't take in any crazy nuns. My Aunt Libby's husband had made a joke once, about a nun that a nunnery sent to Teresa for a check-up. This nun kept hearing harp notes in her ears and a voice saying over and over, 'Alleluia!' Only she wasn't sure, on being closely questioned, whether the voice was saying Alleluia or Arizona. The nun had been born in Arizona. I think she ended up in some asylum.

I tugged my black veil down to my chin and strode in through the wrought-iron gates. I thought it odd that in all the time my father had been buried in this graveyard, none of us had ever visited him. My mother hadn't let us come to his funeral because we were only children then, and he had died in hospital, so the graveyard and even his death, had always seemed unreal to me.

I had a great yearning, lately, to pay my father back for all the years of neglect, and start tending his grave. I had always been my father's favourite, and it seemed fitting I should take on a mourning my mother had never bothered with.

I thought that if my father hadn't died, he would have taught me all about insects, which was his speciality at the university. He would also have taught me German and Greek and Latin, which he knew, and perhaps I would be a Lutheran. My father had been a Lutheran in Wisconsin, but they were out of style in New England, so he had become a lapsed Lutheran and then, my mother said, a bitter atheist.

The graveyard disappointed me. It lay at the outskirts of the town, on low ground, like a rubbish dump, and as I walked up and down the gravel paths, I could smell the stagnant salt marshes in the distance.

The old part of the graveyard was all right, with its worn, flat stones and lichen-bitten monuments, but I soon saw my father must be buried in the modern part with dates in the 1940s.

The stones in the modern part were crude and cheap, and here and there a grave was rimmed with marble, like an oblong bathtub full of dirt, and rusty metal containers stuck up about where the person's navel would be, full of plastic flowers.

A fine drizzle started drifting down from the grey sky, and I grew very depressed.

I couldn't find my father anywhere.

Low, shaggy clouds scudded over that part of the horizon where the sea lay, behind the marshes and the beach shanty settlements, and raindrops darkened the black mackintosh I had bought that morning. A clammy dampness sank through to my skin.

I had asked the salesgirl, 'Is it water-repellent?'

And she had said, 'No raincoat is ever water-*repellent*. It's showerproofed.'

And when I asked her what showerproofed was, she told me I had better buy an umbrella.

But I hadn't enough money for an umbrella. What with bus fare in and out of Boston and peanuts and newspapers and abnormal psychology books and trips to my old home town by the sea, my New York fund was almost exhausted.

I had decided that when there was no more money in my bank account I would do it, and that morning I'd spent the last of it on the black raincoat.

Then I saw my father's gravestone.

It was crowded right up by another gravestone, head to head, the way people are crowded in a charity ward when there isn't enough space. The stone was of a mottled pink marble, like tinned salmon, and all there was on it was my father's name and, under it, two dates, separated by a little dash.

At the foot of the stone I arranged the rainy armful of azaleas I had picked from a bush at the gateway of the graveyard. Then my legs folded under me, and I sat down in the sopping grass. I couldn't understand why I was crying so hard.

Then I remembered that I had never cried for my father's death.

My mother hadn't cried either. She had just smiled and said what a merciful thing it was for him he had died, because if he had lived he would have been crippled and an invalid for life, and he couldn't have stood that, he would rather have died than had that happen.

I laid my face to the smooth face of the marble and howled my loss into the cold salt rain.

I knew just how to go about it.

The minute the car tyres crunched off down the drive and the sound of the motor faded, I jumped out of bed and hurried into my white blouse and green figured skirt and black raincoat. The raincoat felt damp still, from the day before, but that would soon cease to matter.

I went downstairs and picked up a pale blue envelope from the dining-room table and scrawled on the back, in large, painstaking letters: *I am going for a long walk*.

I popped the message where my mother would see it the minute she came in.

Then I laughed.

I had forgotten the most important thing.

I ran upstairs and dragged a chair into my mother's closet. Then I climbed up and reached for the small green strongbox on the top shelf. I could have torn the metal cover off with my bare hands, the lock was so feeble, but I wanted to do things in a calm, orderly way.

I pulled out my mother's upper right-hand bureau drawer and slipped the blue jewellery box from its hiding-place under the scented Irish linen handkerchiefs. I unpinned the little key from the dark velvet. Then I unlocked the strongbox and took out the bottle of new pills. There were more than I had hoped.

There were at least fifty.

If I had waited until my mother doled them out to me, night by night, it would have taken me fifty nights to save up enough. And in fifty nights, college would have opened, and my brother would have come back from Germany, and it would be too late.

I pinned the key back in the jewellery box among the clutter of inexpensive chains and rings, put the jewellery box back in the drawer under the handkerchiefs, returned the strongbox to the closet shelf and set the chair on the rug in the exact spot I had dragged it from.

Then I went downstairs and into the kitchen. I turned on the tap and poured myself a tall glass of water. Then I took the glass of water and the bottle of pills and went down into the cellar.

A dim, undersea light filtered through the slits of the cellar windows. Behind the oil burner, a dark gap showed in the wall at about shoulder height and ran back under the breezeway out of sight. The breezeway had been added to the house after the cellar was dug, and built out over this secret, earth-bottomed crevice.

A few old, rotting fireplace logs blocked the hole mouth. I shoved them back a bit. Then I set the glass of water and the bottle of pills side by side on the flat surface of one of the logs and started to heave myself up.

It took me a good while to heft my body into the gap, but at last, after many tries, I managed it, and crouched at the mouth of the darkness, like a troll.

The earth seemed friendly under my bare feet, but cold. I wondered how long it had been since this particular square of soil had seen the sun.

Then, one after the other, I lugged the heavy, dust-covered logs across the hole mouth. The dark felt thick as velvet. I reached for the glass and bottle, and carefully, on my knees, with bent head, crawled to the farthest wall.

Cobwebs touched my face with the softness of moths. Wrapping my black coat round me like my own sweet shadow, I unscrewed the bottle of pills and started taking them swiftly, between gulps of water, one by one by one.

At first nothing happened, but as I approached the bottom of the bottle, red and blue lights began to flash before my eyes. The bottle slid from my fingers and I lay down.

The silence drew off, baring the pebbles and shells and all the tatty wreckage of my life. Then, at the rim of vision, it gathered itself, and in one sweeping tide, rushed me to sleep.

Chapter Fourteen

It was completely dark.

I felt the darkness, but nothing else, and my head rose, feeling it, like the head of a worm. Someone was moaning. Then a great, hard weight smashed against my cheek like a stone wall and the moaning stopped.

The silence surged back, smoothing itself as black water smooths to its old surface calm over a dropped stone.

A cool wind rushed by. I was being transported at enormous speed down a tunnel into the earth. Then the wind stopped. There was a rumbling, as of many voices, protesting and disagreeing in the distance. Then the voices stopped.

A chisel cracked down on my eye, and a slit of light opened, like a mouth or a wound, till the darkness clamped shut on it again. I tried to roll away from the direction of the light, but hands wrapped round my limbs like mummy bands, and I couldn't move.

I began to think I must be in an underground chamber, lit by blinding lights, and that the chamber was full of people who for some reason were holding me down.

Then the chisel struck again, and the light leapt into my head, and through the thick, warm, furry dark, a voice cried, 'Mother!'

*

Air breathed and played over my face.

I felt the shape of a room around me, a big room with open windows. A pillow moulded itself under my head, and my body floated, without pressure, between thin sheets.

Then I felt warmth, like a hand on my face. I must be lying in the sun. If I opened my eyes, I would see colours and shapes bending in upon me like nurses.

I opened my eyes.

It was completely dark.

Somebody was breathing beside me.

'I can't see,' I said.

A cheery voice spoke out of the dark. 'There are lots of blind people in the world. You'll marry a nice blind man some day.'

The man with the chisel had come back.

Why do you bother?' I said. 'It's no use.'

'You mustn't talk like that.' His fingers probed at the great, aching boss over my left eye. Then he loosened something, and a ragged gap of light appeared, like the hole in a wall. A man's head peered round the edge of it.

'Can you see me?'

'Yes.'

'Can you see anything else?'

Then I remembered. 'I can't see anything.' The gap narrowed and went dark. 'I'm blind.'

'Nonsense! Who told you that?'

'The nurse.'

The man snorted. He finished taping the bandage back over my eye. 'You are a very lucky girl. Your sight is perfectly intact.'

'Somebody to see you.'

The nurse beamed and disappeared.

My mother came smiling round the foot of the bed. She was

wearing a dress with purple cartwheels on it and she looked awful.

A big tall boy followed her. At first I couldn't make out who it was, because my eye only opened a short way, but then I saw it was my brother.

'They said you wanted to see me.'

My mother perched on the edge of the bed and laid a hand on my leg. She looked loving and reproachful, and I wanted her to go away.

'I didn't think I said anything.'

'They said you called for me.' She seemed ready to cry. Her face puckered up and quivered like a pale jelly.

'How are you?' my brother said.

I looked my mother in the eye.

'The same,' I said.

'You have a visitor.'

'I don't want a visitor.'

The nurse bustled out and whispered to somebody in the hall. Then she came back. 'He'd very much like to see you.'

I looked down at the yellow legs sticking out of the unfamiliar white silk pyjamas they had dressed me in. The skin shook flabbily when I moved, as if there wasn't a muscle in it, and it was covered with a short, thick stubble of black hair.

'Who is it?'

'Somebody you know.'

'What's his name?'

'George Bakewell.'

'I don't know any George Bakewell.'

'He says he knows you.'

Then the nurse went out, and a very familiar boy came in and said, 'Mind if I sit on the edge of your bed?'

He was wearing a white coat, and I could see a stethoscope

poking out of his pocket. I thought it must be somebody I knew dressed up as a doctor.

I had meant to cover my legs if anybody came in, but now I saw it was too late, so I let them stick out, just as they were, disgusting and ugly.

'That's me,' I thought. 'That's what I am.'

'You remember me, don't you, Esther?'

I squinted at the boy's face through the crack of my good eye. The other eye hadn't opened yet, but the eye doctor said it would be all right in a few days.

The boy looked at me as if I were some exciting new zoo animal and he was about to burst out laughing.

'You remember me, don't you, Esther?' He spoke slowly, the way one speaks to a dull child. 'I'm George Bakewell. I go to your church. You dated my room-mate once at Amherst.'

I thought I placed the boy's face then. It hovered dimly at the rim of memory – the sort of face to which I would never bother to attach a name.

'What are you doing here?'

'I'm houseman at this hospital.'

How could this George Bakewell have become a doctor so suddenly? I wondered. He didn't really know me, either. He just wanted to see what a girl who was crazy enough to kill herself looked like.

I turned my face to the wall.

'Get out,' I said. 'Get the hell out and don't come back.'

'I want to see a mirror.'

The nurse hummed busily as she opened one drawer after another, stuffing the new underclothes and blouses and skirts and pyjamas my mother had bought me into the black patent leather overnight case.

'Why can't I see a mirror?'

I had been dressed in a sheath, striped grey and white, like mattress ticking, with a wide, shiny red belt, and they had propped me up in an armchair.

'Why can't I?'

'Because you better not.' The nurse shut the lid of the overnight case with a little snap.

'Why?'

'Because you don't look very pretty.'

'Oh, just let me see.'

The nurse sighed and opened the top bureau drawer. She took out a large mirror in a wooden frame that matched the wood of the bureau and handed it to me.

At first I didn't see what the trouble was. It wasn't a mirror at all, but a picture.

You couldn't tell whether the person in the picture was a man or a woman, because their hair was shaved off and sprouted in bristly chicken-feather tufts all over their head. One side of the person's face was purple, and bulged out in a shapeless way, shading to green along the edges, and then to a sallow yellow. The person's mouth was pale brown, with a rose-coloured sore at either corner.

The most startling thing about the face was its supernatural conglomeration of bright colours.

I smiled.

The mouth in the mirror cracked into a grin.

A minute after the crash another nurse ran in. She took one look at the broken mirror, and at me, standing over the blind, white pieces, and hustled the young nurse out of the room.

'Didn't I *tell* you,' I could hear her say.

'But I only . . .'

'Didn't I *tell* you!'

I listened with mild interest. Anybody could drop a mirror. I didn't see why they should get so stirred up.

The other, older nurse came back into the room. She stood there, arms folded, staring hard at me.

'Seven years' bad luck.'

'What?'

'I said,' the nurse raised her voice, as if speaking to a deaf person, 'seven years' bad luck.'

The young nurse returned with a dustpan and brush and began to sweep up the glittery splinters.

'That's only a superstition,' I said then.

'Huh!' The second nurse addressed herself to the nurse on her hands and knees as if I wasn't there. 'At you-know-where they'll take care of her!'

From the back window of the ambulance I could see street after familiar street funnelling off into a summery green distance. My mother sat on one side of me, and my brother on the other.

I had pretended I didn't know why they were moving me from the hospital in my home town to a city hospital, to see what they would say.

'They want you to be in a special ward,' my mother said. 'They don't have that sort of ward at our hospital.'

'I liked it where I was.'

My mother's mouth tightened. 'You should have behaved better, then.'

'What?'

'You shouldn't have broken that mirror. Then maybe they'd have let you stay.'

But of course I knew the mirror had nothing to do with it.

I sat in bed with the covers up to my neck.

'Why can't I get up? I'm not sick.'

'Ward rounds,' the nurse said. 'You can get up after ward

rounds.' She shoved the bed-curtains back and revealed a fat young Italian woman in the next bed.

The Italian woman had a mass of tight black curls, starting at her forehead, that rose in a mountainous pompadour and cascaded down her back. Whenever she moved, the huge arrangement of hair moved with her, as if made of stiff black paper.

The woman looked at me and giggled. 'Why are you here?' She didn't wait for an answer. 'I'm here on account of my French-Canadian mother-in-law.' She giggled again. 'My husband knows I can't stand her, and still he said she could come and visit us, and when she came, my tongue stuck out of my head, I couldn't stop it. They ran me into Emergency and then they put me up here,' she lowered her voice, 'along with the nuts.' Then she said, 'What's the matter with you?'

I turned her my full face, with the bulging purple and green eye. 'I tried to kill myself.'

The woman stared at me. Then, hastily, she snatched up a movie magazine from her bed-table and pretended to be reading.

The swinging door opposite my bed flew open, and a whole troop of young boys and girls in white coats came in, with an older, grey-haired man. They were all smiling with bright, artificial smiles. They grouped themselves at the foot of my bed.

'And how are you feeling this morning, Miss Greenwood?'

I tried to decide which one of them had spoken. I hate saying anything to a group of people. When I talk to a group of people I always have to single out one and talk to him, and all the while I am talking I feel the others are peering at me and taking unfair advantage. I also hate people to ask cheerfully how you are when they know you're feeling like hell and expect you to say 'Fine'.

'I feel lousy.'

'Lousy. Hmm,' somebody said, and a boy ducked his head with a little smile. Somebody else scribbled something on a clipboard. Then somebody pulled a straight, solemn face and said, 'And why do you feel lousy?'

I thought some of the boys and girls in that bright group might well be friends of Buddy Willard. They would know I knew him, and they would be curious to see me, and afterwards they would gossip about me among themselves. I wanted to be where nobody I knew could ever come.

'I can't sleep . . .'

They interrupted me. 'But the nurse says you slept last night.' I looked round the crescent of fresh, strange faces.

'I can't read.' I raised my voice. 'I can't eat.' It occurred to me I'd been eating ravenously ever since I came to.

The people in the group had turned from me and were murmuring in low voices to each other. Finally, the grey-haired man stepped out.

'Thank you, Miss Greenwood. You will be seen by one of the staff doctors presently.'

Then the group moved on to the bed of the Italian woman.

'And how are you feeling today, Mrs . . .' somebody said, and the name sounded long and full of l's, like Mrs Tomolillo.

Mrs Tomolillo giggled. 'Oh, I'm fine, doctor. I'm just fine.' Then she lowered her voice and whispered something I couldn't hear. One or two people in the group glanced in my direction. Then somebody said, 'All right, Mrs Tomolillo,' and somebody stepped out and pulled the bed-curtain between us like a white wall.

I sat on one end of a wooden bench in the grassy square between the four brick walls of the hospital. My mother, in her purple cartwheel dress, sat at the other end. She had her head propped in her hand, index finger on her cheek, and thumb under her chin.

Mrs Tomolillo was sitting with some dark-haired, laughing Italians on the next bench down. Every time my mother moved, Mrs Tomolillo imitated her. Now Mrs Tomolillo was sitting with her index finger on her cheek and her thumb under her chin, and her head tilted wistfully to one side.

'Don't move,' I told my mother in a low voice. 'That woman's imitating you.'

My mother turned to glance round, but quick as a wink, Mrs Tomolillo dropped her fat white hands in her lap and started talking vigorously to her friends.

'Why no, she's not,' my mother said. 'She's not even paying any attention to us.'

But the minute my mother turned round to me again, Mrs Tomolillo matched the tips of her fingers together the way my mother had just done and cast a black, mocking look at me.

The lawn was white with doctors.

All the time my mother and I had been sitting there, in the narrow cone of sun that shone down between the tall brick walls, doctors had been coming up to me and introducing themselves. 'I'm Doctor Soandso, I'm Doctor Soandso.'

Some of them looked so young I knew they couldn't be proper doctors, and one of them had a queer name that sounded like Doctor Syphilis, so I began to look out for suspicious, fake names, and sure enough, a dark-haired fellow who looked very like Doctor Gordon, except that he had black skin where Doctor Gordon's skin was white, came up and said, 'I'm Doctor Pancreas,' and shook my hand.

After introducing themselves, the doctors all stood within listening distance, only I couldn't tell my mother that they were taking down every word we said without their hearing me, so I leaned over and whispered into her ear.

My mother drew back sharply.

'Oh, Esther, I wish you would co-operate. They say you don't co-operate. They say you won't talk to any of the doctors or make anything in Occupational Therapy . . .'

'I've got to get out of here,' I told her meaningly. 'Then I'd be all right. You got me in here,' I said. 'You get me out.'

I thought if only I could persuade my mother to get me out of the hospital I could work on her sympathies, like that boy with brain disease in the play, and convince her what was the best thing to do.

To my surprise, my mother said, 'All right, I'll try to get you out – even if only to a better place. If I try to get you out,' she laid a hand on my knee, 'promise you'll be good?'

I spun round and glared straight at Doctor Syphilis, who stood at my elbow taking notes on a tiny, almost invisible pad. 'I promise,' I said in a loud, conspicuous voice.

The negro wheeled the food cart into the patients' dining-room. The Psychiatric Ward at the hospital was very small – just two corridors in an L-shape, lined with rooms, and an alcove of beds behind the OT shop, where I was, and a little area with a table and a few seats by a window in the corner of the L, which was our lounge and dining-room.

Usually it was a shrunken old white man that brought our food, but today it was a negro. The negro was with a woman in blue stiletto heels, and she was telling him what to do. The negro kept grinning and chuckling in a silly way.

Then he carried a tray over to our table with three lidded tin tureens on it, and started banging the tureens down. The woman left the room, locking the door behind her. All the time the negro was banging down the tureens and then the dinted silver and the thick, white china plates, he gawped at us with big, rolling eyes.

I could tell we were his first crazy people.

Nobody at the table made a move to take the lids off the tin tureens, and the nurse stood back to see if any of us would take the lids off before she came to do it. Usually Mrs Tomolillo had taken the lids off and dished out everybody's food like a little mother, but then they sent her home, and nobody seemed to want to take her place.

I was starving, so I lifted the lid off the first bowl.

'That's very nice of you, Esther,' the nurse said pleasantly. 'Would you like to take some beans and pass them round to the others?'

I dished myself out a helping of green string beans and turned to pass the tureen to the enormous red-headed woman at my right. This was the first time the red-headed woman had been allowed up to the table. I had seen her once, at the very end of the L-shaped corridor, standing in front of an open door with bars on the square, inset window.

She had been yelling and laughing in a rude way and slapping her thighs at the passing doctors, and the white-jacketed attendant who took care of the people in that end of the ward was leaning against the hall radiator, laughing himself sick.

The red-headed woman snatched the tureen from me and upended it on her plate. Beans mountained up in front of her and scattered over on to her lap and on to the floor like stiff, green straws.

'Oh, Mrs Mole!' the nurse said in a sad voice. 'I think you better eat in your room today.'

And she returned most of the beans to the tureen and gave it to the person next to Mrs Mole and led Mrs Mole off. All the way down the hall to her room, Mrs Mole kept turning round and making leering faces at us, and ugly, oinking noises.

The negro had come back and was starting to collect the

empty plates of people who hadn't dished out any beans yet.

'We're not done,' I told him. 'You can just wait.'

'Mah, mah!' The negro widened his eyes in mock wonder. He glanced round. The nurse had not yet returned from locking up Mrs Mole. The negro made me an insolent bow. 'Miss Mucky-Muck,' he said under his breath.

I lifted the lid off the second tureen and uncovered a wodge of macaroni, stone-cold and stuck together in a gluey paste. The third and last tureen was chock-full of baked beans.

Now I knew perfectly well you didn't serve two kinds of beans together at a meal. Beans and carrots, or beans and peas, maybe, but never beans and beans. The negro was just trying to see how much we would take.

The nurse came back, and the negro edged off at a distance. I ate as much as I could of the baked beans. Then I rose from the table, passing round to the side where the nurse couldn't see me below the waist, and behind the negro, who was clearing the dirty plates. I drew my foot back and gave him a sharp, hard kick on the calf of the leg.

The negro leapt away with a yelp and rolled his eyes at me. 'Oh Miz, oh Miz,' he moaned, rubbing his leg. 'You shouldn't of done that, you shouldn't, you reely shouldn't.'

'That's what *you* get,' I said, and stared him in the eye.

'Don't you want to get up today?'

'No.' I huddled down more deeply in the bed and pulled the sheet up over my head. Then I lifted a corner of the sheet and peered out. The nurse was shaking down the thermometer she had just removed from my mouth.

'You *see*, it's normal.' I had looked at the thermometer before she came to collect it, the way I always did. 'You *see*, it's normal, what do you keep taking it for?'

I wanted to tell her that if only something were wrong with

my body it would be fine, I would rather have anything wrong with my body than something wrong with my head, but the idea seemed so involved and wearisome that I didn't say anything. I only burrowed down further in the bed.

Then, through the sheet, I felt a slight, annoying pressure on my leg. I peeped out. The nurse had set her tray of thermometers on my bed while she turned her back and took the pulse of the person who lay next to me, in Mrs Tomolillo's place.

A heavy naughtiness pricked through my veins, irritating and attractive as the hurt of a loose tooth. I yawned and stirred, as if about to turn over, and edged my foot under the box.

'Oh!' The nurse's cry sounded like a cry for help, and another nurse came running. 'Look what you've done!'

I poked my head out of the covers and stared over the edge of the bed. Around the overturned enamel tray, a star of thermometer shards glittered, and balls of mercury trembled like celestial dew.

'I'm sorry,' I said. 'It was an accident.'

The second nurse fixed me with a baleful eye. 'You did it on purpose. I *saw* you.'

Then she hurried off, and almost immediately two attendants came and wheeled me, bed and all, down to Mrs Mole's old room, but not before I had scooped up a ball of mercury.

Soon after they had locked the door, I could see the negro's face, a molasses-coloured moon, risen at the window grating, but I pretended not to notice.

I opened my fingers a crack, like a child with a secret, and smiled at the silver globe cupped in my palm. If I dropped it, it would break into a million little replicas of itself, and if I pushed them near each other, they would fuse, without a crack, into one whole again.

I smiled and smiled at the small silver ball.

I couldn't imagine what they had done with Mrs Mole.

Chapter Fifteen

Philomena Guinea's black Cadillac eased through the tight, five o'clock traffic like a ceremonial car. Soon it would cross one of the brief bridges that arched the Charles, and I would, without thinking, open the door and plunge out through the stream of traffic to the rail of the bridge. One jump, and the water would be over my head.

Idly I twisted a kleenex to small, pill-sized pellets between my fingers and watched my chance. I sat in the middle of the back seat of the Cadillac, my mother on one side of me, and my brother on the other, both leaning slightly forward, like diagonal bars, one across each car door.

In front of me I could see the spam-coloured expanse of the chauffeur's neck, sandwiched between a blue cap and the shoulders of a blue jacket and, next to him, like a frail, exotic bird, the silver hair and emerald-feathered hat of Philomena Guinea, the famous novelist.

I wasn't quite sure why Mrs Guinea had turned up. All I knew was that she had interested herself in my case and that at one time, at the peak of her career, she had been in an asylum as well.

My mother said that Mrs Guinea had sent her a telegram from the Bahamas, where she read about me in a Boston paper. Mrs Guinea had telegrammed, 'Is there a boy in the case?'

If there was a boy in the case, Mrs Guinea couldn't, of course, have anything to do with it.

But my mother had telegrammed back, 'No, it is Esther's writing. She thinks she will never write again.'

So Mrs Guinea had flown back to Boston and taken me out of the cramped city hospital ward, and now she was driving me to a private hospital that had grounds and golf courses and gardens, like a country club, where she would pay for me, as if I had a scholarship, until the doctors she knew of there had made me well.

My mother told me I should be grateful. She said I had used up almost all her money, and if it weren't for Mrs Guinea she didn't know where I'd be. I knew where I'd be, though. I'd be in the big state hospital in the country, cheek by jowl to this private place.

I knew I should be grateful to Mrs Guinea, only I couldn't feel a thing. If Mrs Guinea had given me a ticket to Europe, or a round-the-world cruise, it wouldn't have made one scrap of difference to me, because wherever I sat – on the deck of a ship or at a street café in Paris or Bangkok – I would be sitting under the same glass bell jar, stewing in my own sour air.

Blue sky opened its dome above the river, and the river was dotted with sails. I readied myself, but immediately my mother and my brother each laid one hand on a door handle. The tyres hummed briefly over the grille of the bridge. Water, sails, blue sky and suspended gulls flashed by like an improbable postcard, and we were across.

I sank back in the grey, plush seat and closed my eyes. The air of the bell jar wadded round me and I couldn't stir.

I had my own room again.

It reminded me of the room in Doctor Gordon's hospital – a bed, a bureau, a closet, a table and chair. A window with a screen, but no bars. My room was on the first floor, and the window, a short distance above the pine-needle-padded ground, overlooked a wooded yard ringed by a red brick wall. If I jumped I wouldn't even bruise my knees. The inner surface of the tall wall seemed smooth as glass.

The journey over the bridge had unnerved me.

I had missed a perfectly good chance. The river water passed me by like an untouched drink. I suspected that even if my mother and brother had not been there I would have made no move to jump.

When I enrolled in the main building of the hospital, a slim young woman had come up and introduced herself. 'My name is Doctor Nolan. I am to be Esther's doctor.'

I was surprised to have a woman. I didn't think they had woman psychiatrists. This woman was a cross between Myrna Loy and my mother. She wore a white blouse and a full skirt gathered at the waist by a wide leather belt, and stylish, crescent-shaped spectacles.

But after a nurse had led me across the lawn to the gloomy brick building called Caplan, where I would live, Doctor Nolan didn't come to see me, a whole lot of strange men came instead.

I lay on my bed under the thick white blanket, and they entered my room, one by one, and introduced themselves. I couldn't understand why there should be so many of them, or why they would want to introduce themselves, and I began to think they were testing me, to see if I noticed there were too many of them, and I grew wary.

Finally, a handsome, white-haired doctor came in and said he was the director of the hospital. Then he started talking about the Pilgrims and Indians and who had the land after them, and what rivers ran nearby, and who had built the first hospital, and how it had burned down, and who had built the next hospital, until I thought he must be waiting to see when I would interrupt him and tell him I knew all that about rivers and Pilgrims was a lot of nonsense.

But then I thought some of it might be true, so I tried to sort out what was likely to be true and what wasn't, only before I could do that, he had said good-bye.

I waited till I heard the voices of all the doctors die away. Then I threw back the white blanket and put on my shoes and walked out into the hall. Nobody stopped me, so I walked round the corner of my wing of the hall and down another, longer hall, past an open dining room.

A maid in a green uniform was setting the tables for supper. There were white linen table-cloths and glasses and paper napkins. I stored the fact that there were real glasses in the corner of my mind the way a squirrel stores a nut. At the city hospital we had drunk out of paper cups and had no knives to cut our meat. The meat had always been so overcooked we could cut it with a fork.

Finally I arrived at a big lounge with shabby furniture and a threadbare rug. A girl with a round pasty face and short black hair was sitting in an armchair, reading a magazine. She reminded me of a Girl Scout leader I'd had once. I glanced at her feet, and sure enough, she wore those flat brown leather shoes with fringed tongues lapping down over the front that are supposed to be so sporty, and the ends of the laces were knobbed with little imitation acorns.

The girl raised her eyes and smiled. 'I'm Valerie. Who are you?'

I pretended I hadn't heard and walked out of the lounge to the end of the next wing. On the way, I passed a waist-high door behind which I saw some nurses.

'Where is everybody?'

'Out.' The nurse was writing something over and over on

little pieces of adhesive tape. I leaned across the gate of the door to see what she was writing, and it was E. Greenwood, E. Greenwood, E. Greenwood, E. Greenwood.

'Out where?'

'Oh, OT, the golf course, playing badminton.'

I noticed a pile of clothes on a chair beside the nurse. They were the same clothes the nurse in the first hospital had been packing into the patent leather case when I broke the mirror. The nurse began sticking the labels on to the clothes.

I walked back to the lounge. I couldn't understand what these people were doing, playing badminton and golf. They mustn't be really sick at all, to do that.

I sat down near Valerie and observed her carefully. Yes, I thought, she might just as well be in a Girl Scout camp. She was reading her tatty copy of *Vogue* with intense interest.

'What the hell is she doing here?' I wondered. 'There's nothing the matter with her.'

'Do you mind if I smoke?' Doctor Nolan leaned back in the armchair next to my bed.

I said no, I liked the smell of smoke. I thought if Doctor Nolan smoked, she might stay longer. This was the first time she had come to talk with me. When she left I would simply lapse into the old blankness.

'Tell me about Doctor Gordon,' Doctor Nolan said suddenly. 'Did you like him?'

I gave Doctor Nolan a wary look. I thought the doctors must all be in it together, and that somewhere in this hospital, in a hidden corner, there reposed a machine exactly like Doctor Gordon's, ready to jolt me out of my skin.

'No,' I said. 'I didn't like him at all.'

'That's interesting. Why?'

'I didn't like what he did to me.'

'Did to you?'

I told Doctor Nolan about the machine, and the blue flashes, and the jolting and the noise. While I was telling her she went very still.

'That was a mistake,' she said then. 'It's not supposed to be like that.'

I stared at her.

'If it's done properly,' Doctor Nolan said, 'it's like going to sleep.'

'If anyone does that to me again I'll kill myself.'

Doctor Nolan said firmly, 'You won't have any shock treatments here. Or if you do,' she amended, 'I'll tell you about it beforehand, and I promise you it won't be anything like what you had before. Why,' she finished, 'some people even *like* them.'

After Doctor Nolan had gone I found a box of matches on the window-sill. It wasn't an ordinary-size box, but an extremely tiny box. I opened it and exposed a row of little white sticks with pink tips. I tried to light one, and it crumpled in my hand.

I couldn't think why Doctor Nolan would have left me such a stupid thing. Perhaps she wanted to see if I would give it back. Carefully I stored the toy matches in the hem of my new wool bathrobe. If Doctor Nolan asked me for the matches, I would say I'd thought they were made of candy and had eaten them.

A new woman had moved into the room next to mine.

I thought she must be the only person in the building who was newer than I was, so she wouldn't know how really bad I was, the way the rest did. I thought I might go in and make friends.

The woman was lying on her bed in a purple dress that

fastened at the neck with a cameo brooch and reached midway between her knees and her shoes. She had rusty hair knotted in a schoolmarmish bun, and thin, silver-rimmed spectacles attached to her breast pocket with a black elastic.

'Hello,' I said conversationally, sitting down on the edge of the bed. 'My name's Esther, what's your name?'

The woman didn't stir, she just stared up at the ceiling. I felt hurt. I thought maybe Valerie or somebody had told her when she first came in how stupid I was.

A nurse popped her head in at the door.

'Oh, there you are,' she said to me. 'Visiting Miss Norris. How nice!' And she disappeared again.

I don't know how long I sat there, watching the woman in purple and wondering if her pursed, pink lips would open, and if they did open, what they would say.

Finally, without speaking or looking at me, Miss Norris swung her feet in their high, black, buttoned boots over the other side of the bed and walked out of the room. I thought she might be trying to get rid of me in a subtle way. Quietly, at a little distance, I followed her down the hall.

Miss Norris reached the door of the dining-room and paused. All the way to the dining-room she had walked precisely, placing her feet in the very centre of the cabbage roses that twined through the pattern of the carpet. She waited a moment and then, one by one, lifted her feet over the door-sill and into the dining-room as though stepping over an invisible shin-high stile.

She sat down at one of the round, linen-covered tables and unfolded a napkin in her lap.

'It's not supper for an hour yet,' the cook called out of the kitchen.

But Miss Norris didn't answer. She just stared straight ahead of her in a polite way.

I pulled up a chair opposite her at the table and unfolded a napkin. We didn't speak, but sat there, in a close, sisterly silence, until the gong for supper sounded down the hall.

'Lie down,' the nurse said. 'I'm going to give you another injection.'

I rolled over on my stomach on the bed and hitched up my skirt. Then I pulled down the trousers of my silk pyjamas.

'My word, what all have you got under there?'

'Pyjamas. So I won't have to bother getting in and out of them all the time.'

The nurse made a little clucking noise. Then she said, 'Which side?' It was an old joke.

I raised my head and glanced back at my bare buttocks. They were bruised purple and green and blue from past injections. The left side looked darker than the right.

'The right.'

'You name it.' The nurse jabbed the needle in, and I winced, savouring the tiny hurt. Three times each day the nurses injected me, and about an hour after each injection they gave me a cup of sugary fruit juice and stood by, watching me drink it.

'Lucky you,' Valerie said. 'You're on insulin.'

'Nothing happens.'

'Oh, it will. I've had it. Tell me when you get a reaction.'

But I never seemed to get any reaction. Just grew fatter and fatter. Already I filled the new, too-big clothes my mother had bought, and when I peered down at my plump stomach and my broad hips I thought it was a good thing Mrs Guinea hadn't seen me like this, because I looked just as if I were going to have a baby.

'Have you seen my scars?'

Valerie pushed aside her black bang and indicated two pale

marks, one on either side of her forehead, as if at some time she had started to sprout horns, but cut them off.

We were walking, just the two of us, with the Sports Therapist in the asylum gardens. Nowadays I was let out on walk privileges more and more often. They never let Miss Norris out at all.

Valerie said Miss Norris shouldn't be in Caplan, but in a building for worse people called Wymark.

'Do you know what these scars are?' Valerie persisted.

'No. What are they?'

'I've had a lobotomy.'

I looked at Valerie in awe, appreciating for the first time her perpetual marble calm. 'How do you feel?'

'Fine. I'm not angry any more. Before, I was always angry. I was in Wymark, before, and now I'm in Caplan. I can go to town, now, or shopping or to a movie, along with a nurse.'

'What will you do when you get out?'

'Oh, I'm not leaving,' Valerie laughed. 'I like it here.'

'Moving day!'

'Why should I be moving?'

The nurse went on blithely opening and shutting my drawers, emptying the closet and folding my belongings into the black overnight case.

I thought they must at last be moving me to Wymark.

'Oh, you're only moving to the front of the house,' the nurse said cheerfully. 'You'll like it. There's lots more sun.'

When we came out into the hall, I saw that Miss Norris was moving too. A nurse, young and cheerful as my own, stood in the doorway of Miss Norris's room, helping Miss Norris into a purple coat with a scrawny squirrel-fur collar.

Hour after hour I had been keeping watch by Miss Norris's bedside, refusing the diversion of OT and walks and badminton matches and even the weekly movies, which I enjoyed, and which Miss Norris never went to, simply to brood over the pale, speechless circlet of her lips.

I thought how exciting it would be if she opened her mouth and spoke, and I rushed out into the hall and announced this to the nurses. They would praise me for encouraging Miss Norris, and I would probably be allowed shopping privileges and movie privileges downtown, and my escape would be assured.

But in all my hours of vigil Miss Norris hadn't said a word.

'Where are you moving to?' I asked her now.

The nurse touched Miss Norris's elbow, and Miss Norris jerked into motion like a doll on wheels.

'She's going to Wymark,' my nurse told me in a low voice. 'I'm afraid Miss Norris isn't moving up like you.'

I watched Miss Norris lift one foot, and then the other, over the invisible stile that barred the front doorsill.

'I've a surprise for you,' the nurse said as she installed me in a sunny room in the front wing overlooking the green golf links. 'Somebody you know's just come today.'

'Somebody I know?'

The nurse laughed. 'Don't look at me like that. It's not a policeman.' Then, as I didn't say anything, she added, 'She says she's an old friend of yours. She lives next door. Why don't you pay her a visit?'

I thought the nurse must be joking, and that if I knocked on the door next to mine I would hear no answer, but go in and find Miss Norris, buttoned into her purple, squirrel-collared coat and lying on the bed, her mouth blooming out of the quiet vase of her body like the bud of a rose.

Still, I went out and knocked on the neighbouring door.

'Come in!' called a gay voice.

I opened the door a crack and peered into the room. The

big, horsey girl in jodhpurs sitting by the window glanced up with a broad smile.

'Esther!' She sounded out of breath, as if she had been running a long, long distance and only just come to a halt. 'How nice to see you. They told me you were here.'

'Joan?' I said tentatively, then 'Joan!' in confusion and disbelief.

Joan beamed, revealing her large, gleaming, unmistakable teeth.

'It's really me. I thought you'd be surprised.'

Chapter Sixteen

Joan's room, with its closet and bureau and table and chair and white blanket with the big blue C on it, was a mirror image of my own. It occurred to me that Joan, hearing where I was, had engaged a room at the asylum on pretence, simply as a joke. That would explain why she had told the nurse I was her friend. I had never known Joan, except at a cool distance.

'How did you get here?' I curled up on Joan's bed.

'I read about you,' Joan said.

'What?'

'I read about you, and I ran away.'

'How do you mean?' I said evenly.

'Well,' Joan leaned back in the chintz-flowered asylum armchair, 'I had a summer job working for the chapter head of some fraternity, like the Masons, you know, but not the Masons, and I felt terrible. I had these bunions, I could hardly walk – in the last days I had to wear rubber boots to work, instead of shoes, and you can imagine what *that* did to my morale . . .'

I thought either Joan must be crazy – wearing rubber boots to work, or she must be trying to see how crazy I was – believing all that. Besides, only old people ever got bunions. I decided to pretend I thought she was crazy, and that I was only humouring her along.

'I always feel lousy without shoes,' I said with an ambiguous smile. 'Did your feet hurt much?'

'Terribly. And my boss – he'd just separated from his wife, he couldn't come right out and get a divorce, because that wouldn't go with this fraternal order – my boss kept buzzing me in every other minute, and each time I moved, my feet hurt like the devil, but the second I'd sit down at my desk again, buzz went the buzzer, and he'd have something else he wanted to get off his chest . . .'

'Why didn't you quit?'

'Oh, I did quit, more or less. I stayed off work on sick leave. I didn't go out. I didn't see anyone. I stowed the telephone in a drawer and never answered it . . .

'Then my doctor sent me to a psychiatrist at this big hospital. I had an appointment for twelve o'clock, and I was in an awful state. Finally, at half past twelve, the receptionist came out and told me the doctor had gone to lunch. She asked me if I wanted to wait, and I said yes.'

'Did he come back?' The story sounded rather involved for Joan to have made up out of whole cloth, but I led her on, to see what would come of it.

'Oh yes. I was going to kill myself, mind you. I said "If this doctor doesn't do the trick, that's the end." Well, the receptionist led me down a long hall, and just as we got to the door she turned to me and said, "You won't mind if there are a few students with the doctor, will you?" What could I say? "Oh no," I said. I walked in and found nine pairs of eyes fixed on me. Nine! Eighteen separate eyes.

'Now, if that receptionist had told me there were going to be nine people in that room, I'd have walked out on the spot. But there I was, and it was too late to do a thing about it. Well, on this particular day I happened to be wearing a fur coat . . .'

'In *Aug*ust?'

'Oh, it was one of those cold, wet days, and I thought, my first psychiatrist – you know. Anyway, this psychiatrist kept eyeing that fur coat the whole time I talked to him, and I could just see what he thought of my asking to pay the student's cut-rate instead of the full fee. I could see the dollar signs in his eyes. Well, I told him I don't know whatall – about the bunions and the telephone in the drawer and how I wanted to kill myself, and then he asked me to wait outside while he discussed my case with the others, and when he called me back in, you know what he said?'

'What?'

'He folded his hands together and looked at me and said, "Miss Gilling, we have decided that you would benefit by group therapy."'

'*Group* therapy?' I thought I must sound phoney as an echo chamber, but Joan didn't pay any notice.

'That's what he said. Can you imagine me wanting to kill myself, and coming round to chat about it with a whole pack of strangers, and most of them no better than myself . . .'

'That's crazy.' I was growing involved in spite of myself. 'That's not even *hu*man.'

'That's just what I said. I went straight home and wrote that doctor a letter. I wrote him one beautiful letter about how a man like that had no business setting himself up to help sick people . . .'

'Did you get any answer?'

'I don't know. That was the day I read about you.'

'How do you mean?'

'Oh,' Joan said, 'about how the police thought you were dead and all. I've got a pile of clippings somewhere.' She heaved herself up, and I had a strong horsey whiff that made my nostrils prickle. Joan had been a champion horse-jumper at the annual college gymkhana, and I wondered if she had been sleeping in a stable.

Joan rummaged in her open suitcase and came up with a fistful of clippings.

'Here, have a look.'

The first clipping showed a big, blown-up picture of a girl with black-shadowed eyes and black lips spread in a grin. I couldn't imagine where such a tarty picture had been taken until I noticed the Bloomingdale ear-rings and the Bloomingdale necklace glinting out of it with bright, white highlights, like imitation stars.

SCHOLARSHIP GIRL MISSING. MOTHER WORRIED. The article under the picture told how this girl had disappeared from her home on August 17th, wearing a green skirt and a white blouse, and had left a note saying she was taking a long walk. *When Miss Greenwood had not returned by midnight*, it said, *her mother called the town police.*

The next clipping showed a picture of my mother and brother and me grouped together in our backyard and smiling. I couldn't think who had taken that picture either, until I saw I was wearing dungarees and white sneakers and remembered that was what I wore in my spinach-picking summer, and how Dodo Conway had dropped by and taken some family snaps of the three of us one hot afternoon. *Mrs Greenwood asked that this picture be printed in hopes that it will encourage her daughter to return home.*

SLEEPING PILLS FEARED MISSING WITH GIRL.

A dark, midnight picture of about a dozen moon-faced people in a wood. I thought the people at the end of the row looked queer and unusually short until I realized they were not people, but dogs. *Bloodhounds used in search for missing girl. Police Sgt Bill Hindly says: It doesn't look good.*

GIRL FOUND ALIVE!

The last picture showed policemen lifting a long, limp blanket roll with a featureless cabbage head into the back of an ambulance. Then it told how my mother had been down in the cellar, doing the week's laundry, when she heard faint groans coming from a disused hole . . .

I laid the clippings on the white spread of the bed.

'You keep them,' Joan said. 'You ought to stick them in a scrapbook.'

I folded the clippings and slipped them in my pocket.

'I read about you,' Joan went on. 'Not how they found you, but everything up to that, and I put all my money together and took the first plane to New York.'

'Why New York?'

'Oh, I thought it would be easier to kill myself in New York.'

'What did you do?'

Joan grinned sheepishly and stretched out her hands, palm up. Like a miniature mountain range, large, reddish weals upheaved across the white flesh of her wrists.

'How did you do that?' For the first time it occurred to me Joan and I might have something in common.

'I shoved my fists through my room-mate's window.'

'What room-mate?'

'My old college room-mate. She was working in New York, and I couldn't think of anyplace else to stay, and besides, I'd hardly any money left, so I went to stay with her. My parents found me there – she'd written them I was acting funny – and my father flew straight down and brought me back.'

'But you're all right now.' I made it a statement.

Joan considered me with her bright, pebble-grey eyes. 'I guess so,' she said. 'Aren't you?'

I had fallen asleep after the evening meal.

I was awakened by a loud voice. *Mrs Bannister, Mrs*

Bannister, Mrs Bannister, Mrs Bannister. As I pulled out of sleep, I found I was beating on the bedpost with my hands and calling. The sharp, wry figure of Mrs Bannister, the night nurse, scurried into view.

'Here, we don't want you to break this.'

She unfastened the band of my watch.

'What's the matter? What happened?'

Mrs Bannister's face twisted into a quick smile. 'You've had a reaction.'

'A reaction.'

'Yes, how do you feel?'

'Funny. Sort of light and airy.'

Mrs Bannister helped me sit up.

'You'll be better now. You'll be better in no time. Would you like some hot milk?'

'Yes.'

And when Mrs Bannister held the cup to my lips, I fanned the hot milk out on my tongue as it went down, tasting it luxuriously, the way a baby tastes its mother.

'Mrs Bannister tells me you had a reaction.' Doctor Nolan seated herself in the armchair by the window and took out a tiny box of matches. The box looked exactly like the one I had hidden in the hem of my bathrobe, and for a moment I wondered if a nurse had discovered it there and given it back to Doctor Nolan on the quiet.

Doctor Nolan scraped a match on the side of the box. A hot yellow flame jumped into life, and I watched her suck it up into the cigarette.

'Mrs B. says you felt better.'

'I did for a while. Now I'm the same again.'

'I've news for you.'

I waited. Every day now, for I didn't know how many days,

I had spent the mornings and afternoons and evenings wrapped up in my white blanket on the deck chair in the alcove, pretending to read. I had a dim notion that Doctor Nolan was allowing me a certain number of days and then she would say just what Doctor Gordon had said: 'I'm sorry, you don't seem to have improved, I think you'd better have some shock treatments . . .'

'Well, don't you want to hear what it is?'

'What?' I said dully, and braced myself.

'You're not to have any more visitors for a while.'

I stared at Doctor Nolan in surprise. 'Why that's wonderful.'

'I thought you'd be pleased.' She smiled.

Then I looked, and Doctor Nolan looked, at the waste-basket beside my bureau. Out of the waste-basket poked the blood-red buds of a dozen long-stemmed roses.

That afternoon my mother had come to visit me.

My mother was only one in a long stream of visitors – my former employer, the lady Christian Scientist, who walked on the lawn with me and talked about the mist going up from the earth in the Bible, and the mist being error, and my whole trouble being that I believed in the mist, and the minute I stopped believing in it, it would disappear and I would see I had always been well, and the English teacher I had in high school who came and tried to teach me how to play Scrabble, because he thought it might revive my old interest in words, and Philomena Guinea herself, who wasn't at all satisfied with what the doctors were doing and kept telling them so.

I hated these visits.

I would be sitting in my alcove or in my room, and a smiling nurse would pop in and announce one or another of the visitors. Once they'd even brought the minister of the Unitarian church, whom I'd never really liked at all. He was terribly nervous the whole time, and I could tell he thought I was crazy as a loon, because I told him I believed in hell, and that certain people, like me, had to live in hell before they died, to make up for missing out on it after death, since they didn't believe in life after death, and what each person believed happened to him when he died.

I hated these visits, because I kept feeling the visitors measuring my fat and stringy hair against what I had been and what they wanted me to be, and I knew they went away utterly confounded.

I thought if they left me alone I might have some peace.

My mother was the worst. She never scolded me, but kept begging me, with a sorrowful face, to tell her what she had done wrong. She said she was sure the doctors thought she had done something wrong because they asked her a lot of questions about my toilet training, and I had been perfectly trained at a very early age and given her no trouble whatsoever.

That afternoon my mother had brought me the roses.

'Save them for my funeral,' I'd said.

My mother's face puckered, and she looked ready to cry.

'But Esther, don't you remember what day it is today?'

'No.'

I thought it might be Saint Valentine's day.

'It's your *birth*day.'

And that was when I had dumped the roses in the waste-basket.

'That was a silly thing for her to do,' I said to Doctor Nolan.

Doctor Nolan nodded. She seemed to know what I meant.

'I hate her,' I said, and waited for the blow to fall.

But Doctor Nolan only smiled at me as if something had pleased her very, very much, and said, 'I suppose you do.'

Chapter Seventeen

'You're a lucky girl today.'

The young nurse cleared my breakfast tray away and left me wrapped in my white blanket like a passenger taking the sea air on the deck of a ship.

'Why am I lucky?'

'Well, I'm not sure if you're supposed to know yet, but today you're moving to Belsize.' The nurse looked at me expectantly.

'Belsize,' I said. 'I can't go there.'

'Why not?'

'I'm not ready. I'm not well enough.'

'Of course, you're well enough. Don't worry, they wouldn't be moving you if you weren't well enough.'

After the nurse left, I tried to puzzle out this new move on Doctor Nolan's part. What was she trying to prove? I hadn't changed. Nothing had changed. And Belsize was the best house of all. From Belsize people went back to work and back to school and back to their homes.

Joan would be at Belsize. Joan with her physics books and her golf clubs and her badminton rackets and her breathy voice. Joan, marking the gulf between me and the nearly well ones. Even since Joan left Caplan I'd followed her progress through the asylum grapevine.

Joan had walk privileges, Joan had shopping privileges, Joan had town privileges. I gathered all my news of Joan into a little, bitter heap, though I received it with surface gladness. Joan was the beaming double of my old best self, specially designed to follow and torment me.

Perhaps Joan would be gone when I got to Belsize.

At least at Belsize I could forget about shock treatments. At Caplan a lot of the women had shock treatments. I could tell which ones they were, because they didn't get their breakfast trays with the rest of us. They had their shock treatments while we breakfasted in our rooms, and then they came into the lounge, quiet and extinguished, led like children by the nurses, and ate their breakfast there.

Each morning, when I heard the nurse knock with my tray, an immense relief flooded through me, because I knew I was out of danger for that day. I didn't see how Doctor Nolan could tell you went to sleep during a shock treatment if she'd never had a shock treatment herself. How did she know the person didn't just *look* as if he was asleep, while all the time, inside, he was feeling the blue volts and the noise?

Piano music sounded from the end of the hall.

At supper I had sat quietly, listening to the chatter of the Belsize women. They were all fashionably dressed and carefully made up, and several of them were married. Some of them had been shopping downtown, and others had been out visiting with friends, and all during supper they kept tossing back and forth these private jokes.

'I'd call Jack,' a woman named DeeDee said, 'only I'm afraid he wouldn't be home. I know just where I could call him, though, and he'd be in, all right.'

The short, spry blonde woman at my table laughed. 'I almost had Doctor Loring where I wanted him today.' She widened her starey blue eyes like a little doll. 'I wouldn't mind trading old Percy in for a new model.'

At the opposite end of the room, Joan was wolfing her spam and broiled tomato with great appetite. She seemed perfectly at home among these women and treated me coolly, with a slight sneer, like a dim and inferior acquaintance.

I had gone to bed right after supper, but then I heard the piano music and pictured Joan and DeeDee and Loubelle, the blonde woman, and the rest of them, laughing and gossiping about me in the living room behind my back. They would be saying how awful it was to have people like me in Belsize and that I should be in Wymark instead.

I decided to put a lid on their nasty talk.

Draping my blanket loosely around my shoulders, like a stole, I wandered down the hall toward the light and the gay noise.

For the rest of the evening I listened to DeeDee thump out some of her own songs on the grand piano, while the other women sat round playing bridge and chatting, just the way they would in a college dormitory, only most of them were ten years over college age.

One of them, a great, tall, grey-haired woman with a booming bass voice, named Mrs Savage, had gone to Vassar. I could tell right away she was a society woman, because she talked about nothing but débutantes. It seemed she had two or three daughters, and that year they were all going to be débutantes, only she had loused up their débutante party by signing herself into the asylum.

DeeDee had one song she called 'The Milkman' and everybody kept saying she ought to get it published, it would be a hit. First her hands would clop out a little melody on the keys, like the hoofbeats of a slow pony, and next another melody came in, like the milkman whistling, and then the two melodies went on together.

'That's very nice,' I said in a conversational voice.

Joan was leaning on one corner of the piano and leafing through a new issue of some fashion magazine, and DeeDee smiled up at her as if the two of them shared a secret.

'Oh, Esther,' Joan said then, holding up the magazine, 'isn't this you?'

DeeDee stopped playing. 'Let me see.' She took the magazine, peered at the page Joan pointed to, and then glanced back at me.

'Oh no,' DeeDee said. 'Surely not.' She looked at the magazine again, then at me. 'Never!'

'Oh, but it *is* Esther, isn't it Esther?' Joan said.

Loubelle and Mrs Savage drifted over, and pretending I knew what it was all about, I moved to the piano with them.

The magazine photograph showed a girl in a strapless evening dress of fuzzy white stuff, grinning fit to split, with a whole lot of boys bending in around her. The girl was holding a glass full of a transparent drink and seemed to have her eyes fixed over my shoulder on something that stood behind me, a little to my left. A faint breath fanned the back of my neck. I wheeled round.

The night nurse had come in, unnoticed, on her soft rubber soles.

'No kidding,' she said, 'is that really you?'

'No, it's not me. Joan's quite mistaken. It's somebody else.'

'Oh, say it's you!' DeeDee cried.

But I pretended I didn't hear her and turned away.

Then Loubelle begged the nurse to make a fourth at bridge, and I drew up a chair to watch, although I didn't know the first thing about bridge, because I hadn't had time to pick it up at college, the way all the wealthy girls did.

I stared at the flat poker-faces of the kings and jacks and

queens and listened to the nurse talking about her hard life.

'You ladies don't know what it is, holding down two jobs,' she said. 'Nights I'm over here, watching you . . .'

Loubelle giggled. 'Oh, we're good. We're the best of the lot, and you know it.'

'Oh, *you're* all right.' The nurse passed round a packet of spearmint gum, then unfolded a pink strap from its tinfoil wrapper herself. '*You're* all right, it's those boobies at the state place that worry me off my feet.'

'Do you work in both places then?' I asked with sudden interest.

'You bet.' The nurse gave me a straight look, and I could see she thought I had no business in Belsize at all. 'You wouldn't like it over there one bit, Lady Jane.'

I found it strange that the nurse should call me Lady Jane when she knew what my name was perfectly well.

'Why?' I persisted.

'Oh, it's not a nice place, like this. This is a regular country club. Over there they've got nothing. No OT to talk of, no walks . . .'

'Why haven't they got walks?'

'Not enough em-ploy-ees.' The nurse scooped in a trick and Loubelle groaned. 'Believe me, ladies, when I collect enough do-re-mi to buy me a car, I'm clearing out.'

'Will you clear out of here, too?' Joan wanted to know.

'You bet. Only private cases from then on. When I feel like it . . .'

But I'd stopped listening.

I felt the nurse had been instructed to show me my alternatives. Either I got better, or I fell, down, down, like a burning, then burnt-out star, from Belsize, to Caplan, to Wymark and finally, after Doctor Nolan and Mrs Guinea had given me up, to the state place next-door.

I gathered my blanket round me and pushed back my chair.

'You cold?' the nurse demanded rudely.

'Yes,' I said, moving off down the hall. 'I'm frozen stiff.'

I woke warm and placid in my white cocoon. A shaft of pale, wintry sunlight dazzled the mirror and the glasses on the bureau and the metal doorknobs. From across the hall came the early morning clatter of the maids in the kitchen, preparing the breakfast trays.

I heard the nurse knock on the door next to mine, at the far end of the hall. Mrs Savage's sleepy voice boomed out, and the nurse went into her with the jingling tray. I thought, with a mild stir of pleasure, of the steaming blue china coffee pitcher and the blue china breakfast cup and the fat blue china cream jug with the white daisies on it.

I was beginning to resign myself.

If I was going to fall, I would hang on to my small comforts, at least, as long as I possibly could.

The nurse rapped on my door and, without waiting for an answer, breezed in.

It was a new nurse – they were always changing – with a lean, sand-coloured face and sandy hair, and large freckles polka-dotting her bony nose. For some reason the sight of this nurse made me sick at heart, and it was only as she strode across the room to snap up the green blind that I realized part of her strangeness came from being empty-handed.

I opened my mouth to ask for my breakfast tray, but silenced myself immediately. The nurse would be mistaking me for somebody else. New nurses often did that. Somebody in Belsize must be having shock treatments, unknown to me, and the nurse had, quite understandably, confused me with her.

I waited until the nurse had made her little circuit of my room, patting, straightening, arranging, and taken the next tray in to Loubelle one door farther down the hall.

Then I shoved my feet into my slippers, dragging my blanket with me, for the morning was bright, but very cold, and crossed quickly to the kitchen. The pink-uniformed maid was filling a row of blue china coffee pitchers from a great, battered kettle on the stove.

I looked with love at the line-up of waiting trays – the white paper napkins, folded in their crisp, isosceles triangles, each under the anchor of its silver fork, the pale domes of the soft-boiled eggs in the blue egg cups, the scalloped glass shells of orange marmalade. All I had to do was reach out and claim my tray, and the world would be perfectly normal.

'There's been a mistake,' I told the maid, leaning over the counter and speaking in a low, confidential tone. 'The new nurse forgot to bring in my breakfast tray today.'

I managed a bright smile, to show there were no hard feelings.

'What's the name?'

'Greenwood. Esther Greenwood.'

'Greenwood, Greenwood, Greenwood.' The maid's warty index finger slid down the list of names of the patients in Belsize tacked up on the kitchen wall. 'Greenwood, no breakfast today.'

I caught the rim of the counter with both hands.

'There must be a mistake. Are you sure it's Greenwood?'

'Greenwood,' the maid said decisively as the nurse came in. The nurse looked questioningly from me to the maid.

'Miss Greenwood wanted her tray,' the maid said, avoiding my eyes.

'Oh,' the nurse smiled at me, 'you'll be getting your tray later on this morning, Miss Greenwood. You . . .'

But I didn't wait to hear what the nurse said. I strode blindly out into the hall, not to my room, because that was where they would come to get me, but to the alcove, greatly inferior to the alcove at Caplan, but an alcove, nevertheless, in a quiet corner of the hall, where Joan and Loubelle and DeeDee and Mrs Savage would not come.

I curled up in the far corner of the alcove with the blanket over my head. It wasn't the shock treatment that struck me, so much as the bare-faced treachery of Doctor Nolan. I liked Doctor Nolan, I loved her, I had given her my trust on a platter and told her everything, and she had promised, faithfully, to warn me ahead of time if ever I had to have another shock treatment.

If she had told me the night before I would have lain awake all night, of course, full of dread and foreboding, but by morning I would have been composed and ready. I would have gone down the hall between two nurses, past DeeDee and Loubelle and Mrs Savage and Joan, with dignity, like a person coolly resigned to execution.

The nurse bent over me and called my name.

I pulled away and crouched farther into the corner. The nurse disappeared. I knew she would return, in a minute, with two burly men attendants, and they would bear me, howling and hitting, past the smiling audience now gathered in the lounge.

Doctor Nolan put her arm around me and hugged me like a mother.

'You said you'd *tell* me!' I shouted at her through the dishevelled blanket.

'But I *am* telling you,' Doctor Nolan said. 'I've come specially early to tell you, and I'm taking you over myself.'

I peered at her through swollen lids. 'Why didn't you tell me last night?'

'I only thought it would keep you awake. If I'd known . . .'

'You *said* you'd tell me.'

'Listen, Esther,' Doctor Nolan said. 'I'm going over with you. I'll be there the whole time, so everything will happen right, the way I promised. I'll be there when you wake up, and I'll bring you back again.'

I looked at her. She seemed very upset.

I waited a minute. Then I said, 'Promise you'll be there.'

'I promise.'

Doctor Nolan took out a white handkerchief and wiped my face. Then she hooked her arm in my arm, like an old friend, and helped me up, and we started down the hall. My blanket tangled about my feet, so I let it drop, but Doctor Nolan didn't seem to notice. We passed Joan, coming out of her room, and I gave her a meaning, disdainful smile, and she ducked back and waited until we had gone by.

Then Doctor Nolan unlocked a door at the end of the hall and led me down a flight of stairs into the mysterious basement corridors that linked, in an elaborate network of tunnels and burrows, all the various buildings of the hospital.

The walls were bright, white lavatory tile with bald bulbs set at intervals in the black ceiling. Stretchers and wheelchairs were beached here and there against the hissing, knocking pipes that ran and branched in an intricate nervous system along the glittering walls. I hung on to Doctor Nolan's arm like death, and every so often she gave me an encouraging squeeze.

Finally, we stopped at a green door with ELECTROTHERAPY printed on it in black letters. I held back, and Doctor Nolan waited. Then I said, 'Let's get it over with,' and we went in.

The only people in the waiting-room beside Doctor Nolan and me were a pallid man in a shabby maroon bathrobe and his accompanying nurse.

'Do you want to sit down?' Doctor Nolan pointed at a wooden bench, but my legs felt full of heaviness, and I thought how hard it would be to hoist myself from a sitting position when the shock treatment people came in.

'I'd rather stand.'

At last a tall, cadaverous woman in a white smock entered the room from an inner door. I thought that she would go up and take the man in the maroon bathrobe, as he was first, so I was surprised when she came towards me.

'Good morning, Doctor Nolan,' the woman said, putting her arm around my shoulders. 'Is this Esther?'

'Yes, Miss Huey. Esther, this is Miss Huey, she'll take good care of you. I've told her about you.'

I thought the woman must be seven feet tall. She bent over me in a kind way, and I could see that her face, with the buck teeth protruding in the centre, had at one time been badly pitted with acne. It looked like maps of the craters on the moon.

'I think we can take you right away, Esther,' Miss Huey said. 'Mr Anderson won't mind waiting, will you, Mr Anderson?'

Mr Anderson didn't say a word, so with Miss Huey's arm around my shoulder, and Doctor Nolan following, I moved into the next room.

Through the slits of my eyes, which I didn't dare open too far, lest the full view strike me dead, I saw the high bed with its white, drumtight sheet, and the machine behind the bed, and the masked person – I couldn't tell whether it was a man or a woman – behind the machine, and other masked people flanking the bed on both sides.

Miss Huey helped me climb up and lie down on my back.

'Talk to me,' I said.

Miss Huey began to talk in a low, soothing voice, smoothing the salve on my temples and fitting the small electric buttons on either side of my head. 'You'll be perfectly all right, you won't feel a thing, just bite down . . .' And she set something on my tongue and in panic I bit down, and darkness wiped me out like chalk on a blackboard.

Chapter Eighteen

'Esther.'

I woke out of a deep, drenched sleep, and the first thing I saw was Doctor Nolan's face swimming in front of me and saying, 'Esther, Esther.'

I rubbed my eyes with an awkward hand.

Behind Doctor Nolan I could see the body of a woman wearing a rumpled black-and-white checked robe and flung out on a cot as if dropped from a great height. But before I could take in any more, Doctor Nolan led me through a door into fresh, blue-skied air.

All the heat and fear had purged itself. I felt surprisingly at peace. The bell jar hung, suspended, a few feet above my head. I was open to the circulating air.

'It was like I told you it would be, wasn't it?' said Doctor Nolan, as we walked back to Belsize together through the crunch of brown leaves.

'Yes.'

'Well it will always be like that,' she said firmly. 'You will be having shock treatments three times a week – Tuesday, Thursday and Saturday.' I gulped in a long draught of air.

'For how long?'

'That depends,' Doctor Nolan said, 'on you and me.'

*

I took up the silver knife and cracked off the cap of my egg. Then I put down the knife and looked at it. I tried to think what I had loved knives for, but my mind slipped from the noose of the thought and swung, like a bird, in the centre of empty air.

Joan and DeeDee were sitting side by side on the piano bench, and DeeDee was teaching Joan to play the bottom half of 'Chopsticks' while she played the top.

I thought how sad it was Joan looked so horsey, with such big teeth and eyes like two grey, goggly pebbles. Why, she couldn't even keep a boy like Buddy Willard. And DeeDee's husband was obviously living with some mistress or other and turning her sour as an old fusty cat.

'I've got a let-ter,' Joan chanted, poking her tousled head inside my door.

'Good for you.' I kept my eyes on my book. Ever since the shock treatments had ended, after a brief series of five, and I had town privileges, Joan hung about me like a large and breathless fruitfly – as if the sweetness of recovery were something she could suck up by mere nearness. They had taken away her physics books and the piles of dusty spiral pads full of lecture notes that had ringed her room, and she was confined to grounds again.

'Don't you want to know who it's *from*?'

Joan edged into the room and sat down on my bed. I wanted to tell her to get the hell out, she gave me the creeps, only I couldn't do it.

'All right.' I stuck my finger in my place and shut the book. 'Who from?'

Joan slipped out a pale blue envelope from her skirt pocket and waved it teasingly.

'Well isn't that a coincidence!' I said.

'What do you mean, a coincidence?'

I went over to my bureau, picked up a pale blue envelope and waved it at Joan like a parting handkerchief. 'I got a letter too. I wonder if they're the same.'

'He's better,' Joan said. 'He's out of hospital.'

There was a little pause.

'Are you going to marry him?'

'No,' I said. 'Are you?'

Joan grinned evasively. 'I didn't like him much, anyway.'

'Oh?'

'No, it was his family I liked.'

'You mean Mr and Mrs Willard?'

'Yes,' Joan's voice slid down my spine like a draft. 'I loved them. They were so nice, so happy, nothing like my parents. I went over to see them all the time;' she paused, 'until you came.'

'I'm sorry.' Then I added, 'Why didn't you go on seeing them, if you liked them so much?'

'Oh, I couldn't,' Joan said. 'Not with you dating Buddy. It would have looked . . . I don't know, *funny*.'

I considered. 'I suppose so.'

'Are you,' Joan hesitated, 'going to let him come?'

'I don't know.'

At first I had thought it would be awful having Buddy come and visit me at the asylum – he would probably only come to gloat and hob-nob with the other doctors. But then it seemed to me it would be a step, placing him, renouncing him, in spite of the fact that I had nobody – telling him there was no simultaneous interpreter, nobody, but that he was the wrong one, that I had stopped hanging on. 'Are you?'

'Yes,' Joan breathed. 'Maybe he'll bring his mother. I'm going to ask him to bring his mother . . .'

'His *mother*?'

Joan pouted. 'I like Mrs Willard. Mrs Willard's a wonderful, wonderful woman. She's been a real mother to me.'

I had a picture of Mrs Willard, with her heather-mixture tweeds and her sensible shoes and her wise, maternal maxims. Mr Willard was her little boy, and his voice was high and clear, like a little boy's. Joan and Mrs Willard. Joan . . . and Mrs Willard . . .

I had knocked on DeeDee's door that morning, wanting to borrow some two-part sheet music. I waited a few minutes and then, hearing no answer and thinking DeeDee must be out, and I could pick up the music from her bureau, I pushed the door open and stepped into the room.

At Belsize, even at Belsize, the doors had locks, but the patients had no keys. A shut door meant privacy, and was respected, like a locked door. One knocked, and knocked again, then went away. I remembered this as I stood, my eyes half-useless after the brilliance of the hall, in the room's deep, musky dark.

As my vision cleared, I saw a shape rise from the bed. Then somebody gave a low giggle. The shape adjusted its hair, and two pale, pebble eyes regarded me through the gloom. DeeDee lay back on the pillows, bare-legged under her green wool dressing-gown, and watched me with a little mocking smile. A cigarette glowed between the fingers of her right hand.

'I just wanted . . .' I said.

'I know,' said DeeDee. 'The music.'

'Hello, Esther,' Joan said then, and her cornhusk voice made me want to puke. 'Wait for me, Esther, I'll come play the bottom part with you.'

Now Joan said stoutly, 'I never really liked Buddy Willard. He thought he knew everything. He thought he knew everything about women . . .'

I looked at Joan. In spite of the creepy feeling, and in spite of my old, ingrained dislike, Joan fascinated me. It was like observing a Martian, or a particularly warty toad. Her thoughts were not my thoughts, nor her feelings my feelings, but we were close enough so that her thoughts and feelings seemed a wry, black image of my own.

Sometimes I wondered if I had made Joan up. Other times I wondered if she would continue to pop in at every crisis of my life to remind me of what I had been, and what I had been through, and carry on her own separate but similar crisis under my nose.

'I don't see what women see in other women,' I'd told Doctor Nolan in my interview that noon. 'What does a woman see in a woman that she can't see in a man?'

Doctor Nolan paused. Then she said, 'Tenderness.'

That shut me up.

'I like you,' Joan was saying. 'I like you better than Buddy.'

And as she stretched out on my bed with a silly smile, I remembered a minor scandal at our college dormitory when a fat, matronly-breasted senior, homely as a grandmother and a pious Religion major, and a tall, gawky freshman with a history of being deserted at an early hour in all sorts of ingenious ways by her blind dates, started seeing too much of each other. They were always together, and once somebody had come upon them embracing, the story went, in the fat girl's room.

'But what were they *doing*?' I had asked. Whenever I thought about men and men, and women and women, I could never really imagine what they would be actually doing.

'Oh,' the spy had said, 'Milly was sitting on the chair and Theodora was lying on the bed, and Milly was stroking Theodora's hair.'

I was disappointed, I had thought I would have some revelation of specific evil. I wondered if all women did with other women was lie and hug.

Of course, the famous woman poet at my college lived with another woman – a stumpy old Classical scholar with a cropped Dutch cut. And when I had told the poet I might well get married and have a pack of children some day, she stared at me in horror. 'But what about your *career*?' she had cried.

My head ached. Why did I attract these weird old women? There was the famous poet, and Philomena Guinea, and Jay Cee, and the Christian Scientist lady and lord knows who, and they all wanted to adopt me in some way, and, for the price of their care and influence, have me resemble them.

'I like you.'

'That's tough, Joan,' I said, picking up my book. 'Because I don't like you. You make me puke, if you want to know.'

And I walked out of the room, leaving Joan lying, lumpy as an old horse, across my bed.

I waited for the doctor, wondering if I should bolt. I knew what I was doing was illegal – in Massachusetts, anyway, because the state was cram-jam full of Catholics – but Doctor Nolan said this doctor was an old friend of hers, and a wise man.

'What's your appointment for?' the brisk, white-uniformed receptionist wanted to know, ticking my name off on a note-book list.

'What do you mean, *for*?' I hadn't thought anybody but the doctor himself would ask me that, and the communal waiting-room was full of other patients waiting for other doctors, most of them pregnant or with babies, and I felt their eyes on my flat, virgin stomach.

The receptionist glanced up at me, and I blushed.

'A fitting, isn't it?' she said kindly. 'I only wanted to make sure so I'd know what to charge you. Are you a student?'

'Ye-es.'

'That will only be half-price then. Five dollars, instead of ten. Shall I bill you?'

I was about to give my home address, where I would probably be by the time the bill arrived, but then I thought of my mother opening the bill and seeing what it was for. The only other address I had was the innocuous box number which people used who didn't want to advertise the fact they lived in an asylum. But I thought the receptionist might recognize the box number, so I said, 'I better pay now,' and peeled five dollar notes off the roll in my pocketbook.

The five dollars was part of what Philomena Guinea had sent me as a sort of get-well present. I wondered what she would think if she knew to what use her money was being put.

Whether she knew it or not, Philomena Guinea was buying my freedom.

'What I hate is the thought of being under a man's thumb,' I had told Doctor Nolan. 'A man doesn't have a worry in the world, while I've got a baby hanging over my head like a big stick, to keep me in line.'

'Would you act differently if you didn't have to worry about a baby?'

'Yes,' I said, 'but . . .' and I told Doctor Nolan about the married woman lawyer and her Defence of Chastity.

Doctor Nolan waited until I was finished. Then she burst out laughing. 'Propaganda!' she said, and scribbled the name and address of this doctor on a prescription pad.

I leafed nervously through an issue of *Baby Talk*. The fat, bright faces of babies beamed up at me, page after page – bald babies, chocolate-coloured babies, Eisenhower-faced babies, babies rolling over for the first time, babies reaching for rattles, babies eating their first spoonful of solid food, babies doing all the little tricky things it takes to grow up, step by step, into an anxious and unsettling world.

I smelt a mingling of Pabulum and sour milk and salt-cod-stinky diapers and felt sorrowful and tender. How easy having babies seemed to the women around me! Why was I so unmaternal and apart? Why couldn't I dream of devoting myself to baby after fat puling baby like Dodo Conway?

If I had to wait on a baby all day, I would go mad.

I looked at the baby in the lap of the woman opposite. I had no idea how old it was, I never did, with babies – for all I knew it could talk a blue streak and had twenty teeth behind its pursed, pink lips. It held its little wobbly head up on its shoulders – it didn't seem to have a neck – and observed me with a wise, Platonic expression.

The baby's mother smiled and smiled, holding that baby as if it were the first wonder of the world. I watched the mother and the baby for some clue to their mutual satisfaction, but before I had discovered anything, the doctor called me in.

'You'd like a fitting,' he said cheerfully, and I thought with relief that he wasn't the sort of doctor to ask awkward questions. I had toyed with the idea of telling him I planned to be married to a sailor as soon as his ship docked at the Charlestown Navy Yard, and the reason I didn't have an engagement ring was because we were too poor, but at the last moment I rejected that appealing story and simply said 'Yes'.

I climbed up on the examination table, thinking: 'I am climbing to freedom, freedom from fear, freedom from marrying the wrong person, like Buddy Willard, just because of sex, freedom from the Florence Crittenden Homes where all the poor girls go who should have been fitted out like me, because what they did, they would do anyway, regardless . . .'

As I rode back to the asylum with my box in the plain brown paper wrapper on my lap I might have been Mrs Anybody coming back from a day in town with a Schrafft's cake for her maiden aunt or a Filene's Basement hat. Gradually the suspicion that Catholics had X-ray eyes diminished, and I grew easy. I had done well by my shopping privileges, I thought.

I was my own woman.

The next step was to find the proper sort of man.

213

Chapter Nineteen

'I'm going to be a psychiatrist.'

Joan spoke with her usual breathy enthusiasm. We were drinking apple cider in the Belsize lounge.

'Oh,' I said dryly, 'that's nice.'

'I've had a long talk with Doctor Quinn, and she thinks it's perfectly possible.' Doctor Quinn was Joan's psychiatrist, a bright, shrewd, single lady, and I often thought if I had been assigned to Doctor Quinn I would be still in Caplan or, more probably, Wymark. Doctor Quinn had an abstract quality that appealed to Joan, but it gave me the polar chills.

Joan chattered on about Egos and Ids, and I turned my mind to something else, to the brown, unwrapped package in my bottom drawer. I never talked about Egos and Ids with Doctor Nolan. I didn't know just what I talked about, really.

'. . . I'm going to live out, now.'

I turned in on Joan then. 'Where?' I demanded, trying to hide my envy.

Doctor Nolan said my college would take me back for the second semester, on her recommendation and Philomena Guinea's scholarship, but as the doctors vetoed my living with my mother in the interim, I was staying on at the asylum until the winter term began.

Even so, I felt it unfair of Joan to beat me through the gates.

'Where?' I persisted. 'They're not letting you live on your own, are they?' Joan had only that week been given town privileges again.

'Oh no, of course not. I'm living in Cambridge with Nurse Kennedy. Her room-mate's just got married, and she needs someone to share the apartment.'

'Cheers.' I raised my apple cider glass, and we clinked. In spite of my profound reservations, I thought I would always treasure Joan. It was as if we had been forced together by some overwhelming circumstance, like war or plague, and shared a world of our own. 'When are you leaving?'

'On the first of the month.'

'Nice.'

Joan grew wistful. 'You'll come visit me, won't you, Esther?'

'Of course.'

But I thought, 'Not likely.'

'It hurts,' I said. 'Is it supposed to hurt?'

Irwin didn't say anything. Then he said, 'Sometimes it hurts.'

I had met Irwin on the steps of the Widener Library. I was standing at the top of the long flight, overlooking the red brick buildings that walled the snow-filled quad and preparing to catch the trolley back to the asylum, when a tall young man with a rather ugly and bespectacled, but intelligent face, came up and said, 'Could you please tell me the time?'

I glanced at my watch. 'Five past four.'

Then the man shifted his arms around the load of books he was carrying before him like a dinner tray and revealed a bony wrist.

'Why, you've a watch yourself!'

The man looked ruefully at his watch. He lifted it and shook it by his ear. 'Doesn't work.' He smiled engagingly. 'Where are you going?'

I was about to say, 'Back to the asylum', but the man looked promising, so I changed my mind. 'Home.'

'Would you like some coffee first?'

I hesitated. I was due at the asylum for supper and I didn't want to be late so close to being signed out of there for good.

'A very *small* cup of coffee?'

I decided to practise my new, normal personality on this man who, in the course of my hesitations, told me his name was Irwin and that he was a very well-paid professor of mathematics, so I said, 'All right,' and, matching my stride to Irwin's, strolled down the long, ice-encrusted flight at his side.

It was only after seeing Irwin's study that I decided to seduce him.

Irwin lived in a murky, comfortable basement apartment in one of the rundown streets of outer Cambridge and drove me there – for a beer, he said – after three cups of bitter coffee in a student café. We sat in his study on stuffed brown leather chairs, surrounded by stacks of dusty, incomprehensible books with huge formulas inset artistically on the page like poems.

While I was sipping my first glass of beer – I have never really cared for cold beer in mid-winter, but I accepted the glass to have something solid to hold on to – the doorbell rang.

Irwin seemed embarrassed. 'I think it may be a lady.'

Irwin had a queer, old-world habit of calling women ladies.

'Fine, fine,' I gestured largely. 'Bring her in.'

Irwin shook his head. 'You would upset her.'

I smiled into my amber cylinder of cold beer.

The doorbell rang again with a peremptory jab. Irwin sighed and rose to answer it. The minute he disappeared, I whipped into the bathroom and, concealed behind the dirty, aluminium-coloured Venetian blind, watched Irwin's monk-fish face appear in the door crack.

A large, bosomy Slavic lady in a bulky sweater of natural

sheep's wool, purple slacks, high-heeled black overshoes with Persian lamb cuffs and a matching toque, puffed white inaudible words into the wintry air. Irwin's voice drifted back to me through the chilly hall.

'I'm sorry, Olga . . . I'm working, Olga . . . no, I don't think so, Olga,' all the while the lady's red mouth moved, and the words, translated to white smoke, floated up among the branches of the naked lilac by the door. Then, finally, 'Perhaps, Olga . . . good-bye, Olga.'

I admired the immense, steppe-like expanse of the lady's wool-clad bosom as she retreated, a few inches from my eye, down the creaking wooden stair, a sort of Siberian bitterness on her vivid lips.

'I suppose you have lots and lots of affairs in Cambridge,' I told Irwin cheerily, as I stuck a snail with a pin in one of Cambridge's determinedly French restaurants.

'I seem,' Irwin admitted with a small, modest smile, 'to get on with the ladies.'

I picked up my empty snail shell and drank the herb-green juice. I had no idea if this was proper, but after months of wholesome, dull asylum diet, I was greedy for butter.

I had called Doctor Nolan from a pay phone at the restaurant and asked for permission to stay overnight in Cambridge with Joan. Of course, I had no idea whether Irwin would invite me back to his apartment after dinner or not, but I thought his dismissal of the Slavic lady – another professor's wife – looked promising.

I tipped back my head and poured down a glass of Nuits St George.

'You do like wine,' Irwin observed.

'Only Nuits St George. I imagine him . . . with the dragon . . .'

Irwin reached for my hand.

I felt the first man I slept with must be intelligent, so I would respect him. Irwin was a full professor at twenty-six and had the pale, hairless skin of a boy genius. I also needed somebody quite experienced to make up for my lack of it, and Irwin's ladies reassured me on this head. Then, to be on the safe side, I wanted somebody I didn't know and wouldn't go on knowing – a kind of impersonal, priestlike official, as in the tales of tribal rites.

By the end of the evening I had no doubts about Irwin whatsoever.

Ever since I'd learned about the corruption of Buddy Willard my virginity weighed like a millstone around my neck. It had been of such enormous importance to me for so long that my habit was to defend it at all costs. I had been defending it for five years and I was sick of it.

It was only as Irwin swung me into his arms, back at the apartment, and carried me, wine-dazed and limp, into the pitch-black bedroom, that I murmured, 'You know, Irwin, I think I ought to tell you, I'm a virgin.'

Irwin laughed and flung me down on the bed.

A few minutes later an exclamation of surprise revealed that Irwin hadn't really believed me. I thought how lucky it was I had started practising birth control during the day, because in my winey state that night I would never have bothered to perform the delicate and necessary operation. I lay, rapt and naked, on Irwin's rough blanket, waiting for the miraculous change to make itself felt.

But all I felt was a sharp, startlingly bad pain.

'It hurts,' I said. 'Is it supposed to hurt?'

Irwin didn't say anything. Then he said, 'Sometimes it hurts.'

After a little while Irwin got up and went into the bathroom, and I heard the rushing of shower water. I wasn't sure if Irwin had done what he planned to do, or if my virginity had obstructed him in some way. I wanted to ask him if I was still a virgin, but I felt too unsettled. A warm liquid was seeping out between my legs. Tentatively, I reached down and touched it.

When I held my hand up to the light streaming in from the bathroom, my fingertips looked black.

'Irwin,' I said nervously, 'bring me a towel.'

Irwin strolled back, a bath towel knotted around his waist, and tossed me a second, smaller towel. I pushed the towel between my legs and pulled it away almost immediately. It was half black with blood.

'I'm bleeding!' I announced, sitting up with a start.

'Oh, that often happens,' Irwin reassured me. 'You'll be all right.'

Then the stories of blood-stained bridal sheets and capsules of red ink bestowed on already deflowered brides floated back to me. I wondered how much I would bleed, and lay down, nursing the towel. It occurred to me that the blood was my answer. I couldn't possibly be a virgin any more. I smiled into the dark. I felt part of a great tradition.

Surreptitiously, I applied a fresh section of white towel to my wound, thinking that as soon as the bleeding stopped, I would take the late trolley back to the asylum. I wanted to brood over my new condition in perfect peace. But the towel came away black and dripping.

'I . . . think I better go home,' I said faintly.

'Surely not so soon.'

'Yes, I think I better.'

I asked if I could borrow Irwin's towel and packed it between my thighs as a bandage. Then I pulled on my sweaty clothes. Irwin offered to drive me home, but I didn't see how I could let him drive me to the asylum, so I dug in my pocketbook for Joan's address. Irwin knew the street and went out to start the car. I was too worried to tell him I was still bleeding. I kept hoping every minute that it would stop.

But as Irwin drove me through the barren, snow-banked streets I felt the warm seepage let itself through the dam of the towel and my skirt and on to the car seat.

As we slowed, cruising by house after lit house, I thought how fortunate it was I had not discarded my virginity while living at college or at home, where such concealment would have been impossible.

Joan opened the door with an expression of glad surprise. Irwin kissed my hand and told Joan to take good care of me.

I shut the door and leaned back against it, feeling the blood drain from my face in one spectacular flush.

'Why, Esther,' Joan said, 'what on earth's the matter?'

I wondered when Joan would notice the blood trickling down my legs and oozing, stickily, into each black patent leather shoe. I thought I could be dying from a bullet wound and Joan would still stare through me with her black eyes, expecting me to ask for a cup of coffee and a sandwich.

'Is that nurse here?'

'No, she's on night duty at Caplan . . .'

'Good.' I made a little bitter grin as another soak of blood let itself through the drenched padding and started the tedious journey into my shoes. 'I mean . . . bad.'

'You look funny,' Joan said.

'You better get a doctor.'

'Why?'

'Quick.'

'But . . .'

Still she hadn't noticed anything.

I bent down, with a brief grunt, and slipped off one of my winter-cracked black Bloomingdale shoes. I held the shoe up, before Joan's enlarged, pebbly eyes, tilted it, and watched her take in the stream of blood that cascaded on to the beige rug.

'My God! What is it?'

'I'm haemorrhaging.'

Joan half-led, half-dragged me to the sofa and made me lie down. Then she propped some pillows under my bloodstained feet. Then she stood back and demanded, 'Who was that man?'

For one crazy minute I thought Joan would refuse to call a doctor until I confessed the whole story of my evening with Irwin and that after my confession she would still refuse, as a sort of punishment. But then I realized that she honestly took my explanation at face value, that my going to bed with Irwin was utterly incomprehensible to her, and his appearance a mere prick to her pleasure at my arrival.

'Oh somebody,' I said, with a flabby gesture of dismissal. Another pulse of blood released itself and I contracted my stomach muscles in alarm. 'Get a towel.'

Joan went out and came back almost immediately with a pile of towels and sheets. Like a prompt nurse, she peeled back my blood-wet clothes, drew a quick breath as she arrived at the original royal red towel, and applied a fresh bandage. I lay, trying to slow the beating of my heart, as every beat pushed forth another gush of blood.

I remembered a worrisome course in the Victorian novel where woman after woman died, palely and nobly, in torrents of blood, after a difficult childbirth. Perhaps Irwin had injured me in some awful, obscure way, and all the while I lay there on Joan's sofa I was really dying.

Joan pulled up an Indian hassock and began to dial down the long list of Cambridge doctors. The first number didn't answer. Joan began to explain my case to the second number, which did answer, but then broke off and said 'I see' and hung up.

'What's the trouble?'

'He'll only come for regular customers or emergencies. It's Sunday.'

I tried to lift my arm and look at my watch, but my hand was a rock at my side and wouldn't budge. Sunday – the doctor's paradise! Doctors at country clubs, doctors at the seaside, doctors with mistresses, doctors with wives, doctors in church, doctors in yachts, doctors everywhere resolutely being people, not doctors.

'For God's sake,' I said, 'tell them I'm an emergency.'

The third number didn't answer and, at the fourth, the party hung up the minute Joan mentioned it was about a period. Joan began to cry.

'Look, Joan,' I said painstakingly, 'call up the local hospital. Tell them it's an emergency. They'll have to take me.'

Joan brightened and dialled a fifth number. The Emergency Service promised her a staff doctor would attend to me if I could come in to the ward. Then Joan called a taxi.

Joan insisted on riding with me. I clasped my fresh padding of towels with a sort of desperation as the cabby, impressed by the address Joan gave him, cut corner after corner in the dawn-pale streets and drew up with a great squeal of tyres at the Emergency Ward entrance.

I left Joan to pay the driver and hurried into the empty, glaringly lit room. A nurse bustled out from behind a white screen. In a few swift words, I managed to tell her the truth about my predicament before Joan came in the door, blinking and wide-eyed as a myopic owl.

The Emergency Ward doctor strolled out then, and I climbed, with the nurse's help, on to the examining table. The nurse whispered to the doctor, and the doctor nodded and began unpacking the bloody towelling. I felt his fingers start to probe, and Joan stood, rigid as a soldier, at my side, holding my hand, for my sake or hers I couldn't tell.

'Ouch!' I winced at a particularly bad jab.

The doctor whistled.

'You're one in a million.'

'What do you mean?'

'I mean it's one in a million it happens to like this.'

The doctor spoke in a low, curt voice to the nurse, and she hurried to a side table and brought back some rolls of gauze and silver instruments. 'I can see,' the doctor bent down, 'exactly where the trouble is coming from.'

'But can you fix it?'

The doctor laughed. 'Oh, I can fix it, all right.'

I was roused by a tap on my door. It was past midnight, and the asylum quiet as death. I couldn't imagine who would still be up.

'Come in!' I switched on the bedside light.

The door clicked open, and Doctor Quinn's brisk, dark head appeared in the crack. I looked at her with surprise, because although I knew who she was, and often passed her, with a brief nod, in the asylum hall, I never spoke to her at all.

Now she said, 'Miss Greenwood, may I come in a minute?'

I nodded.

Doctor Quinn stepped into the room, shutting the door quietly behind her. She was wearing one of her navy blue, immaculate suits with a plain, snow-white blouse showing in the V of the neck.

'I'm sorry to bother you, Miss Greenwood, and especially at this time of night, but I thought you might be able to help us out about Joan.'

For a minute I wondered if Doctor Quinn was going to blame me for Joan's return to the asylum. I still wasn't sure how much Joan knew, after our trip to the Emergency Ward, but a few days later she had come back to live in Belsize, retaining, however, the freest of town privileges.

'I'll do what I can,' I told Doctor Quinn.

Doctor Quinn sat down on the edge of my bed with a grave face. 'We would like to find out where Joan is. We thought you might have an idea.'

Suddenly I wanted to dissociate myself from Joan completely. 'I don't know,' I said coldly. 'Isn't she in her room?'

It was well after the Belsize curfew hour.

'No, Joan had a permit to go to a movie in town this evening, and she's not back yet.'

'Who was she with?'

'She was alone.' Doctor Quinn paused. 'Have you any idea where she might be likely to spend the night?'

'Surely she'll be back. Something must have held her up.' But I didn't see what could have held Joan up in tame night Boston.

Doctor Quinn shook her head. 'The last trolley went by an hour ago.'

'Maybe she'll come back by taxi.'

Doctor Quinn sighed.

'Have you tried the Kennedy girl?' I went on. 'Where Joan used to live?'

Doctor Quinn nodded.

'Her family?'

'Oh, she'd never go there . . . but we've tried them, too.'

Doctor Quinn lingered a minute, as if she could sniff out some clue in the still room. Then she said, 'Well, we'll do what we can,' and left.

I turned out the light and tried to drop back to sleep, but Joan's face floated before me, bodiless and smiling, like the face of the Cheshire cat. I even thought I heard her voice, rustling and hushing through the dark, but then I realized it was only the night wind in the asylum trees . . .

Another tap woke me in the frost-grey dawn.

This time I opened the door myself.

Facing me was Doctor Quinn. She stood at attention, like a frail drill sergeant, but her outlines seemed curiously smudged.

'I thought you should know,' Doctor Quinn said. 'Joan has been found.'

Doctor Quinn's use of the passive slowed my blood.

'Where?'

'In the woods, by the frozen ponds . . .'

I opened my mouth, but no words came out.

'One of the orderlies found her,' Doctor Quinn continued, 'just now, coming to work . . .'

'She's not . . .'

'Dead,' said Doctor Quinn. 'I'm afraid she's hanged herself.'

Chapter Twenty

A fresh fall of snow blanketed the asylum grounds – not a Christmas sprinkle, but a man-high January deluge, the sort that snuffs out schools and offices and churches, and leaves, for a day or more, a pure, blank sheet in place of memo pads, date books and calendars.

In a week, if I passed my interview with the board of doctors, Philomena Guinea's large black car would drive me west and deposit me at the wrought-iron gates of my college.

The heart of winter!

Massachusetts would be sunk in a marble calm. I pictured the snowflakey, Grandma Moses villages, the reaches of swampland rattling with dried cat-tails, the ponds where frog and hornpout dreamed in a sheath of ice, and the shivering woods.

But under the deceptively clean and level slate the topography was the same, and instead of San Francisco or Europe or Mars I would be learning the old landscape, brook and hill and tree. In one way it seemed a small thing, starting, after a six months' lapse, where I had so vehemently left off.

Everybody would know about me, of course.

Doctor Nolan had said, quite bluntly, that a lot of people would treat me gingerly, or even avoid me, like a leper with a warning bell. My mother's face floated to mind, a pale, reproachful moon, at her last and first visit to the asylum since my twentieth birthday. A daughter in an asylum! I had done that to her. Still, she had obviously decided to forgive me.

'We'll take up where we left off, Esther,' she had said, with her sweet, martyr's smile. 'We'll act as if all this were a bad dream.'

A bad dream.

To the person in the bell jar, blank and stopped as a dead baby, the world itself is the bad dream.

A bad dream.

I remembered everything.

I remembered the cadavers and Doreen and the story of the fig-tree and Marco's diamond and the sailor on the Common and Doctor Gordon's wall-eyed nurse and the broken thermometers and the negro with his two kinds of beans and the twenty pounds I gained on insulin and the rock that bulged between sky and sea like a grey skull.

Maybe forgetfulness, like a kind snow, should numb and cover them.

But they were part of me. They were my landscape.

'A man to see you!'

The smiling, snow-capped nurse poked her head in through the door, and for a confused second I thought I really was back in college and this spruce white furniture, this white view over trees and hills, an improvement on my old room's nicked chairs and desk and outlook over the bald quad. 'A man to see you!' the girl on watch had said, on the dormitory phone.

What was there about us, in Belsize, so different from the girls playing bridge and gossiping and studying in the college to which I would return? Those girls, too, sat under bell jars of a sort.

'Come in!' I called, and Buddy Willard, khaki cap in hand, stepped into the room.

227

'Well, Buddy,' I said.

'Well, Esther.'

We stood there, looking at each other. I waited for a touch of emotion, the faintest glow. Nothing. Nothing but a great, amiable boredom. Buddy's khaki-jacketed shape seemed small and unrelated to me as the brown posts he had stood against that day a year ago, at the bottom of the ski run.

'How did you get here?' I asked finally.

'Mother's car.'

'In all this snow?'

'Well,' Buddy grinned, 'I'm stuck outside in a drift. The hill was too much for me. Is there anyplace I can borrow a shovel?'

'We can get a shovel from one of the groundsmen.'

'Good.' Buddy turned to go.

'Wait, I'll come and help you.'

Buddy looked at me then, and in his eyes I saw a flicker of strangeness – the same compound of curiosity and wariness I had seen in the eyes of the Christian Scientist and my old English teacher and the Unitarian minister who used to visit me.

'Oh, Buddy,' I laughed. 'I'm all right.'

'Oh, I know, I know, Esther,' Buddy said hastily.

'It's you who oughtn't to dig out cars, Buddy. Not me.'

And Buddy did let me do most of the work.

The car had skidded on the glassy hill up to the asylum and backed, with one wheel over the rim of the drive, into a steep drift.

The sun, emerged from its grey shrouds of cloud, shone with a summer brilliance on the untouched slopes. Pausing in my work to overlook that pristine expanse, I felt the same profound thrill it gives me to see trees and grassland waist-high under flood water – as if the usual order of the world had shifted slightly, and entered a new phase.

I was grateful for the car and the snowdrift. It kept Buddy from asking me what I knew he was going to ask, and what he finally did ask, in a low, nervous voice, at the Belsize afternoon tea. DeeDee was eyeing us like an envious cat over the rim of her teacup. After Joan's death, DeeDee had been moved to Wymark for a while, but now she was among us once more.

'I've been wondering . . .' Buddy set his cup in the saucer with an awkward clatter.

'What have you been wondering?'

'I've been wondering . . . I mean, I thought you might be able to tell me something.' Buddy met my eyes and I saw, for the first time, how he had changed. Instead of the old, sure smile that flashed on easily and frequently as a photographer's bulb, his face was grave, even tentative – the face of a man who often does not get what he wants.

'I'll tell you if I can, Buddy.'

'Do you think there's something in me that *drives* women crazy?'

I couldn't help myself, I burst out laughing – maybe because of the seriousness of Buddy's face and the common meaning of the word 'crazy' in a sentence like that.

'I mean,' Buddy pushed on, 'I dated Joan, and then you, and first you . . . went, and then Joan . . .'

With one finger I nudged a cake crumb into a drop of wet, brown tea.

'Of course you didn't do it!' I heard Doctor Nolan say. I had come to her about Joan, and it was the only time I remember her sounding angry. 'Nobody did it! *She* did it!' And then Doctor Nolan told me how the best of psychiatrists has suicides among their patients, and how they, if anybody, should be held responsible, but how they, on the contrary, do not hold themselves responsible . . .

'You had nothing to do with us, Buddy.'

'You're sure?'

'Absolutely.'

'Well,' Buddy breathed. 'I'm glad of that.'

And he drained his tea like a tonic medicine.

'I hear you're leaving us.'

I fell into step beside Valerie in the little, nurse-supervised group. 'Only if the doctors say yes. I have my interview tomorrow.'

The packed snow creaked underfoot, and everywhere I could hear a musical trickle and drip as the noon sun thawed icicles and snow crusts that would glaze again before night-fall.

The shadows of the massed black pines were lavender in that bright light, and I walked with Valerie a while, down the familiar labyrinth of shovelled asylum paths. Doctors and nurses and patients passing on adjoining paths seemed to be moving on casters, cut off at the waist by the piled snow.

'Interviews!' Valerie snorted. 'They're nothing! If they're going to let you out, they let you out.'

'I hope so.'

In front of Caplan I said good-bye to Valerie's calm, snowmaiden face behind which so little, bad or good, could happen, and walked on alone, my breath coming in white puffs even in that sun-filled air. Valerie's last, cheerful cry had been 'So long! Be seeing you.'

'Not if I know it,' I thought.

But I wasn't sure. I wasn't sure at all. How did I know that someday – at college, in Europe, somewhere, anywhere – the bell jar, with its stifling distortions, wouldn't descend again?

And hadn't Buddy said, as if to revenge himself for my digging out the car and his having to stand by, 'I wonder who you'll marry now, Esther.'

'What?' I'd said, shovelling snow up on to a mound and blinking against the stinging back-shower of loose flakes.

'I wonder who you'll marry now, Esther. Now you've been,' and Buddy's gesture encompassed the hill, the pines and the severe, snow-gabled buildings breaking up the rolling landscape, 'here.'

And of course I didn't know who would marry me now that I'd been where I had been. I didn't know at all.

'I have a bill here, Irwin.'

I spoke quietly into the mouthpiece of the asylum pay phone in the main hall of the administration building. At first I suspected the operator, at her switchboard, might be listening, but she just went on plugging and unplugging her little tubes without batting an eye.

'Yes,' Irwin said.

'It's a bill for twenty dollars for emergency attention on a certain date in December and a check-up a week thereafter.'

'Yes,' Irwin said.

'The hospital says they are sending me the bill because there was no answer to the bill they sent to you.'

'All right, all right, I'm writing a cheque now. I'm writing them a blank cheque.' Irwin's voice altered subtly. 'When am I going to see you?'

'Do you really want to know?'

'Very much.'

'Never,' I said, and hung up with a resolute click.

I wondered, briefly, if Irwin would send his cheque to the hospital after that, and then I thought, 'Of course he will, he's a mathematics professor – he won't want to leave any loose ends.'

I felt unaccountably weak-kneed and relieved.

Irwin's voice had meant nothing to me.

231

This was the first time, since our first and last meeting, that I had spoken with him and, I was reasonably sure, it would be the last. Irwin had absolutely no way of getting in touch with me, except by going to Nurse Kennedy's flat, and after Joan's death Nurse Kennedy had moved somewhere else and left no trace.

I was perfectly free.

Joan's parents invited me to the funeral.

I had been, Mrs Gilling said, one of Joan's best friends.

'You don't have to go, you know,' Doctor Nolan told me. 'You can always write and say I said it would be better not to.'

'I'll go,' I said, and I did go, and all during the simple funeral service I wondered what I thought I was burying.

At the altar the coffin loomed in its snow-pallor of flowers – the black shadow of something that wasn't there. The faces in the pews around me were waxen with candlelight, and pine boughs, left over from Christmas, sent up a sepulchral incense in the cold air.

Beside me, Jody's cheeks bloomed like good apples, and here and there in the little congregation I recognized other faces of other girls from college and my home town who had known Joan. DeeDee and Nurse Kennedy bent their kerchiefed heads in a front pew.

Then, behind the coffin and the flowers and the face of the minister and the faces of the mourners, I saw the rolling lawns of our town cemetery, knee-deep in snow now, with the tombstones rising out of it like smokeless chimneys.

There would be a black, six-foot-deep gap hacked in the hard ground. That shadow would marry this shadow, and the peculiar, yellowish soil of our locality seal the wound in the whiteness, and yet another snowfall erase the traces of newness in Joan's grave.

I took a deep breath and listened to the old brag of my heart.

I am, I am, I am.

The doctors were having their weekly board meeting – old business, new business, admissions, dismissals and interviews. Leafing blindly through a tatty *National Geographic* in the asylum library, I waited my turn.

Patients, with accompanying nurses, made their rounds of the stocked shelves, conversing, in low tones, with the asylum librarian, an alumna of the asylum herself. Glancing at her – myopic, spinsterish, effaced – I wondered how she knew she had really graduated at all, and, unlike her clients, was whole and well.

'Don't be scared,' Doctor Nolan had said. 'I'll be there, and the rest of the doctors you know, and some visitors, and Doctor Vining, the head of all the doctors, will ask you a few questions, and then you can go.'

But in spite of Doctor Nolan's reassurances, I was scared to death.

I had hoped, at my departure, I would feel sure and knowledgeable about everything that lay ahead – after all, I had been 'analyzed'. Instead, all I could see were question marks.

I kept shooting impatient glances at the closed boardroom door. My stocking seams were straight, my black shoes cracked, but polished, and my red wool suit flamboyant as my plans. Something old, something new . . .

But I wasn't getting married. There ought, I thought, to be a ritual for being born twice – patched, retreaded and approved for the road. I was trying to think of an appropriate one when Doctor Nolan appeared from nowhere and touched me on the shoulder.

'All right, Esther.'

I rose and followed her to the open door.

Pausing, for a brief breath, on the threshold, I saw the silver-haired doctor who had told me about the rivers and the Pilgrims on my first day, and the pocked, cadaverous face of Miss Huey, and eyes I thought I had recognized over white masks.

The eyes and the faces all turned themselves towards me, and guiding myself by them, as by a magical thread, I stepped into the room.